L[...]

Mary S. Sheridan

Munchausen by Proxy
Identification, Intervention, and Case Management

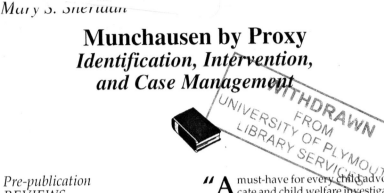

Pre-publication
REVIEWS,
COMMENTARIES,
EVALUATIONS . . .

"Through detailed case studies and analysis, the authors take readers into the lives and minds of people whose obsessive craving for attention compels them to fake illness, sometimes to the point of death. A unique perspective into many case accounts is provided, bringing the reader deep into this disturbing disorder and offering clear and practical methods for identifying, reporting, and intervening. A valuable resource for anyone working with [MBP] cases, this book is a must-read for clinical professionals and anyone with a suspicion of MBP in their own families. It is easily the leading resource available today for MBP identification and intervention."

Mason America, PhD
Director, Asher Meadow
(<www.AsherMeadow.com>
supporting the Munchausen by Proxy
Syndrome Community)

"A must-have for every child advocate and child welfare investigator . . . a well-written, pragmatic, what-to-do and how-to-do-it. This book will save lives, guaranteed."

Janice Wolf, JD
Child Advocate,
Honolulu, Hawaii

"The detailed information in this book will benefit all persons involved in the medical, psychological, and social welfare of children. It should be required reading during the training and education of physicians, psychologists, nurses, and social workers. The organized and systematic approach makes the book especially suitable and user-friendly. Lasher and Sheridan have written a book that will have a significant impact on the identification and protection of victims of MBP. I will be sure to place it on my office bookcase alongside other major pediatric textbooks."

Lynda M. Stidham, MD
Pediatrician, Century-Airport
Pediatrics, New York

More pre-publication
REVIEWS, COMMENTARIES, EVALUATIONS . . .

"Lasher and Sheridan's book is a must for social workers and child protection workers who are the frontline workers charged with the challenging task of managing the difficult and contentious issues involved in MBP investigations. They review the seminal thinking on this disorder and then contribute highly detailed and practical guidelines, protocols, and recommendations that will be invaluable for child protection workers, whether experienced in this field or new to this work. This is a welcome addition to the existing literature on MBP and should contribute a great deal to a thoughtful, fair, and strong approach to protecting children from this type of abuse."

Judith A. Libow, PhD
Co-author of *Hurting for Love:*
Munchausen by Proxy Syndrome;
Coordinator of Psychological Services,
Department of Psychiatry, Children's
Hospital and Research Center
at Oakland, California

"This book is an excellent resource for professionals from all disciplines who may be confronted with this misunderstood disorder. Any question—from the initial identification to assisting victims with treatment—is thoroughly addressed. Each chapter provides quick step-by-step guidelines that can be used by all members of a mulitagency multidisciplinary team. The included Risk Assessment Work Sheet is a valuable tool for MSP practitioners. This book is a must for every professional involved in MBP investigations."

Larry C. Brubaker, MA
FBI Special Agent (Retired)

"This book is a fascinating journey into the underworld of MBP. The authors, by means of case presentations and their own extensive clinical experience, weave a tapestry that provides the reader with a deeper insight into MBP. The book offers an approach on how to evaluate cases sytematically with a logical sequence of questions, and it presents a comprehensive approach to management of the victim and the perpetrator. Because the condition is rare, individual practitioners are unlikely to gain a great deal of personal experience. This book will help them expand their knowledge of this complicated psychiatric disorder."

Michael J. Light, MD
Professor of Clinical Pediatrics,
University of Miami

"A must-read and a must-have for every family law, criminal, and prosecuting attorney as well as every judicial officer who hears cases involving MBP child maltreatment. Every attorney and judicial officer dealing with these types of cases should be required to obtain education on this troubling behavior and how it affects everyone involved in such cases from the children and parents to attorneys, court staff, experts, judges, and witnesses. An outstanding job by the authors—I look forward to more from them in the future."

Jean A. Cotton, JD
Owner, Cotton Law Offices,
Elma, Washington

Munchausen by Proxy
Identification, Intervention, and Case Management

Munchausen by Proxy
Identification, Intervention, and Case Management

Louisa J. Lasher
Mary S. Sheridan

HMTP

The Haworth Maltreatment and Trauma Press®
An Imprint of The Haworth Press, Inc.
New York • London • Oxford

Published by

The Haworth Maltreatment and Trauma Press®, an imprint of The Haworth Press, Inc., 10 Alice Street, Binghamton, NY 13904-1580.

PUBLISHER'S NOTE
Identities and circumstances of individuals discussed in this book have been changed to protect confidentiality.

Cover design by Jennifer M. Gaska.

Library of Congress Cataloging-in-Publication Data

Lasher, Louisa J.
   Munchausen by proxy : identification, intervention, and case management / Louisa J. Lasher, Mary S. Sheridan.
      p. cm.
   ISBN 0-7890-1217-0 (Hard : alk. paper)—ISBN 0-7890-1218-9 (Soft : alk. paper)
   1. Munchausen syndrome by proxy. I. Sheridan, Mary S. II. Title.
RC569.5.M83L37 2004
616.85'8223—dc22

                                                                                2003026566

CONTENTS

ABOUT THE AUTHORS

Louisa J. Lasher, MA, is an internationally recognized Munchausen by proxy (MBP) maltreatment expert and has authored several MBP maltreatment articles. In 1997 she left her position as a state-wide child maltreatment consultant with the State Office of the Georgia Division of Family and Children Services to undertake a full-time forensic practice in the area of MBP. She provides MBP case consultation, technical assistance, expert witness services, and educational programs throughout the world. Participants in her MBP maltreatment workshops and/or for whom she provides expert services include a wide range of professionals from the multiagency-multidisciplinary community. She maintains an MBP maltreatment Web site at <www.mbpexpert.com>. She is a member of the American College of Forensic Examiners.

Mary S. Sheridan, PhD, ACSW, is Professor and Program Chair for Social Work at Hawaii Pacific University, where she was Teacher of the Year in 2003. Author/editor of numerous books and articles, she previously served as a medical social worker at hospitals in Illinois and Hawaii. She is a member of many university committees and community organizations, and was voted 2003 Social Worker of the Year in Professional Education by the Hawaii Chapter of the National Association of Social Workers.

Foreword

Laura, the young woman who provided the poignant passage that follows, is one of perhaps 600 individuals who have felt safe enough to share their personal concerns about Munchausen by proxy (MBP) with me since I established a related Web site in the "ancient" days of the World Wide Web (ca. 1996). She writes,

> When I became aware of Munchausen by proxy, I was so surprised that there is actually a name for this problem. I had always been told that I was a very sick child—and believed it. It was only when I went away to boarding school, and noticed that I never needed to go to the doctor when my mother wasn't around, that I began to suspect that she had been fabricating my illnesses. I stopped using the inhaler that one of my many doctors had prescribed for my "breathing problems," and I felt fine. I can't tell you how many times I have been in an emergency room. I have been to physical therapists, allergists, neurologists, internists, and the list goes on and on. I began to wonder why my mother's stories about my childhood ailments and injuries seemed to change over the years. I began to intentionally expose myself to foods I was "allergic" to only to find that I had no allergic reaction at all. I have never confronted my mother about this; the thought of doing so is too unpleasant.

In most cases involving Internet reports, I have never obtained the requisite records or interviewed any witnesses, and thus could not verify or dispel the allegations. Instead, I have usually suggested further reading as an initial step, and then pecked among the articles and books of the day for a resource that would be relevant and approachable. That task has always been formidable, in that the bulk of the literature has consisted of jargon-filled publications that have been destined for the bookshelf, not ready use.

Despite that fact, the escalating number of inquiries speaks to the public's burgeoning awareness of MBP. That some of the most basic questions asked of me come from health care professionals in active practice—social workers, nurses, physicians, therapists, and even child protection personnel themselves—speaks to their own growing curiosity, but also to the powerful need for more education about essentially every aspect of MBP. In this respect, *Munchausen by Proxy: Identification, Intervention, and Case Management,* is a breakthrough in the field of child abuse and neglect. Having had the privilege of following along as Louisa Lasher and Mary Sheridan fashioned their early draft into a shimmering jewel, I can state clearly that this is the finest book on MBP that has ever been published. Why? Because of its sheer practicality. It not only talks the talk; it teaches the skills. Like a divining rod, each human endeavor about which words can be written eventually finds its classics. MBP has finally found its own.

Today, in many, perhaps even most parts of the world, child maltreatment remains the most taboo of topics. Professional caregivers from countries ranging from Brazil to Nigeria to Saudi Arabia have bewailed the total lack of social and legal mechanisms to curtail abuse and neglect within their borders. When these physicians and others cannot help but diagnose battering or incest, they find the family unit impenetrable, deified by laws that put them—not the abusers—at risk of community denunciation and even civil or criminal liability. As was true in the United States less than fifty years ago, it is sadly easier to bury one's head, ostrichlike, than acknowledge painful truths about the harm that can be inflicted on a child, whether actively or passively.

The challenges, already onerous, are monumentally greater in MBP maltreatment. The unusual term "Munchausen" can itself evoke misgivings. The claim that a parent would inflict serious harm through the feigning or production of illness can seem not only profoundly counterintuitive, but flatly impossible. Who would like to have forced on them a mental picture of a mother, with cool premeditation, administering unnecessary insulin to a three-week-old girl for the thrill of an ambulance ride to the emergency department? How about a babysitter suffocating a six-month-old boy in order to be lauded as the clear-thinking neighborhood savior? No one, of course, and yet these two scenarios were among the earliest I had to confront when it became known that I had some interest in the topic. In essence, I was drafted into battle. I was required to think the unthinkable and explain the inexplicable. Like so many reluctant soldiers, I have sometimes been attacked for doing so.

In the first MBP case in which I ever testified, I had to leave my two-day-old daughter, who was stricken with a respiratory ailment and nestled in the plastic womb of a hospital incubator. "Can't the hearing please be postponed?" I begged. "No," the judge replied with obvious irritation: "I've never heard of 'Munkowsen syndrome and proxy,' or whatever hooey it is, and if you don't show up I'm throwing out the case." I knew that a previous child in this same family had died after a series of unexplained interruptions in his breathing. I also knew that their new baby required constant resuscitation—until he was removed from his mother's custody, at which point he became the epitome of cheery, chubby health. I left my daughter and testified. Despite the judge's continuing refusal to believe a mother could deliberately suffocate her child for intangible reasons, the outcome was a positive one. When the coroner and I independently spoke of the former death as a probable maternal homicide (based on the exact duplication of symptoms in the new child), the mother essentially entered the verdict herself. Her lawyer suddenly stood up and asked, as she nodded, that the baby be placed in the permanent custody of her estranged husband. I have since learned that there is a very disturbing bargain—usually unspoken—in the majority of MBP cases: if the mother gives up custody, she will not undergo criminal prosecution.

Soon afterward, I received a letter from the child's father:

> When I saw my son for the first time, I cannot tell you how I felt. He was so small. He had just had a spinal tap and he looked miserable. For the next ten days, he remained in the hospital, and the doctors put him through every test known to man, but couldn't find anything wrong with him. They thought his problem might be due to an infection, but they found no infection. They thought it had something to do with the shape of his heart; there was nothing wrong with his heart. They tested his blood; everything checked normal. They did sleep studies on him, and they performed an amazing number of other tests. Finally, they sent him home.
>
> Within two weeks, he was back in the hospital. He remained in intensive care hooked up to monitors and undergoing another round of tests. No abnormalities were discovered, and eventually he was sent home again. When the next call came telling me

that my son was once again in the hospital, I walked in to see him with a gauze helmet on and he looked totally miserable. I said, "Son, I'm going to take care of you." I was determined that something was going to be done.

Part of that "something" was calling on me. The pain of leaving my daughter (now a healthy ten-year-old) was countered by the positive outcome and this moving letter.

Anyone who has encountered MBP wishes it were indeed an impossibility—an invention, perhaps, of people who crave excitement and exotica as fervidly as the literary Baron von Münchhausen. Yet, it is the perpetrators of this covert maltreatment who seek such emotional rewards. Although they represent merely the tip of the iceberg of MBP prevalence, over 550 published case reports from nearly thirty countries attest to the reality and relative commonality of MBP. Still, even in Western countries, it remains perhaps the most difficult form of maltreatment to pursue. The telltale bruises and broken bones most people associate with harm to children are typically absent in MBP. Also, the perpetrators often have the ability to hire attorneys, mobilize the media, launch malpractice suits, and wage campaigns of deceit to discredit those who would bring them to justice and their children to safety. In contrast, the victims are silent due either to their tender age or their impotence against an adult whose behavior they may not understand themselves. This disparity is why I believe the word "collusion" should never be used to refer to older children who are victims of MBP and fail to "fight." The word "collusion" implies choice, and victims face even greater bodily and emotional threats if they shatter the wall of secrecy. Like all abused children, they may also believe that they somehow "deserve" the maltreatment, or they may fail to discern the relationship between events, such as being forced to swallow "medicine" and later becoming frighteningly ill.

The history behind the MBP rubric has colorful elements that belie the horror of the maltreatment it represents. Baron Karl Friedrich Hieronymus Freiherr von Münchhausen (1720-1797) was a brave Prussian cavalry officer who, after his retirement to his estate in 1760, often regaled his guests with tales of his exploits in the Russo-Turkish War. The baron's stories were essentially true. However, a German thief named Rudolph Erich Raspe (1737-1794), who fled to England and knew of the baron, anonymously published a forty-nine-page pamphlet of adventure stories so outlandish as to be utterly laughable.

Sadly for the baron, Raspe titled his 1785 work, *Baron von Münchausen's Narrative of His Marvellous Travels and Campaigns in Russia.* The small book eventually became a sensation, but one that forever equated the anglicized name "Munchausen" with wild falsehoods. The book enlarged as writers added new stories, spawning over 200 editions. It has been transmogrified into at least six movies, a card game, a role-playing game, and even a type of candy bar (slogan: "Munch the Munchausen!"). The baron failed in a lawsuit against Raspe and, now the subject of derision, became depressed, a state worsened by the death of his wife. He remarried and his new wife had a child by another man. The child, Maria Wilhelmina, died in infancy near the German town of Polle. Baron Münchhausen divorced his wife and lived unhappily thereafter.

Although the baron, and his literary incarnation, never claimed or exaggerated illness, British physician Richard Asher coined the term Munchausen syndrome in 1951 to refer to individuals who sought the "sick role" by fabricating dramatic physical ailments in themselves. Pediatrician Roy Meadow, in turn, created Munchausen syndrome by proxy in 1977 when he recognized that parents (or, as we now know, others in loco parentis) sometimes manufactured or induced sickness in another person to meet their own needs for attention, nurturance, and perverse control.

This foray into history and nomenclature is more important than it might seem. Once it was clear that Munchausen syndrome by proxy was a validated subtype of abusive and/or neglectful behavior, not simply a constellation of symptoms, the word "syndrome" was dropped by many in the field, including me. MBP or, as in this book, *Munchausen by proxy,* became a clearer way of referencing behavior that, like the self-inflicted version, sometimes involves misrepresentations of emotional or behavioral, not just physical, maladies. Along the line, alternative terms such as *Meadow's syndrome* and *Polle's syndrome* have been offered, but they have no evident advantages. Most recently, a small group of experts has advocated for a veritable alphabet soup of acronyms, simultaneously using PCF *(pediatric condition falsification),* FDP *(factitious disorder by proxy),* and MBP to depict different elements of the phenomenon. My conviction, which I share with Lasher and Sheridan, is that MBP is a form of illness-based maltreatment and that the term is best used alone or denoted with the precise harmful behaviors that have occurred. Otherwise, judges and juries who must act in these cases, and who are responsible for children who almost always lack the potent advocacy engineered by the perpetrators, will find themselves as befuddled as many of the clinicians who write to me about "this Munchausen thing."

Lasher and Sheridan are not the first to produce a book about MBP. Academic tomes, including my own, have multiplied during the past decade, along with books (generally by nonclinicians) that purport to debunk the "myth" of MBP. Books in the latter category become the fodder for the guilty, who see a way out through the navel-gazing philosophy and pseudoscience on which these publications are based. Books in the former category may eruditely review the professional literature and incorporate limited recommendations, but they fail to teach skills that can be applied on a day-to-day basis. It is the skills-based and pragmatic approach—rich in case examples, sample forms, and representative management plans—that makes *Munchausen by Proxy* the small miracle that it is. Eminently readable, it has immediate applicability from the moment that MBP enters fuzzily into the realm of diagnostic possibility through potential confirmation, case management, and treatment for any underlying psychiatric problems among perpetrators and for the victims. Primary care physicians have had their Harrison's and Cecil (textbooks). At last, child advocates have their Lasher and Sheridan.

Marc D. Feldman, MD
Clinical Professor of Psychiatry
University of Alabama, Tuscaloosa

Preface and Acknowledgments

I (Louisa) first became interested in Munchausen by proxy (MBP) in 1989, when I was a child protective services investigator. A mother reported that her seven-year-old daughter was bleeding from the mouth and vagina. MBP was confirmed after it had been proven that the mother had deliberately placed blood on the child's panties and elsewhere, and after it had been established that the behavior did qualify as MBP. Since then I have been involved in over 400 suspected and/or confirmed MBP cases. I have learned that MBP is not rare. Rather, it is underidentified due to a lack of public awareness and professional knowledge and skills for appropriate investigation and confirmation/disconfirmation. MBP is very different from other kinds of maltreatment. For example, investigative methods and activities, confirmation/disconfirmation, victim risk assessment, out-of-home placement, visitation and other contact supervision, case planning, and case management in MBP cases all require specialized knowledge, activities, and techniques. Yet physicians and other physical and mental health care providers, social services, child protective agencies, law enforcement, and other professionals usually do not have the correct basic MBP education necessary for even rudimentary involvement in suspected or confirmed MBP cases.

In 1997 I left my position with the state office of the Georgia Division of Family and Children Services (DFCS) to devote myself full time to private practice related to MBP. I present educational programs, provide case consultation and technical assistance, and serve as an expert witness. One major goal when I left DFCS was to complete this book. It is intended as a guide to understanding MBP and to working with suspected or confirmed cases. Because this book is designed for workers in a variety of professions who need the information for practice, we have tried to keep the writing simple, direct, and practical.

I am grateful to Georgia DFCS consultant Jim Hansen who first mentioned the term "Munchausen by proxy" to me and convinced me that this kind of maltreatment really exists; to Judy Libow who provided so much education and support from the beginning; to my mentor and colleague Marc Feldman for his kindness, inspiration, and willingness to always be available to assist; and finally to my friend and co-author Mary Sheridan, without whom my growth and development in this field would never have happened.

I have never before experienced the career satisfaction of these past few years. I know that I have made a positive difference in the lives of maltreated children. I wanted to write this book so that other professionals can also make a difference. This book is dedicated to the many MBP victims waiting to be identified and protected.

I (Mary) became involved in MBP in the mid-1980s when I was apnea coordinator at a children's hospital, responsible for working with infants who had or were at risk of breathing pauses (apnea). Most of these babies were at home on monitors that would sound an alarm if they stopped breathing or their heart rate dropped. Our team was involved with several families who were certainly falsely reporting prolonged apnea, and some who were probably inducing it as well. My experience with apnea had taught me to trust parents' intuition and reports. Other experiences had convinced me that health care professionals are often too quick to discount symptoms or attribute them to "psychosomatic" causes. So I was reluctant to admit that these apparently exemplary parents might be deceiving us or harming their children. In retrospect, and from the best motives, I committed many of the errors I now caution other professionals against.

When I was in social work school, MBP had not been discovered. Today, we still know relatively little about it. Although I offer training in MBP and consultation on specific cases, my major interest has always been in knowing and understanding more. "How" and especially "why" are the questions that still fascinate me.

In 1995, Louisa Lasher asked me to assist her in writing this book, based on the training and consultation she provides to people interested in MBP. The majority of the practical information is hers; my contribution has been to assist with the literature, theory, and writing. I am grateful to her for her friendship and support. I am also grateful to Dr. Michael Light for collaboration during the difficulties that MBP cases present. Our disagreements, learning, and testing the facts always took place in a climate of mutual respect. He never said, "I told you so." I would also like to acknowledge the contribution of Sir Roy Meadow to the field of MBP. It has taken courage to identify and publicize this form of maltreatment. He has quietly supported my efforts to learn and understand, and I suspect he does the same for many others.

I join in Louisa's dedication of this book to the victims, particularly those not yet discovered. They are the reason that we, and others, study and practice in a part of child maltreatment that everyone wishes would go away, and that many still deny. In addition, Louisa and I would like to commemorate those close to us who died during the years we were working on this book: her mother, Mildred Ross Lasher; my mother, Betty G. Stoebe; my husband Harold Sheridan; and my stepdaughter, Carole A. Sheridan.

Louisa and I would like to thank Dr. Robert Geffner of The Haworth Press for his help in bringing this book to "life," and for challenging us to delve deeper into the literature and our experience to make the book more complete. We would also like to thank Dr. Constance J. Dalenberg for her careful work in editing and her useful suggestions.

AUTHOR'S NOTE

The information contained in this book represents our experience and, we believe, the state of knowledge about MBP and its management as of the time of publication. Readers are responsible for considering local conditions and situations as they apply it to practice. Case studies are disguised and are usually a compilation of situations, with imaginary but typical details. Any use of real names of persons, institutions, or localities is coincidental.

PART I:
MUNCHAUSEN BY PROXY MALTREATMENT

Chapter 1

Defining Munchausen by Proxy

Munchausen by proxy (MBP) is a dangerous kind of maltreatment (abuse and/or neglect) in which caretakers, usually parents, deliberately and repeatedly exaggerate, fabricate and/or induce a problem or problems in someone who is under their care. The problems can be physical and/or psychological and/or behavioral. MBP was first identified by Roy Meadow in 1977. Since that time, awareness of MBP and its dynamics has grown, although much still remains to be learned. The purpose of this book is to present specific and practical approaches to identification, intervention, and management of these difficult cases, within a framework that includes both the knowledge base from the professional literature and clinical experience.

Munchausen by proxy (MBP) is a dangerous kind of maltreatment (abuse and/or neglect) in which caretakers, usually parents, deliberately and repeatedly exaggerates, fabricates, and/or induces a problem or problems in someone who is under their care.

The desired outcome with MBP cases, as in any form of child maltreatment, is the identification and protection of victims and the avoidance of false accusations. It is very important that MBP neither be missed nor falsely confirmed. This is a challenging task because children may genuinely suffer from difficult-to-diagnose problems, and perpetrators can be skilled at deception. This process of discernment begins with a thorough understanding of MBP. As different and puzzling as they can be, MBP cases are also often strikingly similar. The following case example contains many typical elements.

3

Case 1.1

A child protective services (CPS) investigator received a report alleging filthy conditions in the Andrews family home. Following departmental procedure, she made an unannounced home visit. To her surprise, the home was clean and tidy. Mrs. Andrews seemed pleasant, sincere, and puzzled as to why anyone would report her children as abused or neglected. While the investigator was in the house, ten-year-old Nancy Andrews and her twelve-year-old brother Billy arrived home from school. The relationship between mother and children seemed excellent, and both children seemed normal and healthy. Mrs. Andrews seemed glad to see them, fixed a snack, and asked about their day. The investigator watched them eat, then saw them go outside to play with children from the neighborhood. Everything seemed fine. The investigator was about to leave the home, already mentally writing a report on this unfounded allegation, when Mrs. Andrews began talking about Nancy's health problems. Nancy, she said, was spewing blood from her mouth and vagina every day. With mounting excitement and in dramatic detail the mother told of Nancy's seven hospitalizations in recent months. She vividly recounted the numerous tests and medical procedures Nancy had been subjected to in attempts to discover what was wrong. She thanked the social worker for listening to her, explaining that many doctors did not recognize the seriousness of her daughter's condition, and that she had been through dozens of incompetent providers. She said that the cause of Nancy's bleeding was still a mystery, and that the child was soon to be admitted to a specialized medical facility in another state for even more tests and procedures. Mrs. Andrews also said that she suspected Nancy might be emotionally disturbed because of Nancy's bizarre behavior—unprovoked screaming in the middle of the night, and attacks of rage in which she became violent and seemed disoriented.

The investigator listened to the account of Nancy's mysterious problems, the painful and embarrassing examinations and tests she had been through, the list of family friends and relatives who had become involved in the situation, and the church and other community groups who were lending emotional and financial support. She couldn't help but think: "What a sad situation. What a wonderful mother, so unrelenting in her quest to find out what is wrong. And now to be the target of an anonymous report to CPS—this family is going through terrible times!"

Although the Andrews family had medical insurance, there were still large expenses. "What might our agency do to assist?" the investigator asked herself. When she returned to the office, she couldn't help discussing the sad situation with her supervisor and co-workers. All were impressed by Mrs. Andrews' courage, and were brainstorming about various sources of funding when a visiting consultant asked the investigator more questions about the discrepancy between how healthy Nancy looked and the long list of physical and behavioral problems she was supposed to have. When the investigator described this paradox, the consultant asked, "I wonder if this could be a case of Munchausen by proxy?" None of the investigators had ever heard the term before. They thought it must be a joke of some kind. But the consultant explained that MBP is a form of maltreatment in which a perpetrator repeatedly creates or feigns symptoms of illness or other problems in a dependent person such as a child. The consultant pointed to several "red flags" in the Andrews family: Mother's dramatic involvement in the symptoms, the fact that many specialists were confused while mother pressed on for a diagnosis, and the observation that Nancy appeared completely active and healthy in spite of supposedly heavy bleeding almost every day.

The investigator was shocked at the idea that this apparently exemplary mother might be harming her child. MBP sounded bizarre. Did such a thing really exist? Could the consultant have become too cynical and suspicious after many years in child protective practice, so that this was an example of "blaming the victim"? The investigator went to the library for more information. Not only did the medical and child protective literature support the existence of MBP as a form of maltreatment, but the investigator found a published case in a medical journal that was very similar to the Andrews family. The consultant had not exaggerated the danger: one review of the literature suggested a 9 percent death rate among child victims of MBP (Rosenberg, 1987). Other articles suggested that survivors could suffer severe emotional and physical harm (Bools, Neale, and Meadow, 1993; Libow, 1995).

From her reading, the worker learned the importance of collateral information as part of her investigation. Had anyone other than Mrs. Andrews seen the dramatic events at their onset? Was there truly no medical explanation? Did the bleeding ever occur when the mother was not present? Mrs. Andrews had readily given a list of people who, she said, would "vouch for her being a good mother and keeping a clean house." She also said that everyone on the list had helped the family in one way or another with Nancy's medical problems. They had all, Mrs. Andrews said, seen the blood. As the investigator interviewed these collateral contacts, numerous friends, neighbors, and relatives agreed that they had seen the blood—in the toilet, on Nancy's clothing, on the floor or furniture, and in various other places. But no one had actually seen blood coming out of Nancy's mouth or vagina.

The literature suggested that separating the alleged victim and perpetrator can be a way to determine if, over an appropriate period of time, the described problems actually exist. Or, if they do exist, will they improve during the separation? Action to remove a child from the home is undertaken when a child protective agency believes it is necessary for the safety of a child. At this stage, the investigator knew it was highly unlikely that she had enough information to convince a court to intervene. What judge would believe that this well-dressed, articulate, seemingly caring woman could be harming her child by deliberately subjecting her to unnecessary medical treatment?

After a good deal of thought, the investigator developed a plan. Mrs. Andrews had said that Nancy was exhibiting severe behavioral problems. Neither the investigator nor the school had seen any evidence of emotional disturbance. Could Mrs. Andrews be falsifying both physical and behavioral symptoms? The investigator suggested that Nancy be admitted to a children's mental health facility for monitoring and evaluation.

Nancy remained in the facility for six weeks. For the first five weeks, although staff monitored carefully, no one saw blood on her body, clothes, or bedding. There were also no behavior problems. During the sixth week, Mrs.

Andrews was allowed an unsupervised visit. During that visit, she told a nurse that there was blood on Nancy's panties. The panties were sent to the law enforcement crime laboratory for analysis. There was blood—but it matched Mrs. Andrews', not Nancy's. There was no one else in the room at the time that the "bleeding" occurred, and a physical examination of Nancy did not reveal any bleeding. Mrs. Andrews had "planted" the blood in an attempt to "prove" that Nancy had bleeding problems. CPS then had sufficient evidence to remove Nancy from her mother on the basis of MBP. Knowing that Nancy was not physically or mentally ill, Mrs. Andrews had subjected her to repeated physical examinations, mental health evaluations, and medical diagnostic and therapeutic procedures that involved pain and risk, including hospitalizations. Mrs. Andrews' false stories and planting of false evidence had led to actions that violated Nancy's privacy, interfered with her sense of bodily integrity, and caused her to miss school and other normal childhood experiences. They constituted physical abuse, emotional abuse, and neglect (failure to provide necessary health care, education, etc.). After CPS's evidence was presented in court, protective custody of Nancy was granted to the agency. Nancy was placed in a foster home. There were no more reports of bleeding or behavior problems.

The investigator realized that, in this case, she had been able to fulfill her agency's mission in protecting a child. She could not help but wonder, however, how many other MBP cases she and other professionals had missed.

ELEMENTS OF THE DEFINITION

Although scholars in the field debate some of the subtleties, the definition given at the beginning of this chapter reflects the authors' view and the medical/social science literature as a whole. Each element of this definition is important and is related to what is known about MBP.

Munchausen by proxy is dangerous.

The literature of MBP cases includes numerous children who have endured poisonings and undergone unnecessary surgeries, invasive diagnostic procedures, and feeding tube insertions (Levin and Sheridan, 1995). Video- and audiotaping has documented parents exaggerating, fabricating, and inducing problems in their children, although most cases are confirmed by other methods such as records analysis and specialized interviews. Documented behavior has included smothering, poisoning, and inducing infections (Southall et al., 1997). A recent review of the medical and social science literature found that

6 percent, or 27/451 MBP victims died (Sheridan, 2003). All victims were judged to have suffered at least short-term harm, and 33 (7.3 percent) had suffered long-term or permanent disability. In addition, fifty-three of the victims' siblings (25 percent of identifiable siblings) were known to be dead, and 130 (61.32 percent) of the known siblings had symptoms of illness. The cause(s) of these symptoms were impossible to determine, but the symptoms were often similar to those of the victim.

In Case 1.1, Mrs. Andrews reported that Nancy—a healthy child— had serious physical and behavior problems. She subjected her to numerous unnecessary and invasive tests, procedures, and examinations. Many of these were unpleasant, some were painful, and most had potential side effects. In addition, this girl, just at the brink of adolescent development, had a great deal of unwelcome attention focused on her genitals. Nancy also missed normal life experiences because her mother said that she was "sick." Instead of being in school, she was in the hospital. Instead of going out with friends, she went to the doctor's office. Her mother's attention was focused only on her health. She was embarrassed in front of her peers when she went to the mental hospital, and she now carries that stigma—unfairly—for life. She lost the opportunity to live in her own home. Other parents have burned, suffocated, infected, or poisoned their children to create the appearance of illness. They have severely limited their children's diets or activities. They have subjected their victims to unnecessary medications. The medical literature suggests that some children subjected to MBP grow up to perpetuate an obsession with illness in themselves and their children.

MBP is maltreatment.

Because the patterns associated with MBP are different from the beatings, sexual injury, malnutrition, and other conditions commonly seen in maltreated children, some people have been unsure whether MBP constitutes child maltreatment. Child maltreatment includes both abuse and neglect. Abuse is defined as the causing of harm to a victim; something is actually done that is hurtful. Neglect is the failure to do something that is required, such as provide appropriate care. MBP can include both abuse and neglect. Therefore, professionals in the field believe that, whatever other factors may be included in MBP, it is a form of maltreatment (Mitchell et al., 1993). Feldman and Lasher state (1999):

> Knowing there is no reason to suspect or believe that the victim has problems, the typical perpetrator misleads others. Understandably, health care providers rely upon this information in establishing the diagnosis and offering treatment. As a result, the victim is subjected unnecessarily to examinations, tests, medications, surgeries, and other interventions, with the attendant risks. Thus, MBP constitutes emotional, and usually physical abuse even if the perpetrator has not directly harmed the victim. . . . To the extent that a perpetrator deliberately fails to meet the child's physical or psychological needs, MBP may instead involve maltreatment through neglect. MBP may be manifested through both abuse and neglect in specific cases. (p. 27)

In Case 1.1, Nancy was clearly abused through unnecessary physical and psychological examinations and treatment. Her mother also neglected to provide her with a normal environment for healthy psychological growth and development. Because of the focus on supposed vaginal bleeding, and the examinations that this necessitated, a case could also be made that Nancy was sexually abused.

Because MBP is a form of maltreatment, it must be reported to child protective authorities wherever this is required by law. Child maltreatment must be reported in all fifty of the United States. Feldman and Ford state, "Not every case of child abuse is Munchausen by Proxy, but every case of Munchausen by Proxy is child abuse" (1994, p. 147). MBP also occurs with adults as victims; most often these adults are physically or emotionally dependent on the perpetrator. Whether anything can be done to conduct a thorough investigation and confirmation/disconfirmation process and to protect adult victims depends on local reporting and intervention laws and policies, the ability to consult with experts for advice, the dynamics of the situation, and the ability of concerned professionals to design appropriate and effective interventions.

MBP is a specific form of maltreatment.

Although MBP can include elements of physical, emotional, and sexual abuse and neglect, it is a separate category of maltreatment. Nancy was abused and neglected, but not in ways that the investigator was used to seeing. A defining feature of MBP is the perpetrators' deliberate and usually repeated attempt to create the appearance of a victim with physical, emotional, or behavioral problems, and the appearance of themselves as conscientious caretakers who do not know the reasons for the problems. The creation of the problem or problem story does not serve simply to cover up or explain maltreatment that has occurred in other contexts. Mrs. Andrews, for example, fabricated the story of Nancy's bleeding and created false "evidence" of bleeding because she wanted people to think that Nancy had this problem. This was not a case in which Nancy bled because she had been sexually abused or beaten, and a parent gave a false story to physicians to deflect suspicion. Nor was it a situation in which an overwhelmed caretaker needed respite, or the parent of a truly sick child persisted in seeking help. In MBP, there is a lack of external incentives as the primary reason for creating or reporting the problem.

The challenges of dealing with MBP are different from those associated with other forms of abuse and neglect. Although many pathways may lead to MBP, common elements are also often found in cases. The patterns and deceptive elements of MBP require specialized identification, intervention, and case management activities and skills—as do MBP legal and related activities.

MBP is deliberate behavior.

Often, professionals find it difficult to believe that MBP is a conscious and chosen behavior. They feel that it must occur because parents are mistaken about their children's symptoms or under the sway of mental illness. These dynamics do occur—but they are not MBP. When the details of MBP are uncovered, there is often clear evidence of calculation and advanced planning. For example, one mother deceptively obtained the name of a teenage patient from the local Cystic Fibrosis (CF) Association. She contacted the patient, identified herself as a health care professional, and requested a sputum sample "for research." Once she had obtained the sample, the mother presented it to the staff of the hospital where her own child was being treated, as "proof" the child had CF (Orenstein and Wasserman, 1986). In other cases, parents have tampered with medical equipment to make it appear that infants were having prolonged breathing pauses (apnea), created emergencies only when a physician or spouse was out of town, or used an electric mixer to create a caustic cream that could be applied to the child's skin to create a "rash." (Cases known or described to authors.) In Case 1.1, Mrs. Andrews showed no signs of disorientation or mental illness when she reported physical or behavioral problems with Nancy, or when she placed her own blood on Nancy's panties.

Many other common elements in MBP cases also speak to deliberateness and calculation, but the most telling evidence comes from parents themselves: In a retrospective study, MBP perpetrators remembered exactly what they had done and stated that it was conscious, deliberate behavior (Meadow, 1990). Parnell (1998) also reports that perpetrators whom she has interviewed described deliberate actions.

MBP is deliberate but this does not mean that it is benign. In general, MBP perpetrators use children as objects to meet their own needs. They lack the internal "stop signs" that keep normal parents from ever thinking of abusing their children in this way.

MBP is repeated behavior.

One characteristic of MBP cases is that the behavior is not a single, isolated event. This may or may not be apparent in the initial stages of investigation, but usually emerges as further information is gathered and analyzed. Victims of MBP often accumulate stacks of physical and/or mental health care records because they are so frequently in doctors' offices, emergency rooms, or inpatient facilities. Some children have spent more of their lives in the hospital than at home. It is hard to imagine public ambulances refusing to respond to the report of a life-threatening emergency—but this has occurred in MBP cases after they received daily calls for weeks. In the case of Nancy Andrews, the fabrication of symptoms was repeated over many months.

MBP includes exaggeration and/or fabrication and/or induction of problems. It may include an unpredictable and changing combination of all three. It may coexist with noninduced ("real") problems.

Exaggeration

Exaggeration means that a genuine physical, psychological, or behavioral condition exists, but not to the extent reported by the perpetrator. For example, a child may have a temperature of 99.9° (F) and be fussy. Over a period of several days, the mother contacts the pediatrician a number of times claiming that the fever has reached 104.5° and that the child is screaming from pain. Another child may be normally active; the mother tells a psychologist that he is uncontrollably hyperactive. An infant has brief, normal irregularities in breathing; a sitter calls emergency medical services to report prolonged breathing pauses (apnea) requiring cardiopulmonary resuscitation (CPR).

Some practitioners have objected to the inclusion of exaggeration in the definition of MBP. For example, Morley (1995) feels that exaggeration is part of common language: "he always . . . ," "a million times. . . ." Sometimes parents will exaggerate a child's condition in order to gain an earlier or more convenient clinic appointment. Feldman and Ford (2000) suggest that exaggeration may be a way that parents call attention to concerning symptoms that the health care provider is ignoring. Masterson (1988), however, believes that "extreme illness exaggeration" does constitute at least a variant of MBP. The authors of this book believe that deliberate exaggeration is a method used in MBP maltreatment. Hyperbole, figures of speech, and practical motivations (such as the earlier appointment) can be separated from MBP behavior. For example, a parent exaggerating as a figure of speech would likely admit this if questioned carefully. The key is to consider the results of the language and the pattern of behavior as a whole.

Fabrication

Fabrication means that the perpetrator makes up a symptom or illness, and/or makes it look as if a symptom/illness exists when it does not. It can be verbal or behavioral. This was the primary method used in the case of Nancy Andrews. For example, health care providers may be told that an infant has suffered a seizure requiring cardio-pulmonary resuscitation (CPR) when, in fact, nothing has happened. A school may be told that the child has been diagnosed with hyper-activity, when this is not the case. Beyond false reports, however, perpetrators may also use a wide variety of actions to create the false appearance of problems. In the case of Nancy Andrews, the mother placed her own blood on the child's panties. Other examples include cases in which thermometers have been manipulated to simulate fe-vers, laboratory samples have been contaminated, or records have been altered.

Induction

Induction means the perpetrator causes a real symptom or illness to exist. Sheridan (2003) found that 57 percent of MBP cases in the medical literature included induced symptoms. Perpetrators have used many methods to make children ill. Common ones include poi-soning with salt or medications prescribed for someone else, smoth-ering to the point of transient or permanent brain damage, exposure to infectious agents, and subtle provocation of abnormal behavior. De-liberate inaction or withholding of physical/mental health treatment or food can also produce or intensify illness. For example, perpetra-tors can withhold medications prescribed for genuine asthma, so that the child is then treated for the resulting "resistant" wheezing.

Exaggeration, fabrication, and induction may all be present at vari-ous times in a single case. Each of these behaviors may cause serious harm (Rosenberg, 1995). Exaggeration and fabrication are not neces-sarily less harmful than induction. A well-told lie, for example, could cause a child to be placed on medications with serious side effects, subjected to invasive medical tests, or even taken to surgery. MBP does not appear to progress along a defined trajectory or continuum. All forms may be present, or may appear in any order. The distinc-tions among the methods may not be clear-cut. MBP may also coexist with a genuine problem or problems. Just as "even paranoids have en-emies," even children who are victims of MBP come down with colds, flu, and other noninduced illness. The occurrence of such "real" problems does not prove that MBP is not present.

Munchausen by proxy may involve physical, psychological, or behavioral symptoms, or a combination.

The majority of identified MBP cases have involved physical symptoms. An increasing number of cases, however, include psychological or behavioral features. Sometimes, as part of the deception, perpetrators falsely claim that the victim has suffered other forms of abuse. Case 1.1 involved false allegations of both physical and behavioral symptoms.

Sheridan's review of the MBP literature (2003) found that the average number of symptoms reported per victim was 3.25 (range unstated to 19). The problems most frequently encountered were: apnea (26 percent of cases), anorexia/feeding problems (24.6 percent), diarrhea (20 percent), seizures (17.5 percent), cyanosis (11.7 percent), behavior (10.4 percent), asthma (9.3 percent), allergy (9.3 percent), fevers (8.6 percent), and pain (8.0 percent).

Many problems are exaggerated, fabricated, or induced, but often they share certain characteristics:

1. *Problems reported may be of types that cannot be independently confirmed.* Often, the symptoms claimed in MBP are those that leave no verifiable evidence. Examples include breathing disorders, pain, and behavioral problems. The occurrence or nonoccurrence of these symptoms cannot be proven, although patterns or circumstances may be able to suggest whether occurrence or nonoccurrence was likely. For example, breathing pauses in infants (apnea) do not leave any "markers." However, if a recording monitor has been prescribed for an infant because of apnea, yet the parents only report episodes when the baby is not on the monitor, this may raise suspicion that the reports are false.

2. *Problems may be dramatic.* The symptoms often connote, at least to the lay observer, a medical emergency or life-and-death situation. Apnea, seizures, cyanosis (turning blue from lack of oxygen), asthma, fevers, and pain are all dramatic. Bleeding, although not among the most frequent, is another example of a dramatic symptom that is often claimed by MBP perpetrators. Alternatively, symptoms may have a bizarre quality beyond what is usually expected. For example, one mother claimed that

her son was so hyperactive that he ate his books and papers if she did not watch over him.

3. *Problems cannot be ignored.* One of the manipulative elements of MBP is that the health care provider must take the parent's reports of such symptoms seriously. Even if professionals are suspicious about reported breathing pauses or bleeding, for example, they cannot simply tell the parents to "go home and don't worry." If the symptoms are real, there is no guarantee that they will not recur. The child could die. Few professionals are willing to bet the child's life or health against their "hunch" that the symptom might not have occurred as reported.

MBP is behavior perpetrated on others.

The name, "Munchausen by proxy" has a colorful history. The Baron von Münchhausen (1720-1790) was a German mercenary who served with the Russians against the Turks. After his return, he became known as a teller of colorful tales. Fantastic stories attributed to the baron were collected and published (later made into movies), and have remained popular throughout the years. In 1951, English physician Richard Asher published his observations on a group of patients who came to hospitals giving false stories about their own illnesses. He gave the name "Munchausen's syndrome" to this phenomenon because the patients went from place to place telling "tall tales." It is probable that the name, rather than the behavior, was novel (Meadow 1995a). When Meadow first reported cases of parents falsely reporting illness in their children (1977), he adapted Asher's terminology to produce the diagnostic label, Munchausen by proxy. This conveyed typical features of the entity as it was then understood: that the parents tended to go from doctor to doctor, hospital to hospital, telling false tales, but on behalf of their children.

Most of the world's known cases of MBP involve children. However, there are some known cases of animal victims (Feldman, 1997) and adult victims (Sigal and Altmark, 1995). There are also instances of professionals causing problems in patients so that they can respond heroically (Sheridan, 1995). Since the study of MBP is relatively recent, it is probable that other forms are yet to be discovered. This book will focus only on MBP involving children as victims.

***The primary purpose of MBP appears to be some form
of intangible gratification for the perpetrator through
the problems of someone else.***

The primary purpose of MBP behavior is getting internal "psycho-logical" needs met. These needs are described by Lasher and Feld-man (2001):

> The perpetrator's principal motivation is usually to attract atten-tion, sympathy, care, and concern as the parent of a child with problems. She may be motivated by other "internal" goals as well, such as the desire to control and manipulate others, includ-ing a spouse or a high-status medical professional. For example, in a troubled marriage, the perpetrator may create "problems" intended to avert the spouse's leaving home or finding a new partner. In this example, the perpetrator may intend to gain the spouse's attention, interfere with the new relationship, or obtain revenge.

When attention or a feeling of importance is the primary motive, these may come from mental or physical health providers, a spouse, other family members, friends, the media, etc. Each case will be dif-ferent. The attention or other gratification probably strengthens the perpetrator's shaky identity, alleviates feelings of low self-esteem, or fills some other psychological void. The manipulative elements of the deception may also allow perpetrators to work out feelings of anger toward others. In Case 1.1, Mrs. Andrews' motives were unclear, but did not appear to be primarily the seeking of material gain.

Mental health clinicians distinguish Munchausen syndrome from a related condition called malingering—exaggerating, fabricating, or inducing illness primarily for monetary or other material gain. For example, someone who falsely claims a disabling injury in order to collect compensation or insurance benefits is malingering. As ap-plied to another person, a parent who exaggerates a handicapping condition for the primary purpose of collecting Supplemental Secu-rity Income (a welfare benefit) would be "malingering by proxy" (a concept that has not been well-defined). MBP and malingering may occur in the same case. The possibility of MBP should not be ex-cluded if elements of external gain are present in a case. Most impor-tant, uncertainty over primary motive should not take the place of considering and acting upon the possibility of child maltreatment. For child protection and custody purposes, if MBP has been confirmed it is extremely important that the label MBP be formalized to justify appropriate short- and long-term case planning and management. However, Meadow (1995b, p. 538) states, "Whatever term is used, and in whatever way, does not alter the fact that for an individual child who has been abused the most important thing is for the assessors to define accurately what has happened."

If a child is being maltreated, then the forms of maltreatment and their implications must be understood. This may occur only as an investigation develops. Sometimes the behavior is never understood completely. Information from this book and other sources should be applied as useful and appropriate.

TERMINOLOGY ISSUES

There is no single, universally agreed-upon definition or even name for MBP—a fact used by some opponents to impugn the concept. The original term used to describe this pattern of behavior is "Munchausen syndrome by proxy." In addition to that descriptive label, other terms now used interchangeably by many professionals include Munchausen by proxy syndrome, Munchausen's syndrome by proxy, Munchausen by proxy, and factitious disorder by proxy. The authors of this book do not, at this time, draw a distinction between MBP and any of the variants of that label. "Pediatric condition falsification" has been suggested as a descriptor to apply to a child victim, and "factitious disorder by proxy" has been applied to a perpetrator (Ayoub and Alexander, 1998). (For a more extended discussion of terminology, see Fisher and Mitchell, 1995 and Bools, 1996.)

It is very important to understand the difference between factitious disorder (including the subtype Munchausen syndrome), and Munchausen by proxy, and to use these terms correctly. They are two different entities, although they sound alike and have some commonalities. In referring to MBP it is incorrect—and can be confusing—to shorten the term to "Munchausen" or to use the term "Munchausen syndrome" or refer to a "Munchausen" case. Agency discussions, written records, interview information, court transcripts, etc., are often misinterpreted because of incorrect terminology. Factitious disorder/Munchausen syndrome and MBP do not necessarily have the same dynamics; a professional with expertise in one entity does not necessarily have expertise in the other.

Factitious disorder (including Munchausen syndrome) involves a pattern of exaggerating and/or fabricating and/or inducing a problem or problems *in oneself.* It is a formal diagnosis in the *Diagnostic and Statistical Manual of Mental Disorders,* Fourth Edition (American Psychiatric Association, 1994, p. 472). The DSM-IV (the "Bible" of professional mental health diagnosis) considers Munchausen syndrome to be a subtype of factitious disorder. Feldman and Hamilton (2001) describe both disorders and their incidence:

> The patient's principal goal is to garner gratifications intrinsic to the sick role, such as attention, care, and lenience. The best data indicate that within large general hospitals, factitious disorder is diagnosed in approximately 1 percent of patients on whom psychiatrists consult.
>
> Around 10 percent of factitious disorder patients have Munchausen syndrome. These individuals have a severe, chronic course characterized by perigrination (widespread travel in pursuit of additional medical treatment) and pseudologica fantastica (the creation of a captivating but specious personal history).
>
> Factitious disorder as a whole is more common in females than males. However, in Munchausen syndrome, men prevail. The conditions usually develop during the third or fourth decade of life. Factitious disorder patients often have families and hold responsible jobs, particularly as nurses or nurses' aides. In contrast, Munchausen syndrome is usually incompatible with the individual's maintaining steady employment and family ties. (p. 457)

In contrast with factitious disorder/Munchausen syndrome, MBP involves a pattern of exaggerating and/or fabricating and/or inducing a problem or problems *in someone else* (see Table 1.1). It is not a formal diagnosis in the DSM-IV. Because this is an important issue and is often confused, it will be discussed at some length.

TABLE 1.1. Comparison of Facitious Disorder/Munchausen Syndrome with Factitious Disorder by Proxy/Munchausen by Proxy

	Factitious Disorder Munchausen Syndrome	Factitious Disorder by Proxy Munchausen Syndrome by Proxy (etc.)
Victim	Self	Someone in the care of the perpetrator (child, dependent adult, patient, animal, etc.)
Perpetrator	Self	Someone caring for the victim
Classification	Mental disorder	Maltreatment
Methods	Exaggeration, fabrication, induction	Exaggeration, fabrication, induction
Motives	"Gratifications intrinsic to the sick role, such as attention, care, and lenience." (Feldman and Hamilton, 2001, p. 457)	"The perpetrator's principal motivation is usually to attract attention, sympathy, care, and concern as the parent of a child with problems." (Lasher and Feldman, 2001, p. 2)

MBP (under the term Factitious Disorder by Proxy) is included in the DSM-IV in Appendix B (pp. 725-727) as one of the

> new categories . . . that were suggested for possible inclusion. . . . The DSM-IV Task Force and Work Groups subjected each of these proposals to a careful empirical review and invited wide commentary from the field. The Task Force determined that there was insufficient information to warrant inclusion of these proposals as official categories . . . in DSM-IV. (American Psychiatric Association, 1994, p. 703) (Reprinted with permission from the *Diagnostic and Statistical Manual of Mental Disorders,* Text Revision. Copyright 2000. American Psychiatric Association.)

Professionals from a variety of disciplines have misused information about FDP (factitious disorder by proxy) in Appendix B, particularly since the entry under factitious disorder Not Otherwise Specified (American Psychiatric Association, p. 475) refers the reader to Appendix B. This misuse has taken two forms: claiming that MBP is a mental disorder, and applying the "research criteria" for FDP to clinical situations.

Marc Feldman (personal communication, July 2002) describes the fallacy in the first misuse:

> Appendix B diagnoses are terms and criteria sets still irrefutably under consideration by the American Psychiatric Association and not formalized as mental disorders. If they were, they would be exclusively in the body of the book. The introduction to Appendix B states with admirable clarity that these terms and sets are nothing more than "proposals." . . . I cannot imagine any clearer language. . . . FDP is NOT to be included when diagnosing a patient and it does not have [an] associated code number in Appendix B—as no research diagnosis does. Placing FDP on Axis II [i.e., including it in a formal mental health diagnosis] simply illustrates a total unfamiliarity with the conventions of the DSM iterations to date. It makes a bad situation even worse.
>
> Having been generously asked by the American Psychiatric Association to take primary responsibility in revising the text for FD and FDP in the most recent DSM version (DSM-IV-TR), I am convinced that the inclusion of FDP under FD NOS was an error. . . . The individuals responsible for the castaway mention of FDP under FD NOS, though obviously well meaning, [were] flatly mistaken in referring in the body of the book to a research diagnosis.

The assertion that MBP is a form of mental illness has been used in court cases and elsewhere to argue that a perpetrator should not be held responsible for maltreating a victim. It has also been used to suggest that perpetrators fit only one "pattern" or "profile," and that if this profile is not present, MBP has not occurred. Meadow states (1995b, p. 538):

> There is a danger that applying the term to the perpetrator, rather than to the abuse, will suggest that there is a single cause for the behavior and a possible single remedy. . . . A major disadvantage of [the term MBP] being applied to the perpetrator rather than to the abuse would be if it led to authorities believing that such abuse of children could be diagnosed by psychiatrists, or that an assessment of the perpetrating parent could overrule the clinical and forensic findings made by those involved with the child.

Rand and Feldman (1999, p. 100) add:

> [M]istakes are more likely to occur when MBP is used as a label for the caretaker or the child victim rather than the abuse. . . . Given the legal implications of suspected MBP, it should be noted that psychiatric diagnoses were developed for use in clinical, not forensic contexts. According to DSM-IV, there are significant risks that diagnostic information will be misused or misunderstood when psychiatric categories and criteria are utilized in adversarial legal proceedings. . . . We concur with [Roy] Meadow that the use of the term should be confined to a specific form of abuse in which active deception is involved and the primary motive is emotional gratification. As such, MBP is an objective, verifiable behavior rather than a personal characteristic of parent or child.

MBP may or may not be related to a coexisting mental illness. This is consistent with the way professionals understand other forms of child abuse. The behavior has occurred, and must be dealt with as a behavior. Part of that "dealing with" involves understanding the situation that led to the behavior. Each case must be studied individually to see whether mental illness is present and, if so, what form it takes.

The second misuse of the DSM-IV is applying the suggested "research criteria" for FDP to clinical situations. These research criteria (definitional elements) can be misleading. If they are used to confirm or disconfirm the presence of MBP, they may lead to inappropriate conclusions and activities.

The DSM-IV's suggested research criteria for FDP are:

A. Intentional production or feigning of physical or psychological signs or symptoms in another person who is under the individual's care.
B. The motivation for the perpetrator's behavior is to assume the sick role by proxy.
C. External incentives for the behavior (such as economic gain) are absent.
D. The behavior is not better accounted for by another mental disorder. (American Psychiatric Association, 1994, p. 727) (Reprinted with permission from the *Diagnostic and Statistical Manual of Mental Disorders,* Text Revision. Copyright 2000. American Psychiatric Association.)

The only criterion that the authors of this book accept unreservedly is A. It is close to the definitions that are used throughout the MBP community, although words for the behavior may vary. For example, the words used throughout this book are "exaggerate and/or fabricate and/or induce."

Criterion B is difficult for many professionals to interpret. It limits the behavior to a single, specific motive (Eminson, 2000). As Parnell (1998) points out, it does not explain why perpetrators assume the sick role through others rather than directly in themselves. It may be impossible to demonstrate this specific motive (or any motive) even though there is clear evidence that the child has been maltreated in accordance with Criterion A. Criterion B has been used in court cases and elsewhere to argue that MBP has not occurred, and this can be very damaging to case planning. Eminson states, "The perpetrator's motivations should never assume more importance than the victim's suffering" (2000, p. 32).

Criterion C is not in accord with current understandings of MBP behavior. For example, Sheridan's review (2003) found some signs of external gain in 5.3 percent of MBP cases in the literature. Many unpublished cases also contain elements of external gain. It is more accurate to state that the internal gain is the primary motive.

Criterion D must be carefully applied. Very rarely is a mental health condition directly responsible for MBP-like behavior (Marc Feldman, personal communication, July 2002).

In summary, the authors have four major criticisms of the DSM as it is often used in relation to MBP:

1. MBP is first and foremost a form of maltreatment, and should not be diagnosed as a mental illness. MBP is something that caretakers "do," not a disease that they "have."
2. MBP should not be confirmed or disconfirmed based on the presence of a specific motive.
3. MBP should not be confirmed or disconfirmed on the basis of incidental external gain.
4. MBP, as a form of child maltreatment, may occur in association with a variety of mental disorders. It may also occur without the presence of a diagnosed mental disorder. The role of a mental disorder must be assessed individually in each case.

Neither the definition nor research criteria contained in the DSM-IV should be used to decide if MBP maltreatment is involved. Doing so is a misuse of the DSM-IV and may leave MBP victims unprotected. The following case scenario provides a good example of a situation that is, unfortunately, becoming more common.

Case 1.2
Marshall County Child Protection Service received a report from Connor Medical Center indicating suspicion of MBP. According to the report, Matthew Johnson's mother had, for the third time since he was born, brought the two-month-old to the hospital claiming he had chronic vomiting to the point of dehydration. On all three occasions the infant looked well hydrated and nourished, and took fluids in the emergency room without vomiting. The pediatrician and emergency room staff were puzzled, particularly because a series of tests following previous episodes had all been normal and Matthew was on medication to stop reflux (vomiting), as prescribed by a specialist. On the third occasion, in accordance with previous instructions, the mother brought in a towel that, she said, contained Matthew's vomitus. An alert nurse noted small particles of food inconsistent with the infant's reported diet. When told that the towel would be sent to the lab for testing, Mrs. Johnson said she might have "picked up the wrong towel" and snatched it back. The report to CPS stated that the emergency room staff suspected Mrs. Johnson of fabricating the story and producing false evidence. They felt Matthew had been subjected unnecessarily to medical interventions including medications that had potentially severe side effects.

By the time the CPS investigator arrived for a meeting with hospital staff, the report had been rescinded. The staff had read the DSM-IV research criteria and erroneously believed that they could report suspicion of MBP-type child maltreatment only if it conformed to the DSM-IV research criteria. They felt that they could not be sure that the mother's motivation was "to assume the sick role by proxy." Some staff members felt that she simply wanted attention. Others felt uncomfortable speculating about what her motives might be. A psychiatrist who had interviewed the mother felt that she was depressed. Thus, the psychiatrist felt, the "behavior [might be] better accounted for by another mental disorder."

The CPS investigator explained why MBP should still be suspected, but the hospital staff insisted on their position. They refused to consider that MBP might be involved because they believed the case did not fit the DSM-IV criteria for FDP. With the report rescinded, CPS did not proceed with the case. The CPS investigator was directed to close the case and was later reprimanded by his superiors for "arguing with hospital staff." Inappropriate use of the DSM-IV criteria and the refusal of hospital staff to listen to the CPS investigator interfered with a full investigation and confirmation/disconfirmation process, and possibly with identifying and protecting a child who was being maltreated.

One final terminology problem should be noted. As MBP has become more widely recognized in the popular media, there has been some confusion between MBP and other forms of child maltreatment and child death. For example, there have been cases of child murder in which parents falsely reported that strangers kidnapped their children. These are clear attempts by parents to divert suspicion from their own crime. Instances have been reported in which child murder has been misdiagnosed as sudden infant death syndrome (SIDS) (Firstman and Talan, 1997). The fact that diagnostic mistakes have been made does not mean that SIDS does not exist or that all SIDS deaths are murders. Parents whose infants die through no fault of their own deserve the compassion and support of the community. They are often hurt by publicity and innuendo that suggest otherwise. MBP, other forms of child maltreatment, true illness, and SIDS must all be diagnosed correctly. Great harm can be done by diagnostic confusion. For example, if MBP is erroneously confirmed, someone will be falsely accused and the search for a cure of the child's problem(s) may cease. Conversely, if the existence of genuine MBP is not discovered, a victim will suffer and perhaps incur permanent harm.

A CONTROVERSY: DOES MBP EXIST?

So far, MBP has been discussed as though everyone accepts it. However, several lines of argument have been advanced that, according to their authors, call the existence of MBP into question.

Allison and Roberts (1998) are not convinced that MBP exists as a separate diagnostic entity. They are particularly skeptical about some of the psychological hypotheses that have been developed to describe MBP perpetrators and explain their behavior. They see much of the literature of MBP as repeating speculation and reifying observations from a few cases.

> What we have tried to argue against is the institutionalization—indeed, the criminalization—of the disorder by force of taxonomic classification. The alleged MBPS abuser/mother is assigned a set of characteristics, a largely affabulated etiology, and an inadequately conceived psychological profile, and is consequently identified, treated, and punished as a particularly egregious child abuser. . . .

But child abuse entails a far more complicated and dynamic set of behaviors and activities than can ever be expressed, much less understood, in the abbreviated and reductionistic terms of such categorical formulations. . . . Some mothers—and fathers—may use medical instruments or various medications to abuse their children, as is the argument expressed in virtually all the professional literature. Many people may even have seen frightening scenes of mothers on TV being videotaped while trying to smother their own children. But this behavior does not constitute a specified illness; it suggests only that certain people use a specific means or instrumentality to abuse their children. The legitimate category for all these acts is child abuse. (pp. 277-278)

The authors of this book agree with Allison and Roberts that MBP is best understood as a descriptive label for a particular pattern of behavior that forms a type of child maltreatment. They also agree with Allison and Roberts that all the complexities of individual cases must be taken into consideration. However, based on our study and case experience, we believe that MBP has characteristics not shared with other forms of child maltreatment, and thus should be considered unique. Many MBP perpetrators share characteristics that can be identified. These characteristics do not constitute a "profile" as that term is popularly used nor should they be used to confirm or disconfirm MPB maltreatment. However, they can be useful, in combination with other factors, to raise the possibility of MBP or to guide an investigation. We disagree with the assessment that much of the MBP medical, mental health, and social sciences literature is no more than "reductionistic" and derivative; this may reflect the tentativeness and sometimes the blind alleys associated with the growth of any new field of knowledge.

Another objection to MBP is that it exists, but is so rare that it is unlikely to be encountered in practice. Only a few epidemiological studies of MBP have been attempted. The best controlled of these, conducted in Britain, estimated that 1:200,000 children is a victim of MBP, poisoning, or suffocation (McClure et al., 1996). (But Eminson comments that suffocations and poisonings "must be the tip of the iceberg" [2000, p. 31]). In the McClure et al. (1996) study, children were considered victims if the situation was taken to child protective case conference, suggesting a high standard of suspicion that abuse was occurring. Warner and Hathaway (1984) reviewed cases of pediatric allergy and found MBP in 1:100 children treated for allergies overall and 5 percent of those receiving extensive evaluations for suspected food allergies. Light and Sheridan (1990) surveyed infant apnea programs and uncovered fifty-four cases with suspicion indicators among 20,090 monitored infants (0.27 percent, or approximately 1:4,000). Sheridan later surveyed pediatricians and family practitioners in Honolulu County (1995). They estimated that 1 percent of children in their practices might be victims of MBP.

Statistics on some other conditions affecting children may be useful for comparison. For example, serious congenital hearing loss is found in about one infant per thousand; several states mandate screening of all newborn infants for this condition (National Center for Hearing Assessment and Management, 2000) and the National Institutes of Health (National Center for Hearing Assessment and Management, 2000) has recommended that such screening be universal. The annual incidence of Lyme disease, which has been the focus of concern and publicity, is 5.1 per 100,000 persons of all ages, or approximately 1:19,608 (Surveillance for Lyme Disease, 2000). The preliminary Sudden Infant Death Syndrome death rate for 1998 was 64.1/100,000 live births, or about 1:1,560 infants (Guyer et al., 1999).

These findings suggest that significant public and professional concern is expended on conditions that are relatively infrequent, yet potentially serious. Public and professional educational efforts have built awareness as well as knowledge of how to respond. The same "learning curve" is occurring for MBP. Feldman and Lasher state, "MBP is no longer considered rare by most experts, although it still tends to be underrecognized" (1999, p. 28). A steady stream of inquiries to MBP professionals, from other professionals and from concerned family members, lends further support to this belief. At present the field is handicapped by the lack of an effective, broad-based system for gathering epidemiological data. There are many difficulties in obtaining such data, although these can and should be overcome so that these objections can be answered and children protected.

Several commentators on MBP believe that women are disproportionately accused as perpetrators because of their marginalized and discounted status in society (Guerisik, 1997). In this conceptualization, accusations of MBP are an easy "out" for physicians puzzled by difficult-to-diagnose illnesses, or an easy target if the women are too demanding as they seek care for their legitimately ill children.

There is little question that health care professionals have sometimes treated women unfairly (Sheridan, 1992), and that perhaps the number of male perpetrators of MBP has been underrecognized. However, the number of MBP cases in which there is definitive proof argues against the position that MBP is retaliation or "blaming the victim." Their role as primary caretakers to children, and the greater rewards to women from this role, may account for the preponderance of accused women. Robins and Sesan (1991) summarize this line of reasoning:

> [T]he factors that potentially lead to and perpetuate [MBP] include (a) an imbalance in self-care versus other care that leaves a mother with MSP feeling deprived, empty, and angry; (b) sociocultural support for this imbalance that pushes the mother to use indirect solutions to meet her needs; and (c) intergenerational transmission of abuse and oppression and the search to have her needs met through her child. Furthermore, asymmetries in the current heterosexual family unit make women much more vulnerable than men to using their children to satisfy years of unmet needs. When combined with a proclivity to turn to the medical profession to meet socially sanctioned self needs, variations of this disturbing form of child abuse can occur, with mothers as perpetrators. (p. 287)

Jones et al. (1993) suggest that as fathers assume more child care duties, they will experience the same stresses that lead women to perpetrate MBP.

Ultimately, the dispute over the reality and nature of MBP and its perpetrators reduces to questions of fact. Possibilities and alternative scenarios can always be raised, but is there proof that maltreatment has occurred, and proof of who perpetrated it? In many cases, the answer is unequivocally yes, as further chapters of this book will show.

Chapter 2

Perpetrators, Victims, and Others

PERPETRATORS

Some of the most basic and fascinating questions about MBP have to do with perpetrators. How can they commit this behavior? What do they think about as they do it? How can they deceive so successfully? What happened in their lives to make them choose this solution to their problems? Unfortunately, there are no satisfactory answers to these questions. Professionals writing about MBP have often failed to include much information about perpetrator motivations or life experiences. In any case, perpetrators are often so skilled and persistent at deception that it is difficult to believe their explanations. It is also common for perpetrators to become unavailable after they learn they are under suspicion. They may refuse to provide information, but often they flee before they can even be asked. Thus the information in this chapter is tentative. It is based on sources in the literature and on personal experience.

Some Theories About Motive

In order to engage in this behavior, some theorists believe, perpetrators must have a profound lack of empathy—an inability to see their children as individuals with feelings and rights (Rosenberg, 1987). They must also have an overwhelming sense of their own neediness, perhaps anger at those who have hurt them in the past, and probably other motives yet to be discovered. MBP perpetrators, on the surface, often appear loving and sometimes seem to be ideal parents. This is a facade, what Schreier and Libow (1993) call a "masquerade" of mothering. Perpetrators use children as objects to meet their own needs—needs that outweigh the needs or rights of their victims. The defining feature of this kind of maltreatment, according to the literature, is the perpetrators' need to obtain attention or other internal gratification through involvement in the illness or problem of their victims. Every normal person wants attention, love, and approval. MBP perpetrators, however, go far beyond normal behavior to get these needs met. Their need is so strong that perpetrators exaggerate and/or fabricate and/or induce the problem, then build their lives around "caring" for it. Perhaps they do not know better ways of getting the positive regard they so desperately want. Some believe perpetrators identify so closely with the victim that they are "taking on the role of a sick person by proxy" and thus, in a psychological sense, caring for themselves. Criterion B in the Research Criteria for Factitious Disorder by Proxy of the DSM-IV (American Psychiatric Association, 1994) reflects this hypothesis. Creating illness also may be a way that perpetrators can obtain help for themselves without the stigma of admitting personal inadequacy. This may explain why many perpetrators appear so comfortable in hospitals.

Schreier and Libow (1993) believe that women (the most frequent perpetrators) maltreat in this way because they have come from psychologically deprived, often abusive, backgrounds. Their positive experience with an obstetrician may be the first nurturing relationship of their lives, or perhaps the first such experience with a male. It has a price: the need for medical care. After the birth of the baby, these mothers are threatened with loss of the relationship. However, they can establish a comparable relationship with the child's pediatrician or family practitioner. This also, however, has a price: a sick child. The stage may thus be set for the creation of illness "to order."

The creation of a sick or troubled child also has hostile and manipulative elements (Feldman and Lasher, 1999). As perpetrators fool providers with one symptom after another, they are in control. They are "smarter" than these highly educated and apparently successful professionals. If their previous life has left them with anger toward professionals or others, MBP provides a good opportunity for them to express it with few immediate drawbacks.

Others suggest that relationships with persons besides health care providers may be the goal of some MBP. For example, perpetrators may want attention from first responders (police [Schreier, 1996], fire fighters, paramedics) or from spouses/partners. Some perpetrators may come from families in which illness and illness creation were the primary ways in which people received attention and love. In this sense they may simply be repeating what they learned, and sometimes what was done to them. Often, especially early in an MBP case, the motive and underlying psychological factors are unclear. Motivations probably vary from case to case, and may be mixed.

Attention is not, however, the only gain that MBP perpetrators may receive from their behavior. Sheridan (2003) found that 5.3 percent of MBP cases in her review of the literature had some "secondary (external) gain"— financial and tangible benefits from government, medical, and social agencies, etc. Sometimes elements of malingering (feigning illness for gain) and MBP may be mixed. For example, a newspaper reported on a young "cancer survivor" who had never had cancer. Over many years, this young woman and her family had been the recipients of numerous charity donations for medical expenses, "final wish" trips, and cancer camp. The girl herself had been selected as Junior Volunteer of the Year, in part because of her generosity to others in the face of her own serious illness. The deception in this case was on the part of the mother, who had convinced the girl and others that the disease was real. It was never clear how much the mother did this for attention, and how much for the material things that she received. Clearly, however, deception had occurred and a child's whole sense of self was manipulated to meet the mother's needs. This child had been subjected at least to physical and emotional abuse.

Scientific and professional journals are the forum in which practitioners and theoreticians advance ideas, present findings, and debate with one another. The medical and psychosocial literature is, of course, a resource for legal proceedings and other uses, but this is not its chief purpose. As the professional literature about MBP has grown, it has quite naturally included speculations and hypotheses that may or may not stand the "test of time." Undoubtedly, this will continue as long as MBP is studied. The following characteristics often seen in perpetrators are presented in that spirit.

Perpetrator-Consistent Characteristics

MBP perpetrators tend to have characteristics in common. However, each characteristic can also be true of other child maltreaters. No specific combination of personal characteristics or traits can define with certainty whether someone is an MBP perpetrator. Characteristics consistent with MBP perpetrators may add to MBP suspicion and to the investigative process, but do not constitute a profile and should not be used as a profile because the term has legal and forensic connotations. Furthermore, it is sometimes misused to suggest that persons who fit the characteristics must be guilty. Some MBP cases do not "fit the pattern," and the pattern itself is based on cases that have been identified. Different or less serious cases of MBP may show different features. Those who practice in this field have a special obligation to alert colleagues about new manifestations and features of MBP.

The following characteristics are frequently seen with MBP—but not invariably, as perpetrators and their motives and behaviors can be quite varied. Not all of these characteristics will be present in any one case, or known at the time MBP is first suspected. They should be combined with other case information and patterns.

- MBP perpetrators are usually individuals with primary responsibility for the child.
- MBP perpetrators often present initially and on the surface as "normal," "good" caretakers.
- MBP perpetrators are usually accomplished liars, deceivers, and manipulators.
- MBP perpetrators may appear to be overanxious, overprotective, mistaken, or deluded. On closer observation, however, their concern is of a different quality.
- MBP perpetrators may have a background in a health profession, or an unusual degree of preoccupation with health or mental health.
- MBP perpetrators may seek attention from a variety of people.
- MBP perpetrators may deny all or part of what they have done, even when there is overwhelming evidence.
- MBP perpetrators do not necessarily stop their behavior when they are suspected or caught. The behavior may change or the danger to the victim may increase.
- MBP perpetrators may add or change medical or mental health professionals ("doctor shop") and facilities—or they may not.
- MBP perpetrators may have a personal history of symptom/illness exaggeration, falsification, or induction.
- MBP perpetrators' mental health evaluations may be "normal."
- MBP perpetrators may or may not have prior child protective services involvement.

- MBP perpetrators are usually the only ones consistently present at or in association with the onset of symptoms. When they are absent, symptoms and illness are not reported, or may begin to improve.

MBP perpetrators are usually individuals with primary responsibility for the child.

Rosenberg (1987) found that 98 percent of perpetrators were mothers. Sheridan (2003) found 76.5 percent, suggesting that the field is becoming more aware of other presentations of MBP. However, most reports of MBP still involve mothers. Foster mothers, fathers, and other caretakers of children are occasionally identified as perpetrators of MBP maltreatment. Even more rare is perpetration by both parents.

MBP perpetrators often present initially and on the surface as "normal," "good" caretakers—and dynamics between MBP perpetrators and victims usually appear good, even excellent.

Perpetrators may appear to parent appropriately and love their children. One woman who had been named "foster mother of the year" had three children die in her care (Mother of the Year, 1996). Others became mysteriously ill. Perpetrators are sometimes seen as exemplary parents who "live for" their children. Others simply appear to be "normal" or "average." Some are "difficult," either with most other adults or with selected adults. Alternatively, they may be friendly only with specific people so that alliances are formed with some professionals and enemies made of others. This can divide a treatment team.

Relationships between perpetrators and their children usually *appear* good. This is a facade. A closer look usually tells a much different story. For example, when perpetrators know they are being observed with their children, they are often gentle, loving, and attentive. On covert observation or when walked in on unexpectedly they have been observed to be distant, uninvolved, and rough, even when not abusing their children (Southall et al., 1997).

Often, there is an excessive quality to parent-child relationships in MBP that looks like devotion, but is not. For example, MBP perpetrators are often reluctant to separate from their hospitalized children, insisting on remaining at the bedside day and night. Although many normal parents want to be with their children, often at some sacrifice, MBP perpetrators often seem more comfortable in the hospital than outside. They may not appear to "have a life" separate from the child's problems. They may insist that no one else can provide the required quality of care

This appearance of good parenting creates one of the biggest problems to overcome when working with suspected or confirmed MBP. Involved professionals, family, and friends may simply not believe that the caretaker could have perpetrated the maltreatment.

It is commonly believed that mothers naturally love their children, and that they will nurture, protect, and sacrifice for them. It is extremely difficult to allow oneself to suspect that any mother would deliberately cause physical or emotional harm to her child in this calculating and subtle way. Schreier and Libow state (1993, p. 52):

> What differentiates MBP abuse from other forms of child abuse is the false perception on the part of others that the abusive parents are deeply caring and concerned about their children. Apparent good or even exemplary parenting, when combined with none of the usual signs of child abuse, and no obvious indications of a disturbed parent-child relationship, make it quite difficult to even entertain the possibility of MBP.

MBP perpetrators do not "love" their children in the way most people understand love. They use their children as objects. Their feelings may be strong, but are more related to the child as an image, an "it" that meets their own needs. They disregard moral values and the welfare of their children to get what they need.

MBP perpetrators are usually accomplished liars, deceivers, and manipulators.

Perpetrators can be extremely believable. When questioned, their answers are at least superficially convincing. Presumably as a manipulative ploy, they are sometimes the first to express a fear that they will not be believed. They can excel at concocting seemingly plausible reasons for their behavior and asserting that others "misinterpret" their motives and deeds. All these factors make it more difficult to suspect them.

During or after an MBP investigation, nothing perpetrators say should be taken at face value. Information they supply, or which could have originated with them should not be trusted. *Independent corroboration of facts (not spouse, friends, neighbors, and relatives) should be obtained.* It is common for MBP perpetrators to report that physical or mental health care providers in another area have diagnosed a particular condition in their child. They will talk about the tests and treatment convincingly, often using medical or mental health terminology. Or they may make false allegations. The physician was incompetent, the social worker was prejudiced, the nurse was careless and had to blame someone else to save her job, the teacher was frustrated, the ex-husband sexually abused the children, and so on. They will claim that records have been lost or destroyed. They may bring records that seem to confirm their story. When the "diagnosing" professional is contacted, she or he states that she or he has provided only well-child care. When the original records are obtained, they are missing the key information that would confirm the perpetrator's story.

Case 2.1
A foster mother whose foster child had recurrent severe asthma knew that the physician was researching families in which there had been asthma deaths. She told a dramatic story of how her cousin's child in another state had just died of asthma. The story included details of the family rushing the child to the hospital in an ambulance, the inability of the emergency department staff to save the child, and the funeral. This foster mother expressed the wish that her foster child's doctor could have been in the emergency department, since she so admired the physician's skill, dedication, and interest in fatal asthma. By coincidence, and unknown to the foster mother, the physician had trained at the hospital in question. He contacted the emergency department staff and found that no children had died there from asthma in several years. When confronted, the foster mother said that she was only repeating what had been told to her by the family, and suggested that they must have given her the wrong name of the hospital.

MBP perpetrators may appear to be overanxious, overprotective, mistaken, or deluded.

Overanxious, overprotective, mistaken, and deluded parents report an honest but incorrect belief that their child has a problem. They may exaggerate the importance of symptoms, perhaps to obtain prompt or thorough care, but they do not create physical or mental health problems or lie about them. They generally respond well to information and reassurance. They usually hate for their children to go through testing and procedures. They are greatly relieved when test results are negative and procedures are over, although they may find new areas of concern. First-time parents sometimes do not know what to expect from their children, or overestimate their infant's fragility. They also respond to information, reassurance, and experience. People who are deluded have, for psychological reasons, a strong and persistent false belief. They are reporting accurately what they believe to be true, although it is not true. They cannot separate truth from falsehood. Information appropriately gathered and evaluated in cases of overanxious-overprotective, first-time, or deluded parents does not reveal the lies, deception, and inconsistencies that are found in MBP cases.

MBP perpetrators know (although they will not admit) that the child does not have a problem, or a problem of the magnitude reported. They actively create the situation or make false reports. They may voice concern about what their children are going through, or appear worried, but this is a facade. They are less likely than normal or worried parents to show relief or pleasure when nothing is found to be wrong. They will likely argue with staff, perhaps seem disappointed, insist that the problem exists, and demand further testing and intervention. They will claim that they "want to be sure nothing is missed." When caught inducing symptoms, they may say that they did it "just this one time" to minimize the magnitude of their maltreatment or so that health care professionals would believe that the purported problem was real.

MBP perpetrators may have a background in a health profession, or an unusual degree of preoccupation with health or mental health.

Rosenberg (1987) found some background in health care in 30 percent of cases, and Sheridan (2003) found it in 14.16 percent. The most common reported health care experience among perpetrators is in nursing. Regardless of their background, it is not uncommon for MBP perpetrators to have a strong interest in health issues, to have many professional or popular health reference books in the house, or to claim expert knowledge about health care. Sometimes this helps them perpetrate MBP in very sophisticated ways. In other instances, both the knowledge level and methods of perpetration will be simple. For example, it does not take a great deal of sophistication or medical knowledge to concoct a substance that looks like vomitus, place it around a child, then state that the child has "spit up" and show the "proof."

It is a cliché that people often develop an interest in the helping professions because they are seeking help for themselves. With proper education and reasonably good mental health, students are able to understand their own experiences and discipline this desire. Many health care professionals are first attracted to the field because of their own experiences with illness, or their desire to have the admiration that comes from knowing what to do in an emergency. Among reasonably normal people, these motivations can lay the foundation for high levels of service to others. Being a health care professional or being interested in health care is not a sign that one has committed or will commit MBP. Health care consumers are appropriately encouraged to be informed and active in their care. Medical and psychological information is readily available in bookstores, libraries, and on the Internet—as it should be. However, among MBP perpetrators the focus on problems, especially those of the child and perhaps other family members, may approach an obsession.

In this context, knowledge about illness can become one tool that MBP perpetrators use to practice deception. Knowledge and skills become weapons. Perpetrators know or can find out what symptoms will be convincing, and can deduce or learn from the literature how to create them. When they can use a medical or psychiatric vocabulary comfortably, they are more likely to be accepted as "one of us" by other health care providers. This acceptance lowers barriers and suspicions, and often leads to opportunities for further deception. For example, when a child has or appears to have physical or mental health problems, the mother, who is a physical or mental health professional, may be trusted to take temperatures, collect specimens, "hang out" near the medication cart, have access to records, or be closely involved in other ways. She may begin to participate in the gossip or work of the facility, or perhaps to provide support for other parents of children with "problems." She may have access to areas not normally open to parents, either because this is allowed to her or because she knows how to enter them without detection. Her reports, for example, of elevated temperatures and specimens that come back with abnormal results are not questioned. She will not be associated with the drugs or syringes that are missing. Instead, facility personnel and other families will remember her as wonderfully helpful.

MBP perpetrators may seek attention from a variety of people.

The people from whom perpetrators seek attention may or may not be professionals, powerful or authority figures, and may or may not be associated with health care. MBP perpetrators often have a dramatic flair to their stories, or describe dramatic happenings in their lives. MBP perpetrators often live a lifestyle of deceit that goes beyond the child victim. Their lives are often full of inconsistencies, "soap opera" drama, turbulence, and unusual events. They may claim to have been raped, stalked, or robbed under dramatic circumstances (e.g., while visiting the child at the hospital). A review of their past will often show a long pattern of seeking the "spotlight." It may include frequent accusations against others. They may claim to have experienced events that are, in retrospect, improbable in their occurrence, combination, or frequency. They may comment that they are "unlucky," "cursed," or "always in the wrong place at the wrong time." They may claim an ability to predict the future, perhaps expressing a belief that the child is going to die or that problems will occur at a particular time. Such "forewarnings"—which the parent can later use to "prove" that she or he was right—can sometimes be used as evidence of premeditation. They must, however, be distinguished from the sincere and very frightening premonitions that parents sometimes report (Light and Sheridan, 1990).

Case 2.2
English nurse Beverly Allit was found guilty of murdering four children, attempting to murder three children, and of hurting six other children (Davies, 1993). Her probable motive was to appear to be a competent, even heroic nurse. While under suspicion but prior to the trial, Allit moved in with supportive friends. All of a sudden, the house was thrown into chaos. Money and objects disappeared, only to reappear in unexpected places later. The stove "turned itself" on, possessions were destroyed, a fire broke out, and all members of the household including the animals experienced accidents and illnesses. Allit tried to convince the family that a "poltergeist" was at work. She denied, raged, and threatened suicide when evidence suggested that she was the poltergeist. Once she left the home, these incidents stopped.

MBP perpetrators may deny all or part of what they have done, even when there is overwhelming evidence.

Perpetrators have watched videotapes of themselves injuring their children, only to deny that the maltreatment occurred. From time to time those who are convicted and imprisoned for MBP maltreatment are interviewed on television, still convincingly protesting their innocence. When perpetrators do confess, they may admit only to what they were actually caught doing and not to the MBP behavior as a whole. Thus, as already mentioned, they may concede that they did something "just this one time," but will usually give a self-serving reason and insist that the rest of the episodes occurred as previously described.

MBP perpetrators do not necessarily stop their behavior when they are suspected or caught.

The behavior may change or the danger to the victim may increase. Perpetrators still have the same personality and needs when suspicion focuses on them. When they learn that they are suspected, perpetrators may be even more dangerous than before and escalate their perpetration in an attempt to "prove" the victim's "problems." Or they may cease MBP perpetration—at least for a while—or flee to another jurisdiction.

The likelihood of a situation constituting MBP is increased if symptoms decrease or are resolved when perpetrators know they are suspected. Other MBP-consistent behaviors, such as lying, manipulation, and deception, are likely to continue or even escalate. The perpetrators may move to other targets or exaggerate/fabricate/induce illness in themselves. Efforts may continue to convince professionals and others that specific events occurred and that the child really did have the claimed condition. Perpetrators may shift attention to marshalling a defense, perhaps through locating sympathetic "witnesses" or contacting groups that oppose child protective or MBP court action. Other attention-seeking behavior may occur. If the victim is not appropriately protected, the victim and siblings remain at high risk for further maltreatment. This risk may continue for years.

Case 2.3, Part 1

As an infant, Jo Ellen was removed from her mother after the mother repeatedly suffocated her as part of a long process of fabricating and inducing
episodes of apnea. MBP abuse was found by the court, and Jo Ellen was
placed with a foster family. Jo Ellen thrived in foster care, and her mother
completed a child protective case plan that involved counseling and parenting
classes. After a year in placement, Jo Ellen was returned to her parents and
the child protective case was closed. The child protective worker had forgotten about this case when, several years later, she saw a news report. The
featured family alleged that the soil around their house was contaminated by
toxic waste from a factory that had been on the site years before. They had
organized other residents to keep children from playing outside after their
own child became "extremely dizzy" while playing outside. As the worker
watched the broadcast, she recognized Jo Ellen as the child who supposedly was affected by the toxic waste, and Jo Ellen's mother as the leader of
the neighborhood organization. It appeared that Jo Ellen's mother was once
again successful in gaining attention for herself through claiming that Jo Ellen had symptoms.

*MBP perpetrators may add or change medical or mental health
professionals ("doctor shop") and facilities—or they may not.*

"Doctor shopping" is well documented in the literature as one part
of factitious illness (Libow and Schreier, 1986). It occurs for several
reasons. The complex symptoms presented by the victim and the resistance of those symptoms to conventional treatment often result in
referral to a parade of specialists. This serves the interests of perpetrators, because they receive the repeated attention associated with going to new practitioners, and they can vary the story if they wish.
They can also plant hints that the old practitioners were less than fair
and competent, while flattering the new practitioners by saying, e.g.,
"you are my last hope" or "I've heard such good things about you."

Perpetrators may also move from provider to provider until one is
found who is likely to believe their story. In most communities, it is
not difficult to find a practitioner who holds theories that complement
the fabrication. For example, some practitioners believe that food allergies are a major source of behavioral difficulties in children. A perpetrator could manipulate this until the diet is severely limited and behavior monitoring is constant. If the mother, for example, is then
accused of MBP, she can take refuge in the practitioner's theories and
claim that she was only doing as she was told.

Accumulating providers or moving from one to another is not,
however, always present in MBP. If current professionals are behav-

ing as perpetrators wish, and the perpetrators' needs are being met, there may be no reason to change or add providers. In fact, changing or adding providers may pose a risk, since sometimes deception is uncovered when a less credulous or enmeshed practitioner (or one more informed about MBP) takes over the case.

MBP perpetrators may have a personal history of symptom/illness exaggeration, falsification, or induction.

In cases she reviewed, Rosenberg (1987) found that 10 percent of perpetrators had Munchausen syndrome, and 14 percent had some features of it. Sheridan (2003) found 29.3 percent of perpetrators to have some features of factitious illness. Perpetrators' purported symptoms may be similar to, or share the dramatic and subjective characteristics of, the victim's symptoms. In some cases, the victim's condition is the only problem in a family that otherwise appears normal. In other cases, the identified victim may be part of a family in which many members have symptoms, directed by the perpetrator.

Case 2.3, Part 2
   Jo Ellen's mother, Terry, had actually been the subject of a medical journal article when she was a teenager. She had been admitted to the hospital repeatedly complaining of stomach pains. When finally confronted with normal test results, she stated that she was desperate to get out of the home due to her grandfather's abuse. The grandfather adamantly denied the abuse, but moved out of the home. Terry never complained of stomach pains again. It is not known whether she was indeed abused, or whether this was a false accusation.

When Jo Ellen was referred for maltreatment, the child protective investigator was told that Terry's factitious symptoms were far in the past, and only in response to abuse. However, a review of the records showed that she was hospitalized several times during her pregnancy for "intractable vomiting." After giving birth, she began to experience severe dizzy spells that required ambulance calls or emergency room visits. (Note that she claimed that Jo Ellen had dizzy spells.) Terry reported constant worries about dropping the baby, and heroic efforts to overcome the dizziness long enough to make sure that Jo Ellen was safe. She refused admission to the hospital for evaluation of the dizzy spells because she did not want to leave Jo Ellen, and refused to take any medicines because she was breastfeeding.

MBP perpetrators' mental health evaluations may be "normal."

Perpetrators may be interviewed and tested by competent professionals who do not find mental health pathology. Mental health consultants may express admiration for the perpetrator's dedication and strength in difficult times. No mental health evaluation, interview, or test, including polygraph ("lie detector") exists that can show whether or not MBP has occurred. According to Sheridan's (2003) review, when MBP perpetrators do have a mental health diagnosis, it is likely to be Factitious Disorder/Munchausen syndrome, depression, or one of the personality disorders.

MBP perpetrators may or may not have prior child protective services involvement.

In many non-MBP child maltreatment cases, families have been known to agencies over a span of years and for multiple children. This is much less likely with MBP. Even when several children have been victimized, professionals cannot assume that someone would already have recognized and reported MBP maltreatment. Perpetrators' skills at deception, the subtlety of the behavior, the fact that perpetrators are often articulate and middle class, and the lack of knowledge among health care professionals, all work against the identification of MBP. On the other hand, as more child welfare personnel become aware of MBP, they are discovering more potential cases among families who have been involved with the agency and among siblings of identified victims. Suspicious situations have been found among foster and adoptive parents as well as among cases referred for other forms of maltreatment. For this reason, all child welfare personnel should receive basic MBP education.

MBP perpetrators are usually the only ones consistently present at or in association with the onset of symptoms.

When perpetrators are absent, symptoms and illness are not reported, or may begin to improve. On close examination of circumstances, there is usually a striking pattern that demonstrates that only one person had the opportunity to induce symptoms. The investigative and confirmation-disconfirmation process must be done carefully, as people may think (or the perpetrator may contend) that they have witnessed things they have actually *not* seen. For example, one mother reported that her child had turned blue at another child's birthday party, and that this was witnessed by everyone present. Close questioning revealed that the mother had come running out of a bedroom with the child already blue and limp in her arms. Although everyone saw the results, only the mother was present for the beginning of the episode. Even if someone else is present when an episode begins, it should be remembered that MBP perpetrators are clever and manipulative, and have been known to induce symptoms while being watched.

Similarly, when victim and suspected perpetrator are separated and the victim is protected from any manipulation by the perpetrator or those the perpetrator might influence, if MBP maltreatment is involved, the problems should prove to be nonexistent, should no longer occur, or should taper off. This "separation test" can provide strong evidence that the perpetrator is exaggerating and/or fabricating and/or inducing the problem. In Sheridan's (2003) review this was the second most common method of proving the presence of MBP, after videotape. Demonstration that symptoms resolve or improve after separation from the suspected perpetrator is important because a genuine mental or physical health condition will not ordinarily improve because a child has been moved into a hospital or foster home. A genuine problem that has resolved will not ordinarily recur if a caregiver regains access to the child, but problems caused by MBP often will. Recall that Jo Ellen was ill when with her mother, made a complete recovery while in placement, then developed new and suspicious problems when returned to her mother.

Case 2.4

A woman was concerned about her sister's children. Three infants had died, with no final diagnosis. The first child was at home, and the death was attributed to SIDS. The second child was at a baby-sitter's house, with the parents absent, and the death was ruled "cause unknown." The third death occurred at a different sitter's, again with the parents absent, and was labeled "heart rhythm disturbance." The sister's fourth child was at home on a monitor that sounded an alarm if the heart rate dropped too low. The monitor sounded on several occasions. Sometimes this occurred when the father was home and sometimes when the mother was home. After several of these episodes, the parents insisted on referral to a heart specialist. The new doctor diagnosed a rare, hereditary heart condition and started the baby on medication. The baby had no more episodes.

In this instance, the problem was unrelated to MBP. It is extremely rare for a family to experience three infant deaths from physical causes. However, these deaths occurred in different places and with different people present. Two people responded independently to monitor alarms and witnessed what was going on with the baby. The cardiologist offered a reason for the problem, and the problem resolved as soon as the medication was started. The woman was appropriately concerned about whether her sister was an MBP perpetrator. In this instance, the sister was not.

This list of characteristics is specifically designated "perpetrator-consistent" because they are frequently seen in cases of MBP. This is explicitly not a "profile" of the MBP perpetrator. Hopefully, these characteristics will be used as suggestions by health care professionals when investigating possible MBP cases.

VICTIMS

Following is a list of the most common known victim characteristics of Munchausen by proxy:

- MBP may affect one child or several children at a time. There may be a series of victims.
- Identified MBP victims are usually infants or young children.
- Victims of MBP do not fit the stereotype of maltreated children.
- Victims of MBP should not be assumed to be colluding in their maltreatment.
- Victims of MBP may suffer significant physical or psychological/behavioral harm, immediately or later, from their maltreatment.

MBP may affect one child or several children at a time.

In MBP cases there may be a series of victims. Those who are initially suspected are not necessarily the only victims. Most commonly, perpetrators focus on one victim at a time. As with other forms of maltreatment, the child may be selected based on specific characteristics that meet the maltreater's needs; for example, age or gender. However, in some cases several children are abused serially or simultaneously. A close look at case information during an appropriate confirmation-disconfirmation process may reveal multiple health problems, past and/or present among other children or other nuclear or extended family members, and even child deaths. In Rosenberg's (1987) review, 9 percent of known siblings were dead and "several" had problems similar to those of the identified victim. In Sheridan's (2003) review, 25 percent of known siblings were dead and 61 percent had symptoms that suggested MBP. For these and other reasons, information must be gathered in MBP investigations about suspected or confirmed victims, suspected or confirmed perpetrators, other children presently or formerly in the home of the suspected perpetrator, and sometimes others depending on the case situation.

Identified MBP victims are usually infants or young children.

Statistically, among identified cases, infants and toddlers are disproportionately likely to be victims of MBP. The average age of victims at the time of MBP diagnosis was 39.8 months in Rosenberg's (1987) review and 48.65 months in Sheridan's (2003). Younger victims are dependent on their caregivers, easy to manipulate, and unable to contradict the perpetrator's story. When older children are reported as potential victims of MBP, a close look at the history usually reveals that the behavior began when they were younger.

Adult victims are generally in a physically or psychologically dependent situation (Sigal and Altmark, 1995). Animals may be maltreated in this fashion, again because they are dependent, easy to manipulate, and unable to contradict the perpetrator's story (Feldman, 1997).

Victims of MBP do not fit the stereotype of maltreated children.

Victims of MBP do not necessarily come from homes wracked by poverty and drugs. They do not exhibit the common patterns of burns, bruises, neglected health care, or malnutrition often associated with physical abuse and neglect. They are usually not dirty or unsupervised. Their parents usually do not speak to or about them harshly or negatively in public. All forms of child maltreatment can occur in "the last home where you'd expect it." MBP often does.

Victims of MBP should not be assumed to be colluding in their maltreatment.

Rosenberg states (1995, p. 22), "Children who agree they have all the symptoms which their mothers falsely claim they have, whether those are physical or psychiatric, should not be thought of as liars." Children naturally believe what their parents tell them about their health. They accept the medications and treatments their parents tell them have been prescribed by health care professionals. Parnell states (1998, pp. 35-36),

> It is not feasible to expect young children to make differentiations about the illness perspectives of their mothers that even doctors cannot detect. . . . It becomes impossible for children to tell when and if they are sick if their perceptions have constantly been invalidated.

Young children may not be able to separate reality from unreality due to their developmental stage, and older children may have no reason to suspect anything is wrong.

As they grow, children who are subjected to MBP internalize a reality that includes the problem. If a child merely repeats things that are false out of ignorance or coercion, the child should not be considered to be deceptive or participating in the MBP. The child may sincerely believe that the problem exists. In some cases the perpetrator may have taken deliberate steps to induce the child's belief that there is a physical or mental health problem. For example, in Case 1.1, if Mrs. Andrews placed her own blood on Nancy's bedsheets while Nancy was asleep, the girl might have come to believe that she was bleeding and would have told others that she was bleeding.

Some older victims are very aware of what is being done to them and the lies that are being told. This can create a severe conflict for the child, who naturally feels a loyalty to and dependence on the parent, and who may also be the recipient of threats or bribes. The MBP perpetrator's skill at manipulation must be remembered when the child's role is assessed. There are many reasons children "don't tell" (Libow, 1995). Theorists who hold a family orientation to child abuse sometimes speculate about characteristics in victims that lead to their being abused. They sometimes conceptualize child abuse as a form of communication or unconscious collusion between the abuser and abused. This raises an interesting line of future investigation, but at present the authors are not aware of any data on this in relation to MBP. Even if this speculation is true, it does not imply active and conscious consent to the abuse on the part of the victim. It probably represents every child's desire for survival by doing what parents expect, even if it is injurious to the self.

Victims of MBP may suffer significant physical or psychological/ behavioral harm, immediately or later, from their maltreatment.

As already described, Rosenberg (1987) found a death rate of 9 percent and long-term or permanent harm among 8 percent of the victims in her review. Sheridan (2003) found a death rate of 6 percent and long-term or permanent harm among 7 percent of victims in her review. Rosenberg and Sheridan considered all victims to have suffered at least short-term harm. The catalog of maltreatment methods used by MBP perpetrators—including suffocation, poisoning, emotional abuse, use of high doses of unnecessary prescription medication, etc.—suggests the toll on victims. With some of these methods, the "dose" is sufficiently difficult to control or the method so inherently dangerous that injury could hardly be avoided. Child victims also suffer psychological, social, and physical consequences of unnecessary treatment. For example, in a widely publicized case, Jessica Bush, age eight, had her gall bladder, appendix, and part of her intestines removed unnecessarily. She endured more than 200 hospital stays and 40 surgeries.

Feldman and Ford summarize (1994):

> Victims of MBP may be permanently damaged physiologically and/or psychologically, either directly by the mother's manipulations or by the treatments and tests administered. For example, children may develop brain damage or cerebral palsy from induced anoxia (inadequate oxygen to the tissues of the body), or severe damage to internal organs from recurrent infections. Children may miss a lot of school and suffer educationally and socially. They may go on to display intense anxiety or hyperactivity, fearfulness, or passivity and helplessness. Some of these children may develop Munchausen Syndrome themselves or become convinced of their own "invalid" status. (p. 164)

Bools, Neale, and Meadow (1993) found that children maltreated in this fashion later developed emotional disturbances, and that these were worse in children not removed from the perpetrator's home. Libow (1995) interviewed ten adults who, as children, were victims of MBP and concluded that they had suffered (in addition to the maltreatment and unnecessary treatment):

> [S]ignificant emotional and physical problems during their childhoods including problems with growth, eating disorders, nightmares, self-destructive fantasies, high anxiety and school concentration difficulties. . . . For most of the subjects, the [MBP] abuse stopped only when they left home, or in a few cases, when the child was old enough to actively protest and threaten to tell. . . . Many had gone through their adult lives repeatedly questioning their own reality-testing, trying to find something wrong with themselves to explain why they had uniquely been chosen for the bizarre abuse they experienced. As adults, these subjects experienced a significant number of posttraumatic stress symptoms, as well as a long-lasting sense of insecurity, poor self-esteem, and problems in relationships. . . . Many had spent years in [psycho]therapy. . . At least three of the 10 subjects appeared to be consumed with rage towards family members. (p. 1137)

OTHERS

The following list describes the most common characteristics of others involved with MBP cases:

- The nonoffending partners of MBP perpetrators may be emotionally or physically absent, weak, or uncritical.
- Friends, neighbors, and relatives are usually convinced that the problem is real and that the perpetrator is an exemplary parent.
- Alternatively, friends and relatives may be suspicious that something is wrong, but afraid to act.
- Health care providers and other professionals are often the mechanism through which harm occurs to the child. This may occur passively, when problems are not diagnosed, or actively as professionals prescribe unnecessary treatments and procedures that damage or have the potential to damage the victim.

The nonoffending partners of MBP perpetrators may be emotionally or physically absent, weak, or uncritical.

Nonoffending partners may see the perpetrators as good parents, and thus have no reason to suspect or believe they could engage in MBP maltreatment. MBP occurs in single-parent and two-parent families. In single-parent families, some case reports suggest that the primary motive for the MBP was the perpetrator's desire for attention from the partner, ex-spouse, or child's father. In two-parent homes, different patterns may emerge. Sometimes the partner has a job that requires frequent absences, and the falsification occurs during that absence. This may reflect an attempt to manipulate the partner into coming home, perhaps on an emergency basis. The increased perpetration may reflect the perpetrator's need for support in the absence of the partner, or a greater opportunity to act when close observation is absent. However, in many instances MBP occurs in two-parent homes with both parents in residence.

Less is known about the psychodynamics of nonperpetrator fathers than mothers in MBP cases. They are generally described in the literature as passive and uninvolved. This may reflect society's and their own traditional allocation of child rearing and child health care to women. Fathers are sometimes described as having health problems themselves. They may later admit to having had some questions about why the child or children were always sick, but—for whatever reason—closed their eyes or never raised the questions forcefully. Fathers, too, often appear to have been "duped" and victimized by the perpetrator. They often suffer over the sufferings of their children, worry over high medical bills, and do not enjoy a normal family life because of the perpetrator's preoccupations. Occasionally, their reputations are damaged by false allegations, or they may even become targets of MBP perpetration.

Schreier and Libow (1993) point out that health care providers often "collude" with these family dynamics, perhaps because they accept traditional gender roles. The absence of a mother from the hospital or her lack of involvement with health care appointments would be noted and probably commented upon unfavorably. The absence or lesser involvement of fathers is often taken for granted.

Nonoffending partners will often "stand by" the perpetrator even when presented with convincing evidence of what has occurred, but can still provide valuable information for the MBP investigation. If the victim is removed from the perpetrator, spouses/partners are seldom appropriate as caregivers even if not living in the same house because of this lack of belief in the maltreatment.

Friends, neighbors, and relatives are usually convinced that the problem is real and that the perpetrator is an exemplary parent.

People surrounding the nuclear MBP family—grandparents, relatives, neighbors, and so on are also affected by MBP perpetration. They may suffer greatly over the supposed health problems of the victim; for example, if they are informed that a beloved child has a serious or life-threatening condition. It is common for those around the family to accept what they are told by the perpetrator and what they believe they have witnessed about the victim's condition(s). They may have offered to help, and become enmeshed among the perpetrator's "supporters." They will have the same reluctance as professionals to believe that things are not as they seem. If the case later goes to court, these friends and relatives may be enlisted as character witnesses for the defense. They can be quite convincing, especially if the court has not been educated about the dynamics of MBP. For example, in one case, members of a church congregation prayed aloud in the courthouse lobby during the hearing. Had the judge not understood MBP basics, he might have been influenced unduly by this show of support.

For the investigator who is knowledgeable about MBP, friends and family can be a useful source of information. These supportive friends and relatives may later offer to provide temporary care for the victim, but are seldom appropriate for this task.

Alternatively, friends and relatives may be suspicious that something is wrong, but afraid to act.

Sometimes friends and relatives have a vague sense that "something is not right." If they do not know about the existence of MBP, they may not have words or concepts to express this accurately, and may question their own motivations or perceptions (My Sister-in-Law, 1991). They are, therefore, often confused about what to do with their suspicions, about whether anything should be done at all, or about where to turn for help. As long as professionals, child protective agencies, and public sources of information remain relatively ignorant about MBP, even when friends and relatives attempt to report suspicions, their efforts may be futile.

As MBP has become better known through the media and Internet, friends and family members have sometimes turned to MBP consultants for advice. In some situations, grandparents and other relatives have, with assistance, filed for custody. Sometimes the cases they report are clear-cut, but often they present real ethical and procedural difficulties. However, reports from friends and relatives cannot be taken at face value. They must be assessed for their truthfulness and possible hidden agendas.

Health care providers and other professionals are often the mechanism through which harm occurs to the child.

Harm may occur passively, when problems are not diagnosed, or actively as professionals prescribe unnecessary treatments and procedures that damage or have the potential to damage the victim.

Professionals characteristically fail to recognize that a problem exists until the perpetration has been long-standing—Rosenberg's (1987) cases averaged 14.9 months from first symptoms to diagnosis of MBP, and Sheridan's (2003) averaged 21.77 months. This may occur for several reasons, including lack of knowledge about MBP, misplaced trust, professional pride, power issues, fragmentation of care, and avoidance of difficult cases.

Many professionals still know little about MBP. They often have misconceptions and incorrect information. Many MBP cases are missed because professionals who work with children do not recognize its pattern or know how to respond to suspicions. Without correct MBP education, victim identification and protection will not occur.

Health care professionals are trained to trust parents' reports about their children. They may appropriately think of themselves as patient or parent advocates, and have ethics of accepting and not judging others. Unless there are large "holes" in a story, it may never occur to professionals that perhaps they are being conned. If the professionals do doubt the story, their first reaction may be self-blame for failure to live up to their professional ethics and values. It is often easier to search for a rare and elusive diagnosis than to believe something horrible about a parent. These pro-parent attitudes, which generally facilitate professional practice, may delay recognition of MBP.

Professionals are understandably proud of their achievements, intellectual abilities, and competence. In some professional circles, it is still unacceptable to ask for help or admit that one has made a mistake. Some believe (falsely) that they cannot be fooled, or that there are infallible signs that indicate when someone is lying. These attitudes make professionals slow to consider that MBP is occurring, and very reluctant to admit that it has occurred.

Sometimes politics and status disparities work against recognizing or reporting MBP. For example, Firstman and Talan (1997) assert that in the case of Waneta Hoyt, who killed five children, nurses' suspicions went unheard because they did not fit the attending physician's research theories. Key professionals may not "believe" in MBP, or may not want to report child maltreatment (even though this is mandated by law). These situations can create real problems for team members who recognize their legal responsibility to report suspicions to CPS, but who must also continue to work with their colleagues.

By necessity, health care has become specialized. With each new "complication" reported in the illness process, another specialist may enter the picture. Conversations among specialists are often limited. MBP is frequently confirmed only when all pieces of the puzzle are put together and evaluated. If no one is doing this—and it is extremely time-consuming—the pieces may come together slowly, if at all. The involvement of many professionals, all with their own personalities, agendas, and interests, can become a fertile field for parents who wish to sow disinformation, discord, and deceit.

MBP cases are difficult, even traumatic, for professionals (Blix and Brack, 1988). It is very painful to admit that one has been fooled and to continue offering care to someone who has betrayed trust. Professionals may also be frightened by the perpetrator's threats or specters of personal harm or liability if they are incorrect.

In today's litigious world, patients often demand answers, and have been conditioned to believe that a diagnosis and treatment must be "out there" somewhere. In their view, a competent health care professional is one who will not give up the search for an elusive diagnosis, and health care professionals often also share this perception. Patients and parents of patients can regard their health care professionals—or the health care professionals can regard themselves—

as incompetent or even negligent if the search for a diagnosis is abandoned with no answers having been found. For health care professionals to say that nothing is wrong or that the search for diagnosis is pointless is thus very threatening. What if, later, someone more persistent or skilled finds a serious condition? Legal liability as well as loss of status might well result. When the choice is between doing another procedure with some (albeit minimal) chance of success, the temptation is to do rather than not to do.

Until one has consulted on MBP cases, it is hard to believe how reluctant professionals can be to consider the possibility of MBP and—once they have considered it—to take it seriously and act upon their suspicions by instituting a fair information finding and evaluation process. One major initial task of those concerned about MBP is often to focus and refocus involved professionals on the potential diagnosis and its implications. When diagnosis is delayed, the victim is exposed to all the harms and potential harms associated with continued maltreatment. The very professionals who should be protecting the victim are, by closing their eyes, unwittingly participating in the maltreatment (Zitelli, Seltman, and Shannon, 1987). This is a matter of moral, if not legal, responsibility.

When professionals pursue diagnosis and treatment, they ordinarily make examinations, do tests, perform procedures, and prescribe medications. They may also impose limits, such as restricting certain foods, activities, etc. Ordinarily, these actions are undertaken in the expectation that their potential to help will outweigh their risks. Such an expectation is reasonable when a true disease is being addressed. When no illness is present, however, there is no benefit to counter the risk.

Among the unnecessary interventions received by MBP victims are powerful medications, surgeries and attendant anesthesia, permanently implanted feeding tubes, radiation exposure from repeated x-rays, needle sticks, invasive procedures, dietary/environmental restrictions, and inappropriate inpatient and outpatient mental health care. Rosenberg states (1995), "The damage that has already occurred is an estimate of the least possible risk" (p. 31). By this Rosenberg means that there are risks associated with everything done in health care. Ordinarily, we do not think, for example, of all the side effects of drugs and procedures. Even if the victim did not develop these side effects, the victim was *exposed* to them unnecessarily.

Professionals are not responsible for harmful or unnecessary treatments they have prescribed or administered unless they deliberately close their eyes to the possibility of MBP. If health care providers are honestly duped, the maltreatment is the responsibility of the perpetrator. The involved professionals were no more responsible for the injury than a belt is responsible for a child's beating. Professionals must, however, become educated, maintain an appropriate level of suspicion, and use critical thinking skills to prevent their being too-easy targets for deception.

Chapter 3

Integrity in MBP Practice

Formal knowledge about and response to all forms of child maltreatment is relatively recent. Knowledge of MBP maltreatment is more recent. This book reflects today's knowledge and response, which can be expected to change as information and experience accumulate. What does not change, however, is the responsibility of professionals and practice settings to work with integrity—doing the best they can to use their knowledge, values, skills, and resources to discover the truth and to protect children.

Ford (1996) states, "Ethical dilemmas are created when two principles are in conflict" (p. 52). This chapter will consider ethical issues raised by practice with MBP. Every new field generates questions about right and wrong, and even ethical professionals may differ on answers to those questions. Ideas about ethics in professional practice also change; once it was considered a kindness not to tell patients they were dying. Today it is considered unethical in the United States to withhold this information. This chapter will consider ethical issues related to MBP maltreatment: how patients and families are treated, how professionals practice and treat one another, and how systems create the settings in which services are delivered. Important issues will be discussed, however, not all aspects of MBP ethics can be dealt with here. Nor can this chapter provide all answers. At best, it can discuss the different perceptions and opinions that are current in the field.

Some ethical issues associated with MBP include:

- Fairness
- Reporting to child protective services
- Confidentiality

- Personal qualifications to practice in the field
- Safety
- Colleague relationships
- System issues
- Public awareness
- Building a solid knowledge base for MBP theory and practice

FAIRNESS

As professionals and communities appropriately increase their levels of MBP suspicion, MBP should not become an easy conclusion in situations in which a child's problem is elusive or a caretaker is assertive. The allegations that MBP is no more than this were reviewed in Chapter 1. The authors of this book do not agree with them. But there is potential that MBP accusations may be used in the way that critics describe if practitioners are not sensitive to the complexities of confirmation/disconfirmation, or are tempted to take shortcuts.

Two extremes are often encountered when maltreatment is investigated. People—including professionals—often feel guilty when they become suspicious of a child's caretaker. They feel that such thoughts are not fair to someone who appears to be normal or exemplary. We often answer this by saying that a fair (thorough, just, and unbiased) confirmation/disconfirmation process may reveal either guilt or innocence, and it is important to enter an investigation in this open-minded spirit. A basic investigative error is the confirmation bias—the tendency to find only what one is seeking or has already decided is there. Mental openness should characterize all stages of the confirmation/disconfirmation process.

The issue of avoiding premature decision making is particularly important when cross-cultural issues are involved. Although, as Feldman and Brown (2002) have documented, MBP appears similar in all countries where it has been recognized, information about international presentations and variations is limited. In the interest of fairness, it is particularly important that the meanings of/reasons for behaviors be understood when working in a cross-cultural context. Cross-cultural anatomical and epidemiological variations must also be understood before conclusions are drawn that may be erroneous.

Throughout the postconfirmation stages of a genuine MBP case, fairness should mark activities, interactions, and decisions affecting perpetrators, other associated adults, and children. No matter how egregious the abuse, the perpetrator should be seen as a person who has both problems and rights. To the extent possible, the well-being of the perpetrator and associated adults should be considered. This is particularly important during the confrontation (when the perpetrator is told about the MBP confirmation and may herself or himself be at risk), but is also true in the later stages of the case. For example, case plan elements need to be appropriate to MBP, measurable so that judgments are just, and potentially achievable if the perpetrator is capable of making progress. As elements of competent practice, these are operationalizations of fairness. Consistent with child protection, MBP case management should consider the conflicting needs of all parties. Decisions, particularly serious ones such as termination of parental rights, should be based on objective information.

Certain investigative methods, while potentially effective, have raised questions of fairness. Chief among these is covert video surveillance. Opinions have been advanced about whether protection of a potentially endangered child justifies actions that, while legal, are considered by some not to be fully ethical. A number of different strategies have been suggested to try to meet the needs of child protection while honoring the rights of potential perpetrators. There is, as of yet, no consensus within the MBP community about how to do this. It may be that the task is impossible. In this section, this still-developing discussion is summarized.

In health care matters, parents normally exercise total and unchallenged decision making on behalf of their minor children. They have the right of "informed consent"—knowing what is to be done and agreeing to it in advance—on behalf of their children. This is wise and beneficial except when the child's interests conflict with those of the parents. Unfortunately, this is the situation with MBP.

Covert audio/video surveillance is the use of hidden recording devices and/or cameras to try to "catch" perpetrators in MBP-like behavior. It usually occurs in hospitals. The essence of the process is believed to be secrecy: it is assumed that perpetrators will not maltreat if they know they are being observed and recorded. For health care professionals, this raises the issue of informed consent. They find it difficult to justify any procedure that has not been explained in advance to the parents, and to which the parents have not agreed.

Three solutions to this problem appear in the literature: what could be called "blanket" consent, deceptive consent, and observation without consent. In blanket consent, some document such as the hospital's consent for admission form, signed by all patients or their parents/guardians upon admission, contains language permitting audio and/or video recording. If challenged, the hospital can later honestly state that the signer consented to the observation. However, many signers do not read consent forms. Thus some people feel that blanket consents do not allow for true informed consent. Others would argue that parents have the opportunity to read the consent form, and must take the consequences if they do not. In some hospitals, blanket consents are supplemented by signs stating that patients and visitors are potentially subject to audio and video surveillance.

Rosen, Frost, and Glaze (1986) described an instance of deceptive consent. A suspected perpetrator was asked to consent to videotaping of her interaction with her hospitalized child, and did so. She and the child were in a room with a visible video camera. Unbeknownst to her, the room was also monitored by a hidden camera. After some time, a hospital employee entered the room, said that the visible camera was not working, and removed it. Covert surveillance continued, and the mother was taped in the act of smothering her child. Again, some would argue that this solution preserves the letter but not the spirit of informed consent. Others would counter that the mother did consent to the videotaping.

Brown (1997) and Byard and Burnell (1994) have described observation without consent. In the case reported by Brown, an older sister of the index child had died the previous year at the age of eight months of supposed sudden infant death syndrome (SIDS), and in the case reported by Byard and Burnell there had been two previous supposed SIDS deaths over the preceding two years. Both index infants presented with "apnea." In both cases, covert surveillance was reviewed with a team of hospital personnel, with hospital administration, and with law enforcement. This suggests that it was legal, although informed consent was not present.

The issue of consent for covert surveillance is a difficult one, involving questions of professional conduct and defining who is the patient. Many health care professionals are uncomfortable with deceiving patients or their families, seeing it as a violation of trust (Byard and Burnell, 1994; Lloyd and MacDonald, 2000). The right to full information and candor was hard-won by patients and their advocates. Issues of privacy invasion are raised when patients and family members do not know that they are being observed. For example, an adult in a private room with an infant may undress in view of the camera (Facey, 1993). Nurses have reported feeling like "spies" or "detectives" rather than health care providers (Brown, 1997). Others may believe that if covert surveillance is effected with less than full consent, they are allowing the means to justify the ends or encouraging self-incrimination. Professionals may also define their patient as the family or as the parent-child dyad rather than as the infant. In this case, they may feel an ethical obligation to protect the interests of the perpetrator as well as the victim.

In contrast, other professionals see their responsibility as protecting the child, and believe that some deception may be justified to do this. They believe that child maltreatment, a violation of the law, may be occurring, and they use legal standards as their reference point. Their primary focus is on the child at risk, and not on the family. They do not find any ethical problems in covert activity, particularly if a court order has been obtained.

Differences between these two groups of professionals might be compared to those that could occur in a hostage situation. The hostage taker demands money, a helicopter, and passage out of the country. The police use the false promise that the money and helicopter are on the way to lure the hostage taker out of the building and arrest him. Some observers believe that the deception was justified because the hostages were saved. Others believe that the police are not justified in lying, even as a means of saving the hostages.

Covert surveillance should not be undertaken without the involvement of institutional (e.g., hospital) administration, child protective services, and law enforcement. General policies and procedures should be in place in advance of need, and case-specific planning should take place from the time of earliest suspicion. The advice of a hospital ethics committee, or attorney may be necessary. The knowledge and experience of law enforcement, where covert activities, protection of evidence, and criminal investigation are daily processes, will provide vital information for the process. One advantage to convening an MBP-specific multiagency/multidisciplinary team (MMT) at the earliest sign of serious suspicion is that a variety of opinions will be available to help wrestle with questions such as informed consent.

A second ethical issue raised by covert surveillance is its possible violation of the "first do no harm" rule of health care professions. During covert surveillance, the perpetrator has the opportunity to abuse the child. This abuse, recorded on tape and witnessed by an observer, then forms a basis for confirming maltreatment and for subsequent protective activity. However, in the process the child has often experienced maltreatment of the type suspected (e.g., MBP), and other forms of maltreatment (Southall et al., 1997). For example, in one case, a caregiver struck a baby in the face. Another caregiver picked up the infant and dropped her onto the crib while screaming obscenities.

There is general agreement that a recording device should not be used without an observer monitoring, so that harm can be interrupted as necessary. However, in practice, many questions arise about when the interruption should occur, and how quickly it can occur. Child protection considerations may conflict with the need for documentation and "good" evidence. For example, suppose that a perpetrator is suspected of MBP. While being observed, she or he strikes the child sufficiently to cause injury. If surveillance is terminated at that point, maltreatment will be documented but the incident will not confirm MBP-like behavior. If surveillance is not terminated at this point, evidence of MBP-like behavior *may* be obtained (it is not guaranteed), but at the cost of not protecting the child from the maltreatment. This places those investigating MBP in the difficult situation of appearing to condone or at least allow child maltreatment—an accusation that has also been leveled against them by "watchdog" groups. Sometimes, the observer, stationed in the next room, may be unable to intervene in time to prevent serious injury to the child. For example, suppose that instead of striking the child, the mother shakes him or her sufficiently to cause "shaken baby syndrome."

Those who support covert surveillance do so because they believe it is ultimately in the best interest of a child who is in need of protection from a dangerous and powerful adult. They hold that it is ethical and moral if done according to guidelines that protect, as much as possible, the rights and safety of all participants (Shabde and Craft, 1998; Shinebourne, 1996; Southall and Samuels, 1996). Byard and Burnell argue (1994):

We would consider that the apparent infringement of rights of privacy and breach of trust are less important issues in the face of a potentially homicidal parent. . . . The investigation of suspected cases of Munchausen syndrome by proxy requires extremely sensitive handling, consideration of parents' trust and rights of privacy, involvement of a range of health and law professionals, and careful exploration of ethical issues, but rapid diagnosis is vital. (p. 356)

REPORTING TO CHILD PROTECTIVE AGENCIES

Professionals often hesitate to report cases of suspected child maltreatment to public child protective agencies, even when they are legally mandated to do so. Some professionals do not want to acknowledge that MBP might be occurring. They do not want to believe that parents can maltreat their children in this way. Or they do not want to admit that they were fooled and unwittingly participated in the maltreatment. Anyone, including experienced MBP professionals, can be fooled. There is no shame in it, if one has done one's job with reasonable care. The shame is in concealing suspicions from oneself or others in order to "save face" or avoid the difficulties of pursuing an MBP case.

Some mental health professionals fear losing a therapeutic relationship with the perpetrator and/or child(ren) whom they are seeing. Even if they recognize that there is a high probability of MBP, they may feel that the child is at least receiving some care and oversight from these contacts. They fear, often rightly, that reporting MBP suspicions may cause the contacts to be terminated. When deception is a major part of the "therapeutic" process, however, a therapeutic relationship ceases (if it ever existed).

Some professionals find the process of child maltreatment reporting or the prospect of court testimony so unpleasant that they avoid it whenever possible. This may be due to their own lack of skills in testifying, poor previous experiences with child protective services, or the difficulty of taking time from their practice to meet with child protective investigators or go to court. Other professionals feel that they should report child maltreatment, especially MBP, only when they are sure that it has occurred, even though the law generally requires reporting of *suspicion*. These professionals may attempt to pursue a child maltreatment investigation themselves, not recognizing the many facets of this complex task that are outside their expertise. Their focus may only be on the part of the case that has come to their attention, and they have no legal mandate or support for wider activity.

The children at risk in all these situations are not protected. The adults who should be recognizing and attending to their plight are failing to do so. Failure to take action on suspected child maltreatment is an ethical as well as a legal issue and is supported by professional codes of ethics (American Nursing Association, 1995; American Medical Association, 1996; American Psychological Association, 1995; National Association of Social Workers, 1996). The professional who looks the other way incurs legal liability and moral culpability.

A more difficult problem occurs when the child protective agency is perceived as poorly organized or the personnel as poorly trained, so that the professional has little confidence in the agency's ability to handle cases competently. In this situation, the practitioner wants to help the child and family by reporting the maltreatment, but fears that a child protective referral will do more harm than good.

This is a reasonable point of view, because many child protective agencies are seriously troubled. Often this is due to underfunding, politics, lack of training for child protective workers, and a lack of professionals willing to work in the field. A more central cause is the devaluing of children in American society (Sidel, 1992), so that there is more rhetoric than real support to the field of child protection. However, knowledge of these social factors does not solve the dilemma for the individual practitioner trying to decide whether to report a case of suspected MBP.

Corey, Corey, and Callanan (1998) state:

> It is crucial for professionals to know the boundaries of their own competence and to refer clients to other professionals when working with them is beyond their professional training or when personal [or agency] factors would interfere with a productive working relationship.

> The willingness to consult with other professionals demonstrates good faith on the practitioner's part. (pp. 269, 417)

For most professionals suspecting MBP, an MBP investigation and protection of the victim (if suspicion proves justified) are beyond their own competence or the authority of their agency. Professionals may begin an investigation in good faith, only to be delayed or distracted by the other legitimate demands of their practices. Or, their efforts may be thwarted by the suspected perpetrator's refusal to consent to the release of records or by the transfer of the child to another practitioner. Professionals who are contemplating a referral to CPS may believe that they know how the agency will handle the case, and they may turn out to be correct. They may also, however, be "selling short" the agency. Perhaps a worker will be assigned who exceeds the referring professional's expectations. Perhaps recent training or policy changes, of which the referring professional is unaware, have changed the situation. Suspected cases should be reported to CPS as soon as possible. Professionals should work to enhance the capacity and effectiveness of the agency. For example, if a professional is concerned that CPS workers do not understand MBP, the professional can offer to help arrange training. If a professional is concerned about the overall quality and responsiveness of CPS, this should be addressed outside the context of a specific case. When this strategy is taken, the referring professional is demonstrating "good faith" in the legally mandated process, and encouraging the agency to meet its responsibilities. Although there will likely be a number of cases that are not resolved satisfactorily, more children are protected if professionals continue to pressure the system rather than withdrawing from it.

CONFIDENTIALITY

"Keeping faith" (from the Latin roots of "confidentiality") with the client's desires about the sharing of information is a major ethical issue in the helping professions. Corey, Corey, and Callanan (1998) state, "Perhaps the central right of a client is the guarantee that disclosures in therapy sessions will be protected" (p. 155). However, the right to nondisclosure of medical, mental health, and social information is not absolute. Corey, Corey, and Callanan add:

> [H]owever, you cannot make a blanket promise to your clients that *everything* they talk about will *always* remain confidential.

... Landmark court cases have shed new light on the therapist's duty to warn and to protect both clients and others who may be directly affected by a client's behavior. You have both ethical and legal responsibilities to protect innocent people who might be injured by a dangerous client. (p. 155)

Sometimes, under the guise of "confidentiality," professionals refuse to disclose important information to their colleagues who have a need or even a legal right to know. For example, a hospital social worker refused to provide key information to a colleague about the past medical history of a mother, thus significantly delaying the recognition of MBP suspicion indicators. A hospital's staff refused to turn over complete videotapes of MBP-like perpetration to the child protective agency, even though the staff had reported their suspicions and these tapes were an important part of the investigation. These professionals may withhold information for reasons unrelated to the case, perhaps to further a personal or institutional agenda. The result can be a staff split into factions, or an investigation seriously hindered. The resulting delays and ineffectiveness can leave a child unprotected. This is an ethical violation. Professionals have an obligation to uphold confidentiality, but they also have an obligation to provide information that they are permitted to release.

The usual understanding of confidentiality is that it allows discussions with fellow members of a patient care team in an institution, and with supervisors who have a need to know. There is no place in the investigation or management of MBP cases for team members who withhold information, and thus mislead others. Full disclosure is especially important within the MMT convened to gather information and make recommendations on an MBP case. This may need to be discussed initially. Such discussion may counter an expectation that disclosure of confidential information should be as limited as possible, consistent with circumstances (see, for example, American Counseling Association, 1995). In suspected MBP, the circumstances require disclosure of as much as is known about the perpetrator and family. Even apparently small details, when put together with information from others and data from records, may be key to establishing a pattern of honesty or deception.

If the perpetrator enters therapy as part of the case plan or court order, the usual expectations of confidentiality cannot exist and cannot be promised to the perpetrator implicitly or explicitly. The child protective agency must receive full information about what is disclosed in therapy. The perpetrator must know that this will occur. Otherwise, information needed to make key case decisions will not be available. There is also significant danger that the perpetrator may manipulate the therapist, especially if the therapist has not worked with MBP cases before, unless the therapist is regularly reviewing material with others who can see the "whole picture."

An additional consideration relating to confidentiality concerns victims old enough to be questioned. Children generally feel a loyalty to their caretakers, even when those caretakers abuse them. Their caretaker may have told them to keep certain information secret. If they were not told this directly, it has probably been implicit in the caretaker's behavior. Thus, when children are interviewed in the course of a maltreatment investigation, they may feel that they are being asked to betray a central person in their lives. The content of the interview may also include material that is embarrassing to the child, for example, as it relates to medical procedures on the genitals or urinary tract. At the very least, children who are interviewed deserve consideration for their feelings. They should be given age-appropriate explanations for why the information is needed, and told that ordinary rules about family privacy do not extend to extraordinary situations. Their consent should be "informed" in the sense that they should understand from the beginning why they are being interviewed. As reports are prepared or testimony is elicited, the child's feelings about the information should be considered. Sensitive areas that are unrelated to the investigation should remain confidential between the interviewer and the child. No false promises should be made and later broken.

QUALIFICATIONS TO PRACTICE IN THE FIELD

Currently, there are no academic degrees, certification programs, or licenses attesting to the qualifications of practitioners in the field of MBP. In many areas of the country, a person who has been involved in a few cases or perhaps read a few articles in the literature is too often considered to be an "expert." "A little knowledge can be dangerous" in MBP practice, and this is even truer if practitioners overestimate the degree of their expertise.

Professional codes of ethics make clear that practitioners should represent their qualifications honestly and accurately. For example, the American Medical Association's (1998) "E-Principles of Medical Ethics" state, "A physician shall be dedicated to providing competent medical care. . . . A physician shall . . . be honest in all professional interactions . . . obtain consultation, and use the talents of other health professionals when indicated." The *Code of Ethics and Standards of Practice* of the American Counseling Association states (1995):

> Counselors practice only within the boundaries of their competence, based on their education, training, supervised experience, state and national professional credentials, and appropriate professional experience. Counselors will demonstrate a commitment to gain knowledge, personal awareness, sensitivity, and skills pertinent to working with a diverse client population. While developing skills in new specialty areas [i.e., areas that are new to them], counselors take steps to ensure the competence of their work and to protect others from possible harm. . . . Counselors claim or imply only professional credentials possessed and are responsible for correcting any known misrepresentations of their credentials by others. . . . Counselors are reasonably certain that they have . . . the necessary competencies and resources for giving the kind of consulting services needed. (Sections C.2.a, C.2.b, C.4a, D.2.b)

The *Ethical Principles of Psychologists and Code of Conduct* of the American Psychological Association states as one of its "General Principles" (1995):

> Psychologists . . . recognize the boundaries of their particular competencies and the limitations of their expertise. They provide only those services and use only those techniques for which they are qualified by education, training, or experience. . . . In those areas in which recognized professional standards do not yet exist, psychologists exercise careful judgment and take

appropriate precautions to protect the welfare of those with whom they work. (Principle A)

A similar provision is found in the *Code of Ethics* of the National Association of Social Workers (1996): "Social workers practice within their areas of competence and develop and enhance their professional expertise" (Value: Competence). The *Code for Nurses* (American Nursing Association, 1985) also states, "The nurse exercises informed judgment and uses individual competence and qualifications as criteria in . . . accepting responsibilities" (Provision #6).

It is natural for some professionals to become overconfident about information and recommendations, particularly if that person has participated in a few cases that have turned out to be similar. In such a case, the person may not appreciate the full spectrum of the situation and may, with the best of intentions, mislead others. Because MBP is a relatively new area of practice, with many unknowns, a person with a small amount of knowledge can appear to be an "expert." This is where ethics and humility should exert a protective influence. To deliberately inflate or overestimate one's expertise in order to be considered an "expert" is a serious violation of professional ethics. Fooling oneself about one's expertise is also an ethical violation. For example, one of the authors of this book received a phone call from a physician who was scheduled to testify as an expert witness the following day, and who asked for basic MBP training in order to perform this task. In another situation, a therapist held herself out to the community as an MBP expert, but a review of her qualifications revealed no MBP education, experience, or publications.

There is an old saying among physicians in training: "See one, do one, teach one." As a matter of survival, interns and residents have traditionally had to learn quickly, put their new skills to work quickly, and help one another. In many cases of suspected MBP, local conditions will make similar demands. In neither case is this optimal professional practice. In such situations, professionals must be clear, to themselves and others, about their preparation for MBP practice. If they are unsure of their competency, yet required to do the best they can, they should seek consultation or peer support from others with credible experience in the field.

COLLEAGUE RELATIONSHIPS

Because MBP cases are difficult and elicit many emotions, they may take a toll on interpersonal relationships among professionals. The problem of deliberate withholding of information has already been discussed. Problems also occur when professionals ignore or discount what they are told; for example, when a higher-status professional fails to listen to MBP suspicion from a lower-status professional or nonprofessional.

Ethical practice requires respect for others, whether the others are patients, perpetrators, or colleagues. The *Ethical Principles of Psychologists* states (American Psychological Association, 1995): "Psychologists accord appropriate respect to the fundamental rights, dignity, and worth of all people" (Principle B: Integrity). The *Code of Ethics* of the National Association of Social Workers (1996) states, "Social workers respect the inherent dignity and worth of the person," and specifically, "Social workers should treat colleagues with respect" (Value: Dignity and Worth of the Person). The *Principles of Medical Ethics* (AMA, 1996) include, "A physician shall deal honestly with patients and colleagues. . . . A physician shall respect the rights of patients, of colleagues, and other health professionals" (Principles II and IV). Sometimes, MBP suspicions, concerns, or observations have been discounted because of personal considerations. This is especially risky when the discounting is done by someone who is in a position to block serious consideration of MBP, or to discourage a report to CPS. Firstman and Talan (1997) assert that this occurred in the Waneta Hoyt case. They claim that nurses were suspicious that she might be killing her children (as she was), but that the physician was more concerned about his theories and research protocol.

Ethics, experience, and common sense suggest that all suspicions and opinions should be listened to with respect. The people raising them may have correct intuitions, even though they may not have the correct words or professional qualifications. There is room on professional teams, including the MMT, for differences of opinion. Often a better understanding of the situation and better plans come from different views and perspectives. These also offer more thorough protection for the rights of all involved in the situation.

An attitude of mutual support in the search for truth should also characterize those with more experience and knowledge of MBP. "Politics" do not belong in child protection. They are especially harmful in a developing field. Professionals should be open to differences of opinion, the advancing of theories, and the testing of hypotheses. This is how knowledge grows. The field is too small for professional rivalries, claiming or defending of turf, cliquishness, or personal attack. Already, the failure to agree on standardized terminology and definitions has been used by those who want to discount MBP. Addressing these issues through consensus initiatives would be helpful, as long as these are open to a variety of opinions.

SYSTEM ISSUES

Practice in any field is more likely to be ethical if it is supported by organizational policies and structures that facilitate effectiveness and integrity. In the field of MBP, unique policies and procedures are important if professionals are to recognize, investigate, and respond appropriately to this unique form of maltreatment. Unless these structures are institutionalized, time, effort, and perhaps the case will be lost when a report of MBP suspicion is made. Depending on the jurisdiction and agencies involved, some of these changes can be made at the level of policy and procedure. Others require enactment by law. When policy is to be changed at either level, someone who has credible MBP knowledge and experience should assist so that the best possible policies and procedures are written.

Policies to enhance ethical practice include:

- MBP should be recognized as a specific form of maltreatment.
- Time limits may need to be modified in MBP investigations.
- Contacting the family as the first response is inappropriate for MBP.
- In-service education should be provided on MBP.
- Appropriate resources should be available for MBP cases.
- Child protective investigations and case management in MBP cases should be centralized under CPS.

MBP should be recognized as a specific form of maltreatment.

Practice related to MBP will be more effective if it is recognized as a category of maltreatment, just as sexual abuse is. This recognition legitimates the creation of other policies and procedures related to MBP practice, the provision of special training for those who may be involved in cases, the gathering of data, and the implementation of MBP-specific case plans.

Time limits may need to be modified in MBP case investigations.

CPS policy often requires child protective staff to complete an investigation within a specified time after receiving a report of possible maltreatment. Because of the complexity of MBP cases, the amount of information to be reviewed, and the number of forensic interviews that can be necessary, it may not be possible for CPS to conduct a thorough investigation within the time limit. This places CPS staff in an ethical dilemma: should they violate agency policy, and perhaps suffer sanctions for doing a quality job, or should they follow policy but risk making an uninformed decision about a child at risk? Non-CPS professionals who know that an investigation will be "rushed" may be reluctant to report their suspicions for fear that the investigation will not be sufficiently thorough to make a fair confirmation/ disconfirmation. They may attempt to complete most of the investigation themselves, without the resources, access, skills, or ability to protect the child that would come with a CPS referral. This places them in violation of the law if they are mandated reporters. The solution to this problem is to recognize that time limits for investigations need modification in MBP cases.

Contacting the family as the first response is inappropriate for MBP.

Many child protective agencies require that the first response to a report of suspected maltreatment is to contact the family about whom the report has been made. In MBP cases, as is discussed elsewhere in this book, this is inappropriate because it lets the suspected perpetrator know about suspicions before a firm plan is in place for the victim's protection. Perpetrators are more dangerous if they know about the suspicions; they may flee, or they may increase their maltreatment.

Again, child protective workers are caught between agency policy and the protection of the child. Non-CPS professionals who know that the family will be contacted as a first step, and who understand that this significantly heightens risk for the victim, will be reluctant to report. In some jurisdictions, convening of the MMT is allowed to substitute for the immediate contacting of the suspected perpetrator.

In-service education should be provided about MBP.

Unfortunately, today's MBP victims still cannot depend on community child protective agencies to recognize their maltreatment and to intervene in it. Too often, their welfare depends on being in the right place at the right time. If they do not encounter someone who knows about MBP and is willing—sometimes at significant sacrifice—to pursue the case, the maltreatment continues. This is an ethical issue that must be addressed not only by individual practitioners seeking continuing education, but by educational efforts of all agencies that serve children or families, and by institutions offering professional education.

Many health care, legal system, child protective, educational, and other workers who are likely to come into contact with children and families are not familiar with MBP. If they don't know about it, they are unlikely to suspect it and respond appropriately. Alternatively, they may have and act on incorrect information. Until valid information about MBP becomes part of preservice professional education, and as new developments reshape the field, anyone in any agency who works with children should be "brought up to speed." This is the responsibility of individual agencies, but there is potential for multi-agency cooperation and sharing of training resources. Colleges and universities should incorporate information about MBP into their curricula on child maltreatment. Insurance and managed care organizations should promote knowledge about MBP not only because such knowledge has the potential of saving them considerable money, but also to aid in the identification of cases and to generate data for research.

Child protective workers who receive telephone reports, and especially workers who will be working with MBP cases, should have MBP-specific knowledge and skills. In-service education should include identification, intervention, and case management. Thus, providing training for its workers about MBP is part of CPS' mission to protect children. The *Guidelines for a Model System of Protective Services* (American Public Human Services Association, 1999) states, "The CPS agency is responsible for ensuring that its staff has the specialized knowledge and skills necessary to provide quality services. Specialized skills training should be regularly available to staff already employed by the agency" (p. 28).

Those who have gained expertise in the field have an obligation to contribute to knowledge in their communities. Some of this may need to be through pro bono (uncompensated) work.

Appropriate resources should be available for MBP cases.

MBP cases require a significant commitment of resources if they are to be managed appropriately. Child protective staff who are assigned to suspected or confirmed MBP cases must have sufficient time, release from other parts of their caseload, and emotional/supervisory support. Money should be available, if necessary, to pay experts and obtain all needed documentation. Other staff must be helped to understand that these "extras" are not for the sake of the worker, but are required as part of the agency's ethical commitment to protect the victim. Supervisors/administrators in hospitals, police departments, and other fields beyond the child protective agency should also be helped to understand—ideally before the fact—that their staffs' participation in the MMT is a legitimate and time-consuming part of the job.

Child protective investigations and case management in MBP cases should be centralized under CPS.

The present literature of MBP, largely written by health care professionals and published in the medical literature, often suggests that MBP investigation or case management proceed under the direction of health care professionals. For example, doctors and nurses are envisioned as conducting the MBP investigation, confronting the suspected perpetrator, and developing a follow-up plan such as referral to psychotherapy. This is dangerous and may violate state child abuse reporting laws. Investigation, confrontation, case planning, and ongoing case management should be coordinated by CPS with the advice of other professionals who form the MMT. There is much more to an MBP investigation, and much more to case planning and management, than the health care aspects. Today's atmosphere of discomfort between CPS and health care must change if children are to be protected. This will require give and take on both sides.

These policy elements often represent an ideal that is difficult to achieve. In many areas, CPS is perceived as an obstacle rather than a facilitator. In some areas and cases this perception has been correct. This raises ethical issues that can be difficult to resolve. There are many reasons for problems with child protective services. American society is often said to give only lip service to children (Sidel, 1992), and this translates into inadequate funding for child protection. Inadequate funding translates into high caseloads and poorly prepared, poorly supported workers. If children are to be protected, all potentially involved agencies and organizations should cooperate, assist one another with education, and recognize their common case goals and areas of expertise. Organizations should hire and support competent workers. The professional community is a long way from this ideal, but it is extremely important to work toward it. The authors can only repeat that the time to work on this situation is before the next MBP case.

PUBLIC AWARENESS OF MBP

The situation with MBP is similar to the situation with child maltreatment as a whole several decades ago, and with sexual abuse more recently. If a community does not understand this kind of maltreatment, it will not suspect and therefore not report suspicions. Public awareness could theoretically serve as a deterrent to MBP perpetration, since it may be more difficult for perpetrators to get away with their actions.

MBP professionals sometimes encounter resistance to the concept of MBP from the general public, the media, and public officials such as legislators. This resistance is not terribly different from that among professionals, or among people in general, when child maltreatment was first "discovered." As more key people hear about MBP and the media carry more stories about MBP, some disbelief and resistance will fade. So it is important that knowledgeable and responsible professionals should encourage public discussion of MBP and work to make coverage factual and responsible.

Consideration should be given to the safety of those who practice in MBP, especially those who are high profile. Groups opposing the concept of MBP or experts' involvement in MBP cases have become increasingly vocal and active. Members of these groups, some of whom are confirmed MBP perpetrators, are in frequent communication via the Internet. Using this forum, they exchange information and gossip on cases and on MBP researchers/practitioners—literally around the world in a matter of seconds. Such groups are believed to have targeted some professionals for career and reputation assassination, and sometimes issue thinly veiled threats against their personal safety. Participants in these groups, as well as professionals, have rights of free speech and association. However, the effect of such pressure, even though it comes from a small group, cannot be discounted. It is unfortunate when intimidation impinges on the protection of potentially maltreated children. The field of MBP practice must take seriously the potential of threats to its practitioners.

BUILDING A SOLID KNOWLEDGE BASE FOR MBP THEORY AND PRACTICE

At present, practice in the field of MBP has depended on personal experience and a professional literature that most typically presents cases and advances theories. A standardized definition, standardized data collection, and empirically tested theories for intervention would go a long way toward furthering effective practice in the field. Contributing to the building of this knowledge base should be seen as an ethical obligation of those who have reached a high level of competence or seen a large number of cases.

Standardized data collection has not yet been achieved. Knowledge of MBP from the world's medical, psychosocial, and legal literature totals hundreds of cases, but these primarily reflect the individual interests of the authors. They are not necessarily a representative sample of all cases that occur, or even of all identified cases. Case reports are valuable, but they are not sufficient for testing theories. Although the professional literature represents the best source of data available, it naturally focuses on the more remarkable cases. This may have led researchers and practitioners to neglect less dramatic but probably more frequent presentations. Differences in the ways cases are reported among the various journals, and information that cannot be included because of space limitations, reduce the usefulness of published reports for research purposes.

Full case information, collected and reported according to a standard protocol, would provide the best source of data about presentations, interventions, and outcomes in MBP cases. The development of a uniform national (ideally, international) data collection system for MBP would be most effective. What such a system would look like, who would fund and administer it, and how participation would be encouraged are still areas to be worked out. Some preliminary consideration has been given to such a system, and models already exist for collecting information about other forms of child maltreatment. Data should be multidisciplinary in character, collected from all sources where MBP may present (e.g., health care, CPS, courts), and shared among scholars. Although ethical challenges (chiefly related to confidentiality) must be met, an MBP registry could function both for research purposes and to aid in the tracking of perpetrators and victims/potential victims as they move from place to place. MBP should also be shown as a separate category of abuse on national child welfare data reporting systems.

Empirically tested theories for intervention have not yet been developed. Ideally, standardized definitions and data collection should lead to theories and guidelines that can be tested by practitioners in a variety of settings. Such guidelines can never take the place of individualized, thoughtful practice, but are an important step toward providing professionals with the knowledge they need to manage cases appropriately. Outcomes research is particularly important and should address these concerns: What are the long-term results of MBP victimization? Are there situations that do not call for a permanent separation of victim and perpetrator—and, if so under what conditions? What perpetrator characteristics and therapeutic methods permit successful reunification? Today we do not know the answers to these and many other crucial questions about MBP.

One particularly intriguing field for research is prevention. To what extent do potential MBP perpetrators respond to opportunities in the environment? What characteristics in health care providers or even victims might subtly encourage or discourage MBP? What actions by health care providers, equipment manufacturers, and others might deter MBP? Is it, like other forms of child maltreatment, preventable? If so, preventive actions should have high priority.

The information in this book has focused on child victims and perpetrators who are caregivers to children because those cases have been the most commonly identified to date. Research should also be directed toward other forms of MBP. Dependent adults, pets, and hospitalized patients can also be victims of MBP (Feldman, 1997; Sheridan, 1995). How transferable is knowledge about MBP with child victims to these groups? Is there information to be learned from these forms of MBP that would help understanding of MBP with children? These are fruitful areas for inquiry.

Ultimately, professional practice depends on knowledge, and knowledge building arises from and benefits practice. Ideally, practice and research merge in the clinician who observes, tests, and has the courage to articulate new ideas even under difficult circumstances. Dr. Roy Meadow was such a practitioner/researcher when he first concluded that MBP was taking place in one of his child patients.

PART II:
THE CONFIRMATION/
DISCONFIRMATION PROCESS

Chapter 4

Essential Elements in the Confirmation/Disconfirmation Process

The desired outcome with MBP cases is work that is objective and appropriate and leads to the truth—whatever the truth is. If there are children being abused or at risk, the desired outcome is that they are protected. This desired outcome means that MBP is confirmed when MBP is occurring. Of equal importance, it means that MBP is disconfirmed when it is not occurring.

This chapter will introduce the essential elements for work with MBP from initial suspicions through the investigative and decision-making process. If these essential elements are utilized, cases are far more likely to be investigated and decisions are far more likely to be achieved appropriately. Five essential elements are included in the investigative and decision-making process:

1. MBP basic and continuing education;
2. a thorough and appropriate MBP investigation leading to a confirmation/disconfirmation decision;
3. a case-specific multiagency-multidisciplinary team (MMT);
4. an MBP expert who will provide consultation, technical assistance, and expert testimony if needed as part of the investigation; and
5. a competent, correctly MBP-educated attorney to provide legal advice and to take legal action as necessary regarding investigative activities.

MBP cases follow a typical pathway, as shown in the following list:

1. Initial MBP suspicion.*
2. Report MBP suspicion to appropriate authorities and (if applicable) need for immediate victim protection.
3. If immediate victim protection is necessary: gather records and all available decision makers (in person and/or via telephone) at once to discuss case and make recommendations for victim protection and other decisions that cannot wait for full multiagency-multidisciplinary team (MMT) meeting.
4. If necessary: take action to protect victim or request victim protection from appropriate authorities. Place victim in neutral environment for protection and monitoring and to minimize possibility of case being tainted. If request for victim protection is denied, *do not* close case. MMT holds initial meeting and proceeds as follows.
5. Hold full MMT initial meeting. (See Chapter 7)
6. Full investigation and confirmation/disconfirmation process proceeds. Information is gathered, evaluated, and organized. MMT meets to advise on this process and concur in decision making. MBP expert should be closely involved.
7. MBP confirmed/disconfirmed.
   A. If MBP is confirmed, continue MBP case activities.
   B. If MBP is disconfirmed but other form(s) of maltreatment is/are confirmed, continue as appropriate for the maltreatment confirmed.
   C. If MBP and other maltreatment are disconfirmed, process ends.

Variation in the pathway will occur depending on whether the victim is found to need immediate protection. The pathway includes reporting of MBP suspicion to child protective authorities as required by law, immediate victim protection if necessary, and the essential elements of the investigation and confirmation/disconfirmation process.

---

* Initial reports will occasionally be received by child protective agencies in which it is stated that MBP maltreatment has been confirmed. This constitutes an immediate victim protection situation. However, unless a thorough, correct investigation and confirmation/disconfirmation process has been accomplished, the confirmation should be considered provisional until the process is completed.

DESCRIPTION OF THE ESSENTIAL ELEMENTS

MBP Basic and Continuing Education

MBP is very different from other kinds of maltreatment, and requires specialized knowledge and methods for investigation, confirmation/disconfirmation, case planning, and case management. The need for professional education about MBP is supported in the literature (American Public Human Services Association, 1999; Meadow, 1985; Mian, 1995; Thompson and Sullivan, 1995). For example, Yorker and Kahan state (1991):

> Just as the signs and symptoms of sexual abuse have become widely understood by professionals who work with children, the signs and symptoms of MSBP must also become familiar and therefore identifiable. Protective services workers and medical examiners should be particularly aware of the variations this disorder can have and the life-threatening potential in severe cases. . . . Judges and attorneys who prosecute child abuse cases must be aware of the atypical presentation of MSBP perpetrators. . . . There are many creative approaches to this under-recognized form of child abuse. The first and most imperative is education of all those who work with children. (pp. 56-67)

Although information about MBP is more widely disseminated today, many professionals still know little about it (Hochhauser and Richardson, 1994; Kaufman et al., 1989; Ostfeld and Feldman, 1996b) or have incorrect education or misconceptions about it. Discussion, strategizing, and decision making are counterproductive if key players do not have a solid and correct MBP information base. Lack of knowledge often leads to inappropriate, even dangerous, recommendations and decisions.

For success, those involved in an MBP case need a solid understanding of MBP basics. Those involved in a suspected or confirmed MBP case need to know about:

1. basic factitious disorder/ Munchausen syndrome and factitious disorder by proxy/Munchausen syndrome by proxy definitions (see Chapter 1);
2. perpetrator-consistent characteristics (see Chapter 2);

3. investigative and confirmation/disconfirmation activities and methods (see Chapters 6 and 7);
4. specific case planning and management issues (see Part III);
5. the danger when MBP perpetrators realize they are under suspicion (see Chapter 2);
6. the inappropriateness of risk assessment tools developed for other forms of maltreatment (see Chapter 9);
7. the limits of the DSM-IV as applied to MBP (see Chapter 1); and
8. the MBP situational suspicion indicators (see Chapter 5).

Education is the foundation upon which case success or failure rests. Without involved professionals having accurate MBP education, it is unlikely that MBP victims will be identified or protected.

Education in MBP cases must be ongoing. As personnel change, newly involved professionals must receive basic, correct MBP and detailed case information. As knowledge is generated and disseminated about MBP as well as the case, all involved professionals must be updated.

A Thorough and Appropriate MBP Investigation and Confirmation/Disconfirmation Process

Gathering, evaluating, and organizing information is at the heart of determining whether child maltreatment, including MBP, has occurred. Because health care professionals have written so much of the literature about MBP, most published discussions of the investigative phase detail suggested roles for physicians, nurses, and hospital social workers. Although it is appropriate for them to gather preliminary information in order to see if they have reason to suspect MBP, CPS and law enforcement should be notified and become involved when MBP is initially suspected. CPS has the legal mandate to conduct child abuse investigations, and the power to take or recommend action if it is believed that a child is being maltreated or in danger. Law enforcement's role is to investigate possible crime and to prefer charges as appropriate. MBP is both maltreatment and a crime. All agencies involved in an MBP case, and especially CPS and law enforcement, should work together, building on one another's expertise.

Much more is involved in the investigation and confirmation/disconfirmation process than may be apparent to those suspecting MBP. Even when perpetrators are videotaped/audiotaped exaggerating, fabricating, or inducing problems, much investigative work remains to determine whether the behavior constitutes MBP.

In order to confirm MBP maltreatment, there must be proof, through direct and/or circumstantial evidence, that the suspected perpetrator has deliberately exaggerated and/or fabricated and/or induced problems in the child. This proof, or lack thereof, is discovered through an appropriate investigation. There must also be a determination that the MBP-like behavior constitutes MBP rather than something else, such as torture or assault.

CPS and law enforcement will need the expertise of other professionals. Professionals who are not trained investigators with considerable MBP knowledge and experience or who are not assisted by someone who has such training and experience, may inadvertently compromise victim safety or the investigation. Sometimes relationships between CPS, health care facilities, or other community agencies are poor. Improving those relationships, rather than circumventing involvement with CPS, is the most productive long-term strategy.

Sound general investigative procedures must be followed throughout the investigation and confirmation/disconfirmation process. MBP cases seldom have the kinds of evidence often present in other forms of maltreatment. For example, in MBP there is usually not physical evidence of an injury (e.g., a burn or bruise) that could only have been inflicted by an abuser. Unless covert recording has been undertaken, there is usually not visual or auditory evidence of inappropriate actions or care withheld. Physical evidence and testimony may appear to support the perpetrator's claims that the victim has a genuine problem or problems.

For MBP to be confirmed, there must be a provable (through direct and/or circumstantial evidence) pattern of exaggeration and/or fabrication and/or inducing. This pattern is unique to MBP and requires specialized investigative approaches. It is found through gathering and appropriately evaluating documents and interview information. The investigation includes finding out what potential evidentiary sources exist, tracking them down, interviewing witnesses, obtaining written records, deciding what information is reliable and useful, and organizing relevant information in a meaningful way.

This is painstaking and time-consuming work that requires a thorough understanding of MBP and how deception can be accomplished. It is appropriate for the investigator to be released from other responsibilities in order to perform it. It is also appropriate for investigative work to be delegated to the MBP expert. MMT members may be able to assist under the direction of the investigators.

The Case-Specific, Multiagency-Multidisciplinary Team (MMT)

MBP cases almost always require expertise beyond that of a single investigator or agency, making a team approach desirable (American Public Human Services Association, 1999; Meadow, 1985; Mercer and Perdue, 1993; Pasqualone and Fitzgerald, 1999; Southall and Samuels, 1996). Various professionals have their own competencies, as well as unique information given to them by the perpetrator, family, and others. Each professional involved with the family will have a "piece of the puzzle." In order to come to correct conclusions and make sound plans, as many pieces of the puzzle as possible must be put together. For this reason, the best method of working with MBP cases from suspicion onward is through a specially convened team. This is not the permanent child maltreatment team that exists in some institutions and regularly reviews all suspected or confirmed child abuse and neglect cases. The case-specific multiagency-multidisciplinary team (MMT) is composed in response to a specific case in which MBP is suspected. It consists of representatives from all agencies and services involved with the *family*. A team composed only of a particular hospital's personnel or of a CPS agency staff may be more convenient, but does not contain the range of expertise and potential information needed.

Core MMT members should include CPS, law enforcement, and other key professionals involved with the family and case. Additional members may be included as appropriate. If no professional working with the case has extensive and credible MBP knowledge and experience, involve an MBP expert (see next section). When it is not possible for all team members to convene in the same place, arrangements should be made for participation by telephone conference call, speakerphone, or video teleconference.

The following lists reasons why the MMT is recommended:

- Recommendations coming from a knowledgeable MMT are much more powerful and credible than those made by one professional, agency, or organization.

- There is no substitute for involved case professionals convening to share and clarify information and formulate strategy.
- The diversity of MMT members reduces the chance of errors.
- MMTs can allow an efficient division of labor.
- MMTs can be creative.

1. *Recommendations coming from a knowledgeable, multiagency-multidisciplinary team are much more powerful and credible than those made by one professional or one agency or organization.* Recommendations must be as convincing as possible, particularly when they are made to those with little or no knowledge of MBP. For example, a judge (or other designated court official) wakened at midnight is much more likely to authorize a victim's immediate removal from caregivers if the recommendation comes from an MMT, not just a single concerned professional. Later, a confirmation or disconfirmation of MBP, a recommendation against placement with relatives, or details of a case plan will also be more credible and convincing if they are recommended by the MMT.

2. *There is no substitute for involved case professionals convening to share and clarify information and formulate strategy.* Each professional involved with the family has unique information and perspectives. To put the pieces of the case puzzle together, team members must hear from one another firsthand. They need the opportunity to ask questions, clarify information, resolve conflicts, and problem solve together. A single investigator or agency will not be nearly as effective in gathering information, "brainstorming," and making appropriate decisions. Teams can appear to be an expensive and time-consuming approach to investigation and case management, and someone must assume the burden of coordination and logistics. However, in MBP cases, the MMT will save time in the long run, and result in more thorough investigation and better decisions.

3. *The diversity of MMT members reduces the chance of errors.* MMT members come from a variety of agencies and areas of expertise. Each has his or her own knowledge, skills, and professional orientations. These different points of view lessen the possibility that something will be overlooked, and increase the

likelihood of correct conclusions, sound decision making, and appropriate recommendations.

4. *MMTs can allow an efficient division of labor.* MBP cases are extremely complex and time-consuming. Quick action is sometimes necessary to protect a victim. MMTs can divide tasks among members, taking advantage of their expertise and access to resources. Although MMT members should not be allowed to take over the investigation, if they follow through on their assignments, work will be completed more quickly.

5. *MMTs can be creative.* A group of people listening and thinking together often develop ideas and strategies that would not occur to individuals working alone. For example, a question might be posed, "If fabricating or inducing were involved in this case, what might someone be doing in order to produce the symptoms this child is experiencing or seems to be experiencing?" Ideas can then be exchanged and, if necessary, contacts with specialists can be made.

The MMT approach should be used throughout the life of the MBP case. As long as the child protective agency is involved, the MMT should participate at least in a periodic advisory capacity. Major decisions should not be made nor should the case be closed without the input of the MMT. The composition of the MMT may change over time. Basic MBP education and detailed case information will then be needed for new members. However, there should always be at least one member with credible expertise in MBP, and at least one person on the team should have been involved in the case when MBP was confirmed.

The MBP Expert

Because MBP is so different from other kinds of maltreatment, an investigator or MMT may make critical mistakes. An MBP expert can be indispensable, guiding the investigation, providing technical assistance, and testifying as an expert if needed in court hearings that may be part of the investigative process. For example, court testimony may be necessary to obtain an order for the release of certain records. Thompson and Sullivan (1995) recommend that "medical and social professionals . . . utilize the experience of professionals in the community who are familiar with Munchausen syndrome by proxy" (p. 35). Unfortunately, it is unlikely that a professional with considerable, credible MBP knowledge and experience will be found within the local community, and it is often necessary to find an MBP expert elsewhere. Information regarding MBP expert qualifications is discussed in other chapters of this book, especially in Chapter 11.

The MBP expert can perform or assist with many activities, including the following. Most can be accomplished, if necessary, without the MBP expert being on site.

- Provide basic and continuing, theoretical and practical MBP education.
- Review initial case information and provide initial impressions and recommendations.
- Provide an opinion or second opinion about whether MBP is involved.
- Provide ongoing case consultation.
- Provide direct technical and task assistance.
- Make case planning and management recommendations.
- Work closely with the assigned attorney.

1. *Provide basic and continuing, theoretical and practical, MBP education.* This will be necessary for initially involved professionals and those who subsequently join the case process. Education generally includes theory and practical applications. When needed, the MBP expert can demonstrate various case activities and techniques as applied to MBP cases. These could include investigative interviews, chairing MMT meetings, initial postconfirmation confrontation with the perpetrator, interviews, and the specialized process of considering relatives for potential out-of-home placement decision making, and interviews for therapist selection.

2. *Review initial case information and provide initial impressions and recommendations.* MBP is often suspected in good faith by those who do not have significant or correct MBP knowledge and experience. The MBP expert can review and analyze/organize the information that is initially available and give initial impressions and recommendations based on the literature and experience with other cases.

3. *Provide an opinion or second opinion about whether MBP is involved.* Although professionals may have provisionally confirmed MBP, they may not have conducted a complete confirmation-disconfirmation process and/or may not have enough MBP knowledge and experience to make a valid and convincing confirmation. An opinion or second opinion and recommendations by an MBP expert can uncover any case weaknesses and/or strengthen the case.

4. *Provide ongoing case consultation.* The MBP expert should be kept current on all initial and ongoing case activities, developments, and information in order to provide additional education and recommendations. If possible, the MBP expert should participate in periodic case reviews, providing updated MBP information and recommendations over the life of the case. An MBP expert may be brought back to help at any time there are concerns, or at critical points in the case such as the decision of whether to return the victim to the home.

5. *Provide direct technical and task assistance.* The MBP expert has considerable experience in investigative and confirmation/disconfirmation tasks, for example records evaluation, investigative interviews, and chairing MMT meetings. When there is not time for others to complete necessary activities, the MBP expert can be used to complete them.

6. *Make case planning and management recommendations.* MBP case plans should contain specific elements that differ from those in other maltreatment cases. These will be discussed further in Chapter 10. The MBP expert can make sure these elements are included in the recommended case plan and make suggestions for implementing the case plan.

7. *Work closely with assigned attorney.* As the prospective expert witness, and the person with the most direct experience of MBP court cases, the MBP expert can work in partnership with the assigned attorney to determine what court actions are needed, how the court can best be educated about MBP, and what strategies may be used by the other side. This will be discussed further in Chapter 11.

Given the current level of knowledge and experience with MBP in most communities, the expert is usually the only professional with sufficient experience in this specialized area. The expert brings objectivity and perspective, and over time can teach other professionals how to work with suspected and confirmed MBP cases. Thus, agencies that choose to work with an MBP expert are building their competence for future MBP cases. The use of an expert will not be possible in every case. The agency that cannot gain approval or funding for a consultant must do the best it can. That agency is, however, at a significant disadvantage.

A Competent, Correctly MBP-Educated Attorney to Provide Legal Advice and to Take Legal Action As Necessary Regarding Investigative Activities

An attorney should be assigned to the suspected MBP case immediately, and should be a member of the MMT. This attorney is normally one assigned to the child protection agency, and will provide advice to the child protective agency and the MMT. Usually this attorney will also take the lead in dealing with other attorneys who may become involved in the case; for example, attorneys for hospitals, care providers, and suspected perpetrators. As with other MMT members, the attorney should receive basic MBP and detailed case information immediately. The availability of such an attorney to assist with legal questions is a routine part of child protective work, and does not imply that there will be a finding of child maltreatment. The child protective agency may need legal guidance regarding investigative activities. Court orders and motions may be needed; for example, for specific information to be obtained.

Even if the attorney does not serve as a formal member of the MMT, he or she should receive basic MBP education and be kept up to date regarding case activity. Over the life of a suspected MBP case, the attorney is a key participant. The attorney must understand the unique and complex form of child maltreatment that is under consideration, and the kinds of issues that may be raised and tactics that may be employed. Through networks of personal contacts and Internet resources, some suspected or accused perpetrators have become very sophisticated in employing legal tactics. Even if the attorney is experienced and skilled in other forms of child maltreatment, MBP-specific education is vital.

THE ESSENTIAL ELEMENTS FOR MBP CASE SUCCESS APPLIED TO A CASE EXAMPLE

These are the essential elements in the MBP investigation and confirmation/disconfirmation process: basic MBP education, a thorough and MBP-specific investigation and confirmation/disconfirmation process aided by the MMT, an MBP expert, and an attorney who has received MBP education. These components will be reviewed in a specific case situation.

Case 4.1

Annie Martin, age twelve, was referred to the juvenile court by her elementary school due to truancy concerns. This was done in May, after Annie had missed most of her sixth-grade year due to repeated illness. After each absence, Mrs. Martin sent a note saying that Annie was "too sick" or "too tired" to come to school, but no one at the school knew of any physical problems that would account for such extensive absence. The school became especially concerned when the mother hinted that Annie was dying. The school nurse demanded a release of information and called the pediatrician, who denied any knowledge of a terminal condition.

Mrs. Martin's relationship with the school had been difficult for some years. She insisted that Annie was emotionally disturbed, and on several occasions requested evaluation by the special education team. Mrs. Martin reported bizarre symptoms at home, including uncontrollable muscle movements and sudden bursts of profanity. None of these behaviors was observed at school, but the school admitted that Annie might behave differently at home. Annie had seen a number of child psychologists, based on her mother's belief that she had Tourette's syndrome, an inherited disorder involving involuntary movements (tics) and compulsive sound making that may include profanity. She was currently in therapy with a child psychologist who was new to the community who agreed with the mother's diagnosis. At the psychologist's insistence, the pediatrician had prescribed a powerful tranquilizer and the school had placed Annie for part of the day in a special classroom for emotionally disturbed students. The school also sent home detailed daily behavior reports on the recommendation of the psychologist and at the insistence of Mrs. Martin.

Following the practice in this jurisdiction, Annie was assigned her own volunteer guardian *ad litem*, Jackie Lam, for the truancy case. She was an experienced and conscientious retired social worker. She focused on the question of whether Annie was mentally or physically sick. She obtained, through court order, all of Annie's health and school records. This was a major undertaking, as one record led to another until there were stacks of documents from various providers.

These records, taken at face value, would have suggested that Annie had serious health and behavior problems. They recorded repeated ear infections with seizures resulting from high fever when Annie was an infant. At age twelve, Annie was still seeing a neurologist and taking antiseizure medicine because her mother reported "mini seizures" every time the medication was discontinued. She was under treatment for asthma, requiring daily corticosteroids for its control. The mother reported that Annie wheezed whenever the dosage of the steroids was reduced. Annie's weight was above normal, which the mother attributed to "possible Prader-Willi syndrome" (a disorder that includes severely excessive and indiscriminate eating). There was nothing in the record about any terminal illness, but the pediatrician did recall that Mrs. Martin and Annie attended an asthma education program that stressed the dangers of asthma and the necessity for good control. The pediatrician thought that Mrs. Martin "might have misinterpreted" this information because "she's such a conscientious and loving mother, if a little nervous at times."

Annie's first behavior problems had been reported when she was two years old, and she had been followed by various mental health professionals since. There had been a variety of diagnoses and some trials of medication before the Tourette's syndrome was accepted. Annie's psychologist, who also treated Mrs. Martin's depression, felt that Mrs. Martin was coping admirably with difficult circumstances. Ms. Lam also obtained information about the Martin family. Mrs. Martin was fifty-seven years old, and had two children from a previous marriage. She had told several people that her other daughter was dead as the result of a rape/murder in another state. She had no contact with her son. Mrs. Martin had a long history of health problems and difficult life circumstances. Mr. Martin was ten years younger than Mrs. Martin, and had insisted that they try for a child as soon as they were married. (Ms. Lam got the impression that this was much more Mr. Martin's wish than Mrs. Martin's.) When Annie was ten years old, the Martins separated and Mr. Martin went to live with another woman. During the divorce proceedings, Mrs. Martin alleged that Mr. Martin had physically abused Annie, and he was briefly jailed. These charges were later dropped for lack of evidence, although Mrs. Martin continued to insist that Annie was "traumatized" and had nightmares about the abuse. Annie herself became so upset whenever the subject was raised that she was unable to talk about it. Mrs. Martin felt that the Tourette's syndrome became much worse after this purported abuse.

Ms. Lam first encountered the term "MBP" in a note from Annie's previous pediatrician. This physician had asked Mrs. Martin whether she might be exaggerating Annie's symptoms. Mrs. Martin had immediately taken Annie to another physician, threatening to sue for malpractice and defamation of character. No report was made to CPS.

Ms. Lam had never heard of MBP. Through colleagues in a neighboring city, she found an MBP expert, Mr. Johnson, who agreed to work with her. Mr. Johnson recommended a complete review of records. Mr. Johnson's review of the records revealed a consistent pattern of medical treatment based only on Mrs. Martin's reports. Test results and physical examinations were almost always normal with the exception of mild wheezing. In addition, numerous discrepancies emerged as records from various settings were laid side by side. Mrs. Martin often told one practitioner that someone else had made a diagnosis or provided a treatment, when this had not occurred. Her use of correct medical terminology probably made these false reports more believable. Based on these findings, Mr. Johnson agreed that MBP was probable. He and Ms. Lam made a formal report of MBP suspicion to CPS.

Following this report, Mr. Johnson continued to assist all those involved in the case. At Mr. Johnson's suggestion, an MMT was formed. It included the CPS investigator, the CPS attorney, the pediatrician, the psychologist, the school nurse, and Ms. Lam. Mr. Johnson provided basic MBP education and additional reading materials to the members of the MMT (with the exception of the psychologist, who stated that she could not take so much time from her practice). Several initial MMT sessions were held at which all participants put together their information and shared their observations of Mrs. Martin and Annie. The CPS investigator took careful note of this information and used it, along with the information collected by Ms. Lam, as the basis of her investigation. At Mr. Johnson's suggestion, she also followed up on details and was able to analyze additional records. (A court order, obtained by the CPS attorney, was necessary to acquire Mrs. Martin's physical and mental health records.) At each MMT meeting, she summarized the information that had been obtained so far and the information that was newly obtained. Some of these discussions became heated, as the psychologist refused to concur that MBP was occurring. Eventually the MMT, with the exception of the psychologist, came to believe that there was sufficient evidence to support a finding of MBP, and prepared a document to this effect. The psychologist's reservations were included in the report, with an explanation of why the majority of the MMT had come to a different conclusion. At that point, the case could be considered "confirmed."

Case Discussion

1. *Basic MBP and continuing education:* Most of the professionals in this case had only limited information: a sense that something was wrong, a few discrepancies in Mrs. Martin's story, or the term "MBP" encountered in the literature. The specific education Mr. Johnson provided at the beginning of and throughout the case was vital in helping involved case professionals understand what was happening. The psychologist, who did not attend the educational meeting, was the only member of the MMT who did not concur in the finding of MBP.

2. *A thorough, appropriate MBP investigation and confirmation-disconfirmation process:* In this case, Ms. Lam did much of the preliminary information gathering. This was supplemented with later work by the CPS investigator, who took information from all members of the MMT, added to it from other sources, and organized it for presentation to the MMT and court. The CPS investigator was able to use the powers granted to the state agency

to obtain information that was not available to other members of the MMT, so that all possible information could be evaluated. Only when information was assembled and analyzed did the pattern of deception become clear.

3. *The case-specific, multiagency-multidisciplinary team:* The presence of an MMT facilitated work on this case. It greatly increased the probability of success over that of an investigation in which just one person gathered information from each professional. Until all participants met together, none had all the "pieces of the puzzle" to form a comprehensive picture of the situation. As this full picture emerged and each team member heard the same *kinds* of observations from the others (although the details were different), all except the psychologist came to believe that Annie was not genuinely ill in the way that her mother claimed. The concurrence of several professionals was a key factor in convincing the court that custody should be awarded to the state, and later in making the decision that custody should be awarded to Mr. Martin, a man who had been jailed for abuse. Without this concurrence, the psychologist's insistence—probably based on a lack of complete and correct MBP education and overidentification with Mrs. Martin—could have done a great deal of damage.

All members of the MMT except the psychologist found the MBP education and mutual decision-making process valuable. Ms. Lam was especially grateful that, with the help of Mr. Johnson, her concerns were taken seriously. The CPS worker, who was involved in an MBP case for the first time, appreciated the emotional support as well as the easy access to the pediatrician that the MMT provided.

4. *The MBP expert:* Without Mr. Johnson's assistance, it is unlikely that an appropriate investigation and confirmation/disconfirmation process would have occurred. Mr. Johnson provided education, consulted with CPS, chaired the MMT, and helped analyze case information. At every turn, he was available to discuss, help, and suggest next steps. His advice was particularly valuable to Ms. Lam at the beginning of the case, when she had little more than suspicions, and later to the CPS worker who had never before been involved in an MBP investigation.

5. *A competent, correctly MBP-educated attorney to provide legal advice and to take legal action as necessary regarding investigative activities:* The attorney's most specific contribution to the investigative phase of this case was obtaining the court order for the release of Mrs. Martin's records. The attorney, however, was an active part of the discussion, and was able to clarify legal issues as they arose for the MMT. Through participation in the investigative and confirmation/disconfirmation phase, the attorney was also gathering information that could be used if necessary in later case phases.

The correct outcome in this case—protection of Annie—came about because the five essential elements were followed. Neither Ms. Lam nor the CPS investigator began this case knowing very much about MBP. However, through their persistence, the help of Mr. Johnson, and the work of the multidisciplinary team, a fair investigation and confirmation-disconfirmation process was completed that addressed the MBP-specific features of this case. As a result, the MBP maltreatment occurring in this case was confirmed and could be addressed.

Chapter 5

Suspecting and Reporting

Now that the general features of MBP have been discussed, and the essential elements for MBP case success described, consideration will be given to the practicalities of MBP identification, investigation, and management. Each MBP case is different. Each MBP perpetrator is different in behavior and motives. This chapter and the chapters that follow will "walk" readers through many factors found in cases. The information here is meant to provide guidance. Good judgment, local laws and conditions, and specifics of each case and the personnel involved will dictate how to apply it.

SUSPECTING MBP

As is true with other forms of child maltreatment, virtually anyone who encounters children and families may suspect MBP. Reports of MBP suspicion have come from hospitals, mental health facilities, physicians, schools, other community agencies, emergency medical technicians, relatives, friends, and others. A great deal of the MBP literature is found in medical journals and focuses on cases of hospitalized children with physical symptoms. However, MBP may be suspected and identified in a wide variety of settings; for example, in inpatient and outpatient physical and mental health settings, schools, child care centers, social service agencies, support groups, neighborhoods, and even on Internet discussion forums (Feldman, 2000; Feldman, Bibby, and Crites, 1998). It may present as psychological/behavioral problems, physical problems, or both.

People frequently contact MBP experts for advice and assistance after learning—often via the media—that there is such a condition. They may not have become suspicious until long after the maltreatment began, due to lack of public and professional awareness. Sometimes they had a feeling that "something was wrong." Often they believed completely in the story as presented to them. Pasqualone and Fitzgerald state (1999), "In approaching a suspected case of MBPS, one major deterrent must be identified. This is the failure of medical or nursing personnel to even consider the diagnosis." Zitelli, Seltman, and Shannon (1987) call professionals who fail to recognize MBP "unwitting participants" in the maltreatment of the child. This lack of knowledge extends throughout the professional and lay communities.

As concerned persons—potential reporters of MBP maltreatment—begin to recognize that "something is wrong," they often suffer personal emotional conflicts. They may accuse themselves of being unkind, prejudiced, or unconsciously hostile if they doubt a caretaker's story. If the potential reporters have never heard of MBP, the very suspicion can be horrifying. These feelings can result in significant suffering, and be a significant barrier to recognizing MBP and reporting it. Meadow (1985) describes this process:

> The realisation that a child's prolonged illness may have been fabricated tends to come slowly. . . . There is understandable reluctance by medical and nursing staff to believe that a parent may have been deceiving. Part of this stems from a wish to think good of parents, and part from a wish to avoid facing the fact that all one's investigations and treatments have been both inappropriate and harmful, that one has been hoodwinked, and has made a completely wrong diagnosis up to that moment. . . . On the other hand, paediatricians are reluctant to intervene early for fear of being wrong in their accusations. Parents for their part when later accused vary between those who say, "if you suspected it earlier why didn't you tell us so that it could have been stopped," to those who say, "it is outrageous that we should be accused of these things until there is definite proof." (pp. 386-387)

However, persons who suspect maltreatment should be careful to stay within the limits of their competence, or should seek consultation. They should not jump to conclusions without checking the facts.

Sheridan (1989) also discusses the results of a survey of professionals who had experienced MBP cases:

> [If they were] unable to prove their suspicions, they were afraid to alienate a family that might be "crying for help," yet afraid

of what might happen to the unprotected child if they did not intervene. Many respondents [to the survey] had become emotionally close to the families that they later suspected, and recognized that they had participated in a long process of denial. A team member attempting to confront this denial often was the target of significant hostility. (p. 57)

However, if children are to be protected, professionals must overcome these feelings and confront their suspicions.

Following is a list of "red-flag situations," derived from the literature and experience. This list should be used along with the MBP perpetrator-consistent characteristics discussed in Chapter 2. When any of these is present, MBP may be suspected, along with other possibilities. The medical term for this is "added to the differential diagnosis." This means that the condition in question—in this case, MBP—becomes one of several *possible* diagnoses being actively considered. It does not imply that MBP is definitely occurring or that it will eventually be found to be occurring. Any other disorder in the differential diagnosis, or one not yet considered, could become the final diagnosis depending on information that is gathered.

MBP may also occur in the absence of some of these suspicion indicators. For example, not all perpetrators fit the stereotype of the "good caretaker." Not all have the motive of attention from health care providers. For example, attention from or power over a present or former romantic partner may be the goal.

"Suspicion" is used here deliberately. Finding characteristics in a perpetrator and/or situation does not confirm the presence of MBP. That judgment should be made only after a thorough and appropriate investigation and confirmation/disconfirmation evaluation process, and with the guidance and concurrence of a professional who has credible MBP knowledge and experience. The confirmation/disconfirmation process must be conducted objectively and with an open mind. It can exonerate suspected perpetrators as well as identify real perpetrators.

MBP Situational Suspicion Indicators

The following list describes reasons to suspect MBP (MBP situational suspicion indicators):

- Differences exist between reported history and what is seen, or what makes sense physically or psychologically/behaviorally.
- Problems do not respond to treatment as expected.
- Events occur that are (or could be) consistent with exaggeration, fabrication, or induction.
- Problems appear to originate only in association with the care-taker's presence.
- Problems disappear, or begin to improve, when the child is separated from the caretaker.
- Problems recur after the caretaker is told that the child has recovered, is improving, or is soon to be discharged from treatment. Alternatively, problems recur shortly after the child goes home or the course of treatment ends.
- Investigation of the family shows confirmed or alleged unexplained problems, illness, or death of other family members.
- The suspected perpetrator appears to have a pattern of exaggeration, fabrication, or induction.
- Problems show nonrandom patterning, especially in association with known events.
- Problems occur in a context that suggests secondary (external) gain.
- Induction or tampering is observed or suspected. Conditions may make it likely that induction or tampering is occurring.
- Someone is suspicious.

Difference between reported history and what is seen, or what makes sense physically or psychologically/ behaviorally (Jones et al., 1986; Meadow, 1985).

Science, including medicine, operates by making sense out of data. Popular culture loves stories of heroic parents fighting for an answer to their child's problem. In real life, however, such situations are rare. Most patients have disease courses that ultimately fit a known pattern. In most situations, uncertainty and discrepancies either do not occur, or they resolve within a reasonable length of time.

In MBP cases, when sufficient information is known the visible signs and reported symptoms do not fit into known illness patterns (syndromes). They may not be consistent with the functioning of the human body or mind. Alternatively, they may form an illness pattern so rare that MBP is more common. Often the discrepancies include reports of frightening symptoms unconfirmed by physical examination, laboratory tests, X rays, independently obtained records, or professional or lay observers. For example, a grandmother brings an infant to the pediatrician's office saying that he gets severe diarrhea from all forms of milk, including breast milk. But there is a discrepancy: The baby looks well nourished, so he must be retaining some food. On laboratory testing, the baby's electrolytes are normal; they would not be if the diarrhea was severe. Perhaps the grandmother reports that another physician treated the infant for diarrhea, but when that physician is contacted there is no record of diarrhea.

The grandmother insists that X rays be done of the whole digestive track; they are normal. She reiterates that the baby is not taking any nourishment, so he is admitted to the hospital. When the nurses feed him, he eats hungrily. The nurses do not see diarrhea until the grandmother visits. In this instance, the lack of supporting physical, laboratory, and X-ray evidence, combined with the nurses' observations, raise a strong suspicion that the grandmother has been reporting falsely. Knowledge of common methods of MBP perpetration suggests that perhaps the grandmother is administering a laxative to cause the diarrhea.

Sometimes obscure diseases that resemble the situation are found in the professional or lay literature. When this occurs, the situation and the journal article(s) must be evaluated carefully. Does the report appear in a reliable, recent publication? How frequently does the disease occur? Among what groups (e.g., men or women, adults or children, ethnic groups, etc.) is this problem found? How closely do the symptoms in this disease resemble those in the suspect case? Does knowledge of the disease lead to confirmation of the problem or treatment that works? When all elements are put together, is maltreatment more likely than this rare disorder?

In the case example given, suppose that a nursing student locates an Internet Web page that discusses "pan-milk allergy" (fictitious condition) as "the hidden epidemic of our times." Even the authors of the Web page state that the allergy has never been seen among infants, although they believe that it might be possible. No research findings support these assertions, nor can information on this disorder be found in reputable medical publications. Although the possibility of "pan-milk allergy" cannot entirely be dismissed, the information represents opinion, not research. MBP is far more probable than a first pediatric instance of "pan-milk allergy."

*Problems do not respond to treatment as expected
(Meadow, 1985).*

Just as most patients have problems that make sense, most problems eventually respond to professional intervention. This may not be
immediate; practitioners may need to try several approaches to treatment before a satisfactory one is found. For example, most patients
experiencing a particular type of infection may respond to a particular
antibiotic. Those who do not respond to the first drug often respond to
second-line or third-line antibiotics. A good deal of publicity has
been given to situations in which infections are resistant to many
drugs, or even to all available antibiotics. Such situations are rare, and
they are usually obvious through clinical findings and laboratory
tests. They may have other common features, such as occurring prin-
cipally among certain groups of patients or in certain regions.

In the "milk intolerance" case, according to the grandmother,
many different formulas and breast milk had been tried. Supposedly
nothing worked. It is common for infants to have difficulty with one
formula and to need to be changed to another. It is unlikely that an infant would be intolerant to multiple formulas and even breast milk,
especially when the infant still appears well nourished. This element
of the history, even without the nurses' observations that the baby
feeds well, would raise suspicion.

*Events occur that are (or could be) consistent with exaggeration,
fabrication, or induction.*

When an independent observer says that problems did not occur on
a given instance or were not as severe as reported, this strengthens the
possibility that MBP is occurring. When nonprescribed substances
are known to be present in the home, and these substances could produce the child's symptoms, this suggests that MBP must be considered. Similarly, even if a plausible reason is given, when there is evidence of tampering with medical equipment, records, specimens,
etc., and that tampering could be consistent with symptoms, MBP is
more likely. Certain methods of inducing symptoms are also well
documented in the medical literature. For example, laxatives have
frequently been used to create diarrhea. Salt poisoning has been used
to create electrolyte imbalance. Knowing how the symptoms *could*
have been created, and knowing that this method is within the capa-

bility of the suspected perpetrator, strengthens the chain of circumstantial evidence.

*Problems appear to originate only in association
with the caretaker's presence (Meadow, 1985).*

This was discussed extensively in Chapter 3 as a hallmark of MBP. In the milk allergy case, note that diarrhea recurred after the grandmother's visits. Although she was not present when the diarrhea began, it occurred only after she had visited. Thus it was "in association with" the grandmother's presence. Whenever symptoms fit this pattern, MBP must be considered.

*Problems disappear, or begin to improve, when the child
is separated from the caretaker (Jones et al., 1986).*

This was also discussed in Chapter 3, and is related to the appearance of symptoms only in association with the caretaker. In the milk allergy case, the baby ate well and did not have diarrhea when under the care of the nurses and not visited by the grandmother.

*Problems recur after the caretaker is told that the child
has recovered, is improving, or is soon to be discharged
from treatment.*

Often in MBP cases, problems recur shortly after the child goes home or the course of treatment ends. Today, for economic reasons, hospitals focus on early discharge. Health care providers try to give care only and to the extent that it is clearly needed. Honest misjudgments may occur, and problems—and the patient—may return for further care but this occurs relatively infrequently. In MBP, however, a common pattern is that as soon as the problem appears to be solved or under control, it returns. The recurrence or persistence of problems in MBP is often extreme and striking. For example, no sooner is the child approved for discharge than the symptoms are reported again. No sooner has the child arrived at home, than the ambulance is called again. Some victims of MBP have spent more of their lives in physical and/or mental health settings than at home because of repeated readmissions and "emergencies."

Investigation of the family shows confirmed or alleged unexplained problems, illness, or death of other family members.

No family is free from problems. However, in the nuclear or extended families of MBP victims there are frequently other members who are also said to have problems. These are sometimes similar to the problems of the suspected MBP victim. Sometimes these are vague, resistant to diagnosis or treatment, perhaps with a dramatic component. Alternatively, the problems may appear real or ordinary, but they are in such confluence that the combination is unlikely. If such problems are identified or other deaths are associated in any way with the perpetrator, every effort must be made to obtain information about them and to assess the information from the perspective of possible MBP.

The suspected perpetrator appears to have a pattern of exaggeration, fabrication, or induction.

If the suspected perpetrator appears to engage in attention-seeking or deceptive behavior, or has a history of behavior consistent with Munchausen syndrome (factitious disorder), this increases the possibility that deception is also being practiced involving the child. If the suspected perpetrator appears to engage in exaggeration, fabrication, or induction directed toward the child victim or others, even if these are not directly related to the symptoms in question, this is suggestive of MBP. Ostfeld and Feldman (1996a), in discussing the overlap between MBP and Munchausen syndrome in pregnant patients, state, "Each disorder is a risk factor for the other, the diagnosis of one may lead to recognition of the other; the mysterious medical crises in a mother's health may suddenly become understandable when her FDP behavior is detected" (p. 84).

Problems show nonrandom patterning, especially in association with known events.

Any such patterning or periodicity that is unrelated to a disease process raises suspicions that MBP is occurring. For example, sometimes problems occur only on weekends or in the absence of a significant other such as the perpetrator's husband/partner or the primary physician. Victims have been known to "bleed" only on a monthly basis (the perpetrator was using menstrual blood).

Problems occur in a context that suggests secondary (external) gain.

As MBP is currently understood, internal motivations are primary (Feldman and Lasher, 1999). That is, the perpetrator wants it to appear as if a child has problems because of some psychological gratification that this brings. However, falsification and induction of symptoms also occur for other forms of gain. Sometimes various motivations overlap or are unclear. The central question is always, "is this child being maltreated?"

Potential external gains that may lead caretakers to exaggerate, fabricate, or induce problems in their children include: direct economic benefit (e.g., Supplemental Security Income payments, housing allowances while the child is in the hospital, church/organizational fund-raising for medical expenses, etc.), other forms of gain (e.g., "Make-A-Wish" trips), and preferential treatment (e.g., access to facilities for the handicapped). Some professionals who rely on the DSM-IV criteria would not consider such cases to be MBP. These external motivations do not necessarily invalidate a diagnosis of MBP and cases should be investigated regardless of the type(s) of gain that may be involved.

Induction or fabrication is observed or suspected.

If a suspected perpetrator is observed in the act of smothering an infant, administering unauthorized injections, or tampering with medical equipment, records, specimens, etc., suspicions should be raised that this was not an innocent or one-time occurrence. Even if the perpetrator has a convincing excuse, the behavior should be regarded as speaking for itself.

Similarly, some conditions make it highly likely that symptom induction or fabrication of problems is occurring. If the suspected perpetrator of a hospitalized child, for example, waits until staff are outside the room, pulls the curtains around the bed, and the child then "coincidentally" develops symptoms, it is reasonable to be suspicious that the perpetrator has been responsible. If documents have not been received directly from the original source, they should be considered suspect until original source documents have been received or they have been carefully checked with the original source. Records should be obtained directly from the professional or institution that created them. Caretakers of children with genuine problems frequently do hand carry medical records, especially when they are in transit. Because of the risk that MBP suspicions may be wrong, such records cannot be completely disregarded. Verifying such records will be an additional test of how accurately the caretaker is reporting.

Someone is suspicious.

In many situations, the first sign of possible MBP will not be any of the already mentioned indicators. Rather, someone will have a "funny feeling" about the situation, or perhaps feel uncomfortable or even frightened in the presence of the perpetrator. Usually, this behavior is uncharacteristic of the person harboring the suspicions, and it may cause guilt or anxiety. Such suspicions should always be taken seriously and followed up.

Sometimes interpersonal situations hinder serious consideration of someone's suspicions. For example, a higher-status professional might be unwilling to listen to the observations of a lower-status professional or nonprofessional. The person raising suspicions might be disliked by the person who receives the suspicions. There have been many cases in which the person who was silenced or ignored was correct. Again, suspicions—regardless of source—should be taken seriously.

Reports of possible MBP often come from nonprofessional sources. As more information is available in the media and on the Internet, concerned friends, neighbors, and relatives are contacting health care and child maltreatment professionals to discuss suspicions. Sometimes ulterior motives could be posited. However, again, these suspicions should be taken seriously.

All of these situational indicators are "red flags," not confirmation or accusation that a situation is MBP. Any of them can appear in cases that turn out to be true problems. However, the presence of any of them should trigger a closer look, and a consideration of whether the answer to the problem may be MBP.

False accusations of MBP are disastrous. Failure to identify and protect maltreated children is also disastrous. The presence of situational suspicion indicators should raise suspicions, and suspicions mandate a closer look at situations. They also mandate a report to the appropriate child protective authority, as with any other form of suspected child maltreatment.

REPORTING MBP

Report MBP at the Earliest Suspicion

MBP is child maltreatment. It is consistent with the definition and criteria contained in the federal Child Abuse Prevention and Treatment Act (1996, Sec. 111.2):

> [A]t a minimum, any recent act or failure to act on the part of a parent or caretaker, which results in death, serious physical or emotional harm . . . or an act or failure to act which presents an imminent risk of serious harm.

Those who are legally mandated in their jurisdiction, such as health care, educational, and social service professionals, *must* report. Others who suspect maltreatment *should* report. The report should be made to the agency legally designated to receive child maltreatment reports. In the United States, there are public child protective service agencies (CPS) in every state. These are responsible for the investigation of suspected child maltreatment and for the protection of children (Tumlin and Geen, 2000).

If CPS cannot be reached or local procedure allows this alternative, maltreatment suspicion should be reported to law enforcement with a follow-up report to CPS. Reports of MBP suspicion should not wait for "proof." Reports should be made as soon as anyone is suspicious. This allows CPS and law enforcement to become involved and a multiagency-multidisciplinary team (MMT) to organize and begin meeting.

Case 5.1
On the morning of December 22, sixteen-month-old Sherika Kelly was hospitalized at St. Andrew's Medical Center. This was her sixth admission in

the nine months since she and her single mother, Twana Kelly, had moved to the area. Each time, Sherika had severe vomiting and dehydration that resolved within forty-eight hours. After thorough workups, no reason had been found for Sherika's problems.

During Sherika's fifth admission, in late November, Ms. Kelly had removed Sherika from the hospital against medical advice. This occurred after the hospital social worker, Dena Allen, had begun questioning Ms. Kelly about the illnesses. Hospital staff were suspicious that Ms. Kelly might be poisoning her child. They decided that if another incident occurred, the house physician would order toxicology screening. The staff decided not to make a report to CPS until there was "proof" because CPS might "make things worse" or "mismanage" the case.

When Sherika was admitted on December 22, her vomit-covered shirt was sent to the lab for toxicology testing. However, a test for ipecac was not part of the hospital's standard toxicology panel, and no one had thought to make a special request. The hospital staff concluded that they must have been wrong in their suspicions. Several nurses felt quite guilty that their "cynical" or "prejudiced" attitudes had led them to suspect this "devoted" mother.

On Christmas afternoon, the attending physician took the day off and his partner, Dr. Westerley, made hospital rounds during the evening. Dr. Westerley had some familiarity with MBP and, after reading the chart and talking with hospital staff, she suspected MBP. She immediately called the lab to request new tests including an ipecac screen on the original vomitus; however, the lab had already discarded all samples from the time of admission. Dr. Westerley ordered that tests for ipecac be performed immediately on new urine and blood samples. At about 4:00 p.m. she began attempting to call CPS to report her suspicions.

Because of the holiday, only an on-call CPS staff member was available. The phone number was continually busy, and it was nearly 11:00 p.m. before contact was made. Although Dr. Westerley explained her concerns for Sherika's safety because Ms. Kelly continued to have access to her, the worker refused to respond, saying "Sherika is safe because she is in the hospital and this will have to wait until the next business day." Dr. Westerley then contacted law enforcement, who also declined to respond because of a staff shortage over the holiday period. The next morning the lab confirmed that high levels of ipecac, which had not been prescribed, were found in the blood and urine samples. The ipecac had been given during the twelve hours prior to the collection of the samples. During this time, only Ms. Kelly and the hospital staff had access to Sherika. Dr. Westerley again contacted CPS. This time, a CPS response was initiated, appropriate emergency legal action was taken, and Sherika was placed in protective custody pending a probable cause hearing. It was later discovered that Ms. Kelly had come under suspicion at a hospital in the county where she and Sherika previously lived. That hospital's staff had also questioned whether CPS would "handle the case properly," had decided to "wait for proof," and had not reported MBP suspicion.

Sherika Kelly could have died from ipecac poisoning. No involved professional except Dr. Westerley had enough knowledge to handle the situation appropriately. CPS's response was inappropriate; they should not have disregarded a doctor's perception of immediate danger to a child. Lack of prompt reporting by two sets of professionals left a child in danger, as explained in the following section.

1. The first hospital should have reported its suspicions. Had this been done, Sherika might have been spared months of abuse and danger to her life. The hospital's failure to report did not ensure Sherika's safety or keep Ms. Kelly from fleeing. All involved professionals incurred civil liability for not reporting as required by law.

2. St. Anthony's staff should have reported their concerns when they were first suspicious in late November. Had an appropriate report been made at that time, Sherika might have been spared another month of abuse and danger to her life. All involved professionals incurred civil liability for not reporting as required by law.

3. St. Anthony's staff should have reported their suspicions early in the sixth admission. Because St. Anthony's failed to report, professionals involved with the Kelly family missed opportunities to share information with one another as the situation developed, and to receive education about MBP. This process would have, among other things, provided them with information about specifically ordering a test to identify ipecac, and the necessity of keeping original samples.

   Because of the delay, CPS received the case at the worst possible time for them to begin an investigation, gather information from other jurisdictions, and obtain court orders if necessary. Had they been involved earlier, they would have been able to plan a thoughtful response rather than being forced into a reactive mode. Under these circumstances, the chances of appropriate initial action were diminished.

The importance of early reporting cannot be overstated. Members of the community may be correct that lack of education, inappropriate policies and procedures, or general understaffing and mismanagement may prevent appropriate response by child protective agencies.

If so, these community members should take the initiative to help solve these problems before the first or next suspected or confirmed MBP case presents. For example, hospital staff may be reluctant to report suspicion of MBP maltreatment at early suspicion because they feel "CPS does not know enough" or "CPS will mess things up." They should take the initiative of bringing in an MBP expert to provide comprehensive training, or work with all potentially involved agencies in planning multiagency-multidisciplinary procedures for dealing with suspected and confirmed MBP cases.

Reporting: A Two-Way Communication Process

The decision to report child maltreatment, the speed with which the report is made, and information communicated during the initial reporting conversation are all crucial to successful maltreatment investigation and child protection. Information given and received during the initial reporting conversation sets the stage for immediate decision making and lays the foundation for the investigation and confirmation-disconfirmation process that will follow. The quality and quantity of information provided and the care with which information is received and recorded can be of paramount importance, even saving the life or health of a child.

The reporting conversation is a two-way communication process between reporter and suspicion-report receiver. The initial reporting conversation results in a product, a written report or electronic equivalent, that is given to the assigned agency decision maker, usually a supervisor. Based on information contained in the report, child protective or law enforcement professionals must make at least the following decisions:

1. Is there enough information to make informed decisions?
2. Is the situation appropriate for investigation?
3. Will it be investigated?
4. How soon must the investigation be initiated?
5. What initial activity or activities will take place?
6. Who will be assigned to conduct the investigation?

Frequently, the product submitted to the supervisor is incomplete, unclear, or inaccurate. The results of this can be disastrous. If information must be augmented or clarified before decisions are made, time will be lost. MBP cases can move very quickly; minutes can make a difference in the protection of a child.

If information is inaccurate, inappropriate decisions may be made. This can happen for three major reasons: lack of knowledge, carelessness, and inappropriate attitude. Persons making reports may have only limited information, or their information may be of uncertain quality. Reporters may know little about child maltreatment, including MBP. They may not know how to present a case so that a child protective agency is likely to accept it for service or determine appropriate urgency and priority.

Under ideal circumstances, suspicion-report receivers are skilled interviewers who know how to compensate for the reporter's lack of knowledge. Unfortunately, CPS and law enforcement staff who take maltreatment reports are often in entry-level positions. Some have received training in social work or human services; some have not. Some have learned more than the basics about child maltreatment, but others received only a brief orientation to their jobs. At the present time, very few have received training in MBP. If they do not understand the dynamics of maltreatment, MBP, and investigation techniques, they will not know what information is needed for sound decision making. Nor will they be able to identify the pattern and potential harm associated with MBP when it is reported to them. If the reporter does not use the term MBP or FDP, suspicion-report receivers may not recognize what the reporter is describing. They may "screen out" the report because it does not fit usual patterns of child maltreatment, or because a divorce or custody situation is involved. They may not recognize that the situation constitutes a danger to the victim, may omit the label "MBP" from their product, or may assign the case an incorrect priority.

Reporters and receivers of reports *must* listen to one another. If they do not understand one another's terminology, they should ask for clarification. Jargon should be avoided, as terms that are familiar to one profession may be incomprehensible or intimidating to another. If participants in the reporting conversation need additional information about the case or agency's/organization's policies, they should also ask. The atmosphere should be one of mutual respect, for the goal is shared: the protection of a possibly endangered child.

Suggestions for Reporters

The suspicion-report receiver (who may be a child protective, law enforcement, or other employee) is often not the investigator who will be assigned to the case. The procedure will depend on the jurisdiction. Reporters should know what system will be used. If the person receiving the report will not be following up on the case, he or she may be less interested in full details. This is why it is even more important to strive for clarity in the report, since information will have to be conveyed by the suspicion-report receiver to the investigator, perhaps through a supervisor. The following suggestions will help to maximize the quality of the report. Report quality and good communication are particularly important because, in most states, a single person decides whether the case will be accepted for investigation or "screened out" (meaning that it is not investigated).

Suggestions for reporting MBP suspicion include the following:

- Allow enough time.
- Have all information and documents available.
- Contact the correct agency; verify this if necessary.
- Plan the conversation in advance.
- Ask to be contacted as soon as the case is assigned; follow up if necessary.
- Do not assume that the suspicion-report receiver understands MBP.
- Report to CPS even if a report has already been made to law enforcement.

1. *Reporters should allow enough time for the reporting discussion.* The report sets the stage for all subsequent decision-making and investigative activities. Spending sufficient time at the beginning will save time later.

2. *Reporters should ensure that all their case information and documents are close at hand when the report is made.* Lack of important information undermines reporter credibility and wastes time for both the reporter and the suspicion-report receiver.

3. *Reporters should contact the correct agency.* The child protective agency responsible for investigating is generally the one for the county in which the victim lives. This may or may not be the same as

the county(ies) in which the maltreatment is suspected to have occurred. For example, suspected attempts at suffocation may have
occurred at home, and also in a hospital located in another county. If
law enforcement becomes involved, criminal case jurisdiction will
generally be taken by the law enforcement agency for the location(s)
in which the child was maltreated. Several jurisdictions may be involved in one case.

Reporters should not assume that addresses shown in records are
correct. People may use an address other than their residence for
mailing, billing, school, or other purposes. They may fail to update
their address after moving. If a report is made to the wrong jurisdiction, time will be lost, a case will become more complicated, and victim risk will increase. Incorrect addresses have led to children being
taken into protective custody based on court orders from judges who
did not have jurisdiction. If there is any question, reporters should
take steps to verify the child's address before they make contact with
an agency. For example they can ask a caretaker, "where can we reach
you in case of emergency?" Reporters should also verify with the reporting agency that that address is within their jurisdiction. If there is
any question as to the county in which the address is located, assistance should be requested from law enforcement or other official information providers.

4. *Reporters should think through in advance what they will say.*
Reporters should try to imagine themselves in the role of a child protective or law enforcement investigator. What information would increase the likelihood of good decisions and quick response? What information will convey clearly the present situation, or help expedite
the investigation? What information will help eliminate "phone tag"
or assist in quicker contact with others for clarification or additional
information? Professional jargon and acronyms should be avoided.
Box 5.1 shows key questions that are suggested for suspicion-report
receivers. Not all this information may be available (or available to
the reporter) at the time the report is made. However, if the reporter
reviews these questions and is ready to answer them to the extent possible, information will be conveyed in an orderly, coherent fashion.

5. *Reporters should not assume that the suspicion-report receiver
knows what MBP is or has received basic MBP training.* However,
many report receivers will be reluctant to admit this. So reporters
should be ready to explain their concerns (e.g., "We believe the baby-

BOX 5.1.
Questions for Suspected and Confirmed MBP Cases

1. Who is making the report? How can they be reached? What is their position in relation to the case? Do they have any familiarity or expertise with MBP? Are they making the report on their own, or on behalf of another expert, team, etc.?
2. What date is this information received? (Information will be current only as of this date.)
3. Does any individual or group state that they have confirmed or disconfirmed MBP maltreatment? If so:

  • How did they define MBP?
  • How did they decide that MBP was or was not occurring?
  • What specific information was gathered and reviewed in making the decision (e.g., specific records, interviews, tests, consultations, etc.)?
  • What individuals were involved in any part of the process (discussions, team meetings, consultations, etc.)? For each individual, obtain complete contact information. If any individual is considered or claims to be an MBP maltreatment expert, request a resume. If any individual has or claims to have some knowledge or experience relating to MBP, request details (titles/authors of publications reviewed, dates/presenters' names of workshops attended, number of cases involved in, etc.).
  • When were meetings, discussions, consultations, etc., held that contributed to the decision? For each of these, obtain the date, the names of those attending, the name of the individual responsible for documenting the event, and the location of the documentation. Request copies of all documentation for such meetings, discussions, etc.

4. When was MBP maltreatment first suspected in this case? By whom? What specific reasons led to the suspicion?
5. If MBP was confirmed or is suspected:

  • Who is believed to have perpetrated the maltreatment? Why? Who else was considered?
  • Who is believed to be the victim? What other children are in the home or under the care of the perpetrator?
  • What specific physical and/or psychological-behavioral problems are being exhibited by the victim and believed to

have been caused by the perpetrator? What specific examples support belief that the perpetrator has caused the problems? What specific examples refute this belief? What documentation is available? Are there other problems that do not appear to have been caused by the perpetrator?

- Does it appear that the method of creating these problems was exaggeration and/or fabrication and/or induction? Why? What documentation is available?
- What form(s) of maltreatment, as defined in the jurisdiction, does the MBP appear to constitute? (For example, physical abuse, sexual abuse, emotional abuse, medical neglect, etc.) Why?
- What MBP perpetrator-consistent characteristics have been identified? What documentation is available for these? What alternative explanations appear reasonable, and what documentation is available for those?
- What physical and/or psychological-behavioral interventions (office visits, hospitalizations, medications, surgeries, etc.) has the victim been subjected to unnecessarily because of the perpetrator's exaggeration and/or fabrication and/or induction behavior? What harm has occurred because of these? What harm *might* have occurred?
- What other possibilities besides MBP have been considered? Which have been excluded, and why?
- Where is the victim now? What has been done so far to ensure the victim's safety? What plan has been created to continue to monitor and evaluate the victim?

sitter has been poisoning the child") rather than just using the terminology "Munchausen by proxy" (etc.) or MBP. Another tactful approach is to offer an "update" in this "quickly changing" field. If at all possible, the reporter should fax or e-mail the report and any related initially important information (a basic MBP article, for example) in writing to ensure all major points are "in the record." The definition of MBP used by the reporter or MMT should be included in this report. Specific MBP-related concerns of the reporter and reasons for them should be discussed. For example, the reporter can request that the assigned child protective worker contact the reporter before contacting the family. At some point, when more of a relationship has been formed, MBP education and/or information (written or verbal) can be offered to the child protective agency. Depending on the circumstances, this offer may range from helping coordinate a workshop about MBP to the sharing of pertinent books and journal articles. Reporters should reinforce how potentially dangerous all suspected MBP cases are. The suspicion-report receiver can be asked to include these concerns in the suspicion report.

6. *If a first report of MBP suspicion is made to a law enforcement agency, the reporter should not assume that the report will be forwarded automatically to CPS even if this is supposed to be local procedure.* It is far better for the reporter to make a separate CPS report that includes the information that law enforcement has already been notified.

7. *A reporter who is a professional should ask to be contacted as soon as the case is assigned, to provide further information.* The reporter's assistance may be necessary in coordinating the initial multiagency-multidisciplinary team. If not contacted within an appropriate length of time, it is vital that the reporter follow up.

Suggestions for Suspicion-Report Receivers

Suggestions for suspicion-report receivers include the following:

- Allow enough time to take the report.
- Be cautious; clarify what the reporter means.
- Take reports seriously, regardless of context.
- Give MBP cases highest priority.
- If the report is anonymous, explain how this may hamper the investigation. Try to arrange a call-back time.
- Complete reports promptly, accurately, legibly, and thoroughly.

1. *Personnel receiving reports should also allow sufficient time to understand the situation.* Some agencies are known to place time limits on initial reporting conversations, which can result in an incomplete report. Such policies, which may be meant to encourage efficiency, actually work against it. If suspicion-report receivers find themselves getting confused or missing pieces of the information, clarification should be requested.

2. *Personnel receiving reports that allege MBP suspicion should make sure they understand what the reporter means.* There is still confusion about terminology. If the reporter uses terminology such as "Munchausen by proxy," "Munchausen," "MBP," etc., the intake worker should ask what is meant by the term. It is also helpful to ask nonprofessional reporters where they learned the term. This can be done respectfully: "I've found that people use this term in different ways. Can you tell me what it means to you?" or, "Can you describe exactly what is going on?" The MBP-related qualifications of the reporter or other person who originally used the term should also be probed.

3. *Reports of MBP suspicion should be taken seriously regardless of other circumstances that may be occurring.* For example, a report should not be automatically discounted because: a divorce or custody dispute is in progress; the reporter is involved in a disagreement with the alleged perpetrator; previous reports have been made and discounted; or for other reasons that do not speak directly to the occurrence or nonoccurrence of the specific alleged behavior.

4. *Suspected or confirmed MBP cases should be treated with the highest priority.* The high death and injury rate associated with MBP, the cleverness of perpetrators, and the risk of flight (Mercer and Perdue, 1993), all previously discussed, suggest that this is necessary.

5. *Sometimes nonprofessionals, such as friends or relatives of the suspected perpetrator, wish to make an anonymous report.* They have this right, but exercising it means that the agency cannot call them back for clarification or further information. The person receiving the report should explain to the reporter how important follow-up information can be. If the reporter still wishes to remain anonymous, perhaps a time can be set when the reporter will be willing to call back to talk to the person receiving the report, or to the assigned investigator, in case additional information or clarification is needed.

6. *Paperwork relating to the report should be completed promptly, accurately, legibly, and thoroughly.* Decisions will be based on information contained in the written summary. A supervisor or other person will usually assign cases to investigators based on written material received. In turn, investigators base their initial activity on the written material they receive. If information is incomplete or unclear, the suspicion-report receiver should ensure follow-up to obtain what is needed. Although this may lengthen the time before case assign-

ment, time will be saved in the long run and the chances for an appropriate initial response will be increased.

CRITERIA FOR CONFIRMING/DISCONFIRMING MBP

Two questions form the basic criteria for confirming or disconfirming MBP maltreatment. From the suspicion-report onward, efforts should be directed toward a definitive answer to these questions.

1. Does proof exist, through direct and/or circumstantial evidence, that the suspected perpetrator has deliberately exaggerated and/or fabricated and/or induced a problem or problems in another (MBP-like behavior)?
2. Does the behavior constitute MBP maltreatment or something else?

Each of these criteria is important. The first criterion addresses whether there are facts to back up suspicions, and asks whether it can be proved that a specific person has engaged in *deliberate* behavior. It also speaks to the nature of that behavior in terms that are familiar from the definition of MBP: exaggeration, fabrication, induction, or a combination. Criterion 2 is also vital for a confirmation or disconfirmation of MBP. It asks whether the "MBP-like behavior" identified in Question 1 constitutes MBP maltreatment. An easy example would be that a parent might have exaggerated a child's symptoms on a single occasion, but did so for the purpose of obtaining an earlier appointment time or justifying to an insurance company payment for an emergency room visit. Neither of these situations by itself, although involving "MBP-like behavior," would justify a confirmation of MBP.

If MBP maltreatment is suspected, a specialized investigation and confirmation process should be used. If MBP is confirmed, legal activities, case planning, and case management appropriate to MBP maltreatment should be implemented.

Box 5.1 provides a list of "Questions for Suspected and Confirmed MBP Cases" that will be important during the investigative phase and through the legal process, should the case go to court. Use of these questions should begin as soon as MBP is suspected as a possibility. Obtaining the answers will occur during the investigation and confirmation/disconfirmation process, and answers may be updated through the life of the case. However, report receivers should have a sense of what information may be important, and should try to obtain as much information as they can.

Since the suspicion-report receiver's role is not to investigate, documentation should reflect that the information has not been validated. In MBP cases, no one's word should be taken at face value until it is confirmed. For this reason, a good deal of information needs to be obtained—if possible—about the person making the report and about anyone who has contributed to a conclusion that MBP is occurring. The questions are equally useable in situations in which an MMT will already have met and extensive documentation is available, and in situations in which a concerned friend or relative is voicing suspicions for the first time. The extent to which individual questions are pursued, and the way in which they are asked will, of course, differ with each situation. These questions are intended as guidelines, with the exact wording dictated by the principles of good interviewing and the persons involved in the conversation.

Information About the Person Making the Report

Suspicion-report receivers must understand the context in which the report is made. What are the reporter's position, credentials, and reason for involvement? What has been the reporter's role in the case and what is his or her continuing role? For example, will the reporter serve as reporting agency coordinator? How and where can the reporter be reached if more information, clarification, or assistance are needed? (Complete name, title, agency, telephone number, e-mail, fax, mailing address.) Who can be contacted if the reporter is not available, and how can they be contacted (same information needed)? Although it would seem more important to start with the situation, this credibility-building information may determine whether the investigator receiving the report listens to what is said, and to what extent the investigator is able to follow up.

Date

Information may develop rapidly in an MBP case. It may also be useful to compare what was said at one point with what was said at another. Making sure that reports and other documents are dated ensures clarity about how current material is.

Is Anyone Stating That MBP Has Been Confirmed or Disconfirmed?

In some cases, the reporter will state that MBP has already been confirmed. Regardless of how credible the reporter may seem, or what the reporter's credentials are, unless the complete investigation and confirmation/disconfirmation process have occurred, at best the current status should indicate a "provisional" confirmation. For example, there may be direct evidence that a mother has suffocated or poisoned her child. Although this fulfills criterion 1—proof of MBP-like behavior, it does not necessarily mean that the behavior constitutes MBP maltreatment.

In some cases, someone may be expressing a belief that MBP is occurring, or may have discovered a perpetrator in the act of perpetrating MBP-like behavior. Such a process, of course, builds credibility for the report, but the report receiver should listen just as carefully to situations in which this kind of behavior *has not* occurred. There may also be people involved in the case who believe that MBP has been "ruled out." It is important to know "who is saying what," on what basis, how this conclusion was reached, how well it is documented, and how those involved can be contacted for further information.

First Suspicions

After obtaining information about the suspicion reporter and any conclusions that have been drawn, the suspicion-report receiver then turns attention to the details of what happened. It may be necessary to help the reporter tell the story in a coherent fashion. Begin at the beginning. It will probably be necessary to ask additional "probe" questions: What specific behaviors are alleged that have caused MBP suspicion or confirmation? Why are they harmful to the child?

The Current Situation and Events Leading to It

In this section of the interview, the suspicion-report receiver will seek information on what has happened since the first suspicions. It is particularly important to inquire about the immediate situation. Where is the suspected victim? Is the child thought to be in immediate danger? Why or why not? What about other children who may come under the control or influence of the suspected perpetrator?

A full history of the problem that may have been exaggerated, fabricated, or induced will also help the investigation. This includes areas such as:

- Where has the child previously lived, and with whom?
- Where else has the child been hospitalized or treated previously by physical or mental health care practitioners?
- Has the perpetrator had previous children who are dead or who are no longer living with the family? What is known about them?
- Has the perpetrator had other spouses or partners?
- Are there relatives or friends who are particularly close to the perpetrator or family? What is known about them? Where do they reside?

The report receiver should also find out if there is any chance that the perpetrator knows about the suspicions or the report. For example, has anyone talked with the child, suspected perpetrator, family members, or others about the concerns? Has anyone threatened to report the perpetrator? How can those persons be contacted? In what context were these conversations held? These types of conversations should *not* be held at this stage of the case, since this may be dangerous to the child and to the case process. For example, the suspected perpetrator could become aware of the suspicions and flee. However, if conversations have already been held, the agency should know about them and evaluate them in case action is necessary.

Disconfirmation

Throughout both sections 5 and 6 of the questions (Box 5.1), the suspicion-report receiver should think critically and ask about other possibilities. The reporter may be wrong, even if acting from sincere motives. The reporter may also be presenting only one side of a controversial situation. Even if the report is completely accurate, the agency needs to know if another individual or group has reached a different conclusion or claims that they have "proof" that MBP has not occurred. Such claims must be evaluated fairly during the investigative process. Frequently, advocacy groups that do not "believe" in MBP become a significant force in court proceedings. If it is already known that this may occur, the agency receiving the report should know about it from the time of reporting.

It is a good practice to bring the conversation to an end with several general, open-ended questions. For example, the suspicion-report receiver can ask:

- What other information is available?
- What other information is pertinent to an understanding of this case?
- Where might other information or clues to information be found?
- Are there any important things that you have not yet told me?

INITIAL CHILD PROTECTIVE AGENCY RESPONSE TO A REPORT OF MBP SUSPICIONS

The following principles should guide the agency's overall response:

- Take reports seriously.
- Assign appropriate staff.
- Consider case as high risk; determine need for victim protection.
- Do *not* contact the suspected perpetrator, victim, or family as the first response.

1. *Child protective and law enforcement agency staff should take reports of MBP suspicion seriously.* For that to happen, staff must be educated correctly regarding MBP basics. Staff who do not understand MBP basics are likely to dismiss reports, fail to assign them proper priority, make inappropriate decisions, or even fail to identify the described suspicious behavior as possible MBP. Sometimes a reporter may appear to have a vested interest in making the report. Divorce, custody disputes, and other domestic problems should not be

the basis for dismissing a report or ruling out the possibility of child maltreatment. MBP behavior can occur within or be triggered by those contexts.

2. *MBP investigations should be assigned to appropriate staff.* Few investigative professionals or their supervisors have received correct and up-to-date MBP training. Fewer still have experience with MBP cases. Because an MBP investigation and confirmation/disconfirmation process is so different from other kinds of maltreatment investigations in terms of investigative activities and decision making, and because it is so time-consuming and complex, the investigator should be chosen carefully. The assigned worker should, if possible, be a person who enjoys complicated investigations, can master details, and is a team player. The investigator must receive current and correct basic MBP education and be willing to learn. Appropriate adjustments should be made in the investigator's workload to allow sufficient time for the MBP investigation.

Staff members who are known to have MBP knowledge or experience should be considered, but not necessarily chosen. They may not have the temperament for this kind of case, may be burned-out, or may not have had complete or correct MBP information. If a staff member is assigned who has MBP knowledge or experience, that person should receive update information. In many situations, incorrect information about MBP has been used in case after case, resulting in inappropriate investigations and conclusions.

3. *The case should be considered high risk.* Child protective response always depends on the degree of perceived risk to the child. No matter how harmless a suspected MBP case appears at the time of reporting, it should be considered extremely high risk. The situation may not be as benign as it initially appears. At the time of intake and assignment, much information is still unknown. Some information in the report may be incorrect. All may not be as it seems. Because of the high death rate associated with MBP, every suspected victim should be considered a potential fatality, regardless of how the initial presentation is perceived. As in any case of maltreatment, victim protection should be the priority. Some cases will require immediate action to obtain protection, while others may not, or there may not be enough information yet available to justify immediate protection.

4. *The agency receiving a report should not contact the suspected perpetrator, victim, or family as their first response to a possible*

MBP case. The convening of the MMT should be the initial investigative activity. As already discussed, it is the usual policy for CPS investigators initiating an investigation after case assignment to contact the suspected perpetrator and family. Generally, agency policy specifies the number of days within which this contact must occur. In suspected MBP cases, following this policy will significantly heighten victim risk. If perpetrators become aware that they are suspected, two responses are common. First, they may escalate the MBP perpetration in an attempt to "prove" that the child does, indeed, have naturally occurring symptoms. Second, they may leave the area.

Every precaution must be taken to keep the suspected perpetrator from finding out that a report has been made or that suspicion exists. Contact with the perpetrator, family, friends, and others who might "tip off" the perpetrator should not be made until the safety of the child is assured. Child protection, law enforcement, and other agencies should review their policies and procedures and make any necessary revisions to ensure that MBP is exempted from the normal initial contact requirement, or that other substitute actions (e.g., convening of the MMT) satisfy policy requirements.

Chapter 6

Gathering Information:
The MBP Investigation

The MBP investigation and confirmation/disconfirmation process begins when a report of MBP suspicion is received and ends when a decision has been made about the existence or nonexistence of MBP. It consists of four major activities that overlap and interweave:

- information gathering,
- information evaluation,
- information organization, and
- the MBP confirmation/disconfirmation decision.

Information gathering is discussed in this chapter. The other activities are discussed in Chapter 7.

The two purposes of any child maltreatment investigation are to (1) determine whether maltreatment has or has not taken place and, if it has, (2) to lay the foundation for a court case that will have the best chance of yielding desired results. If maltreatment has taken place, there are two major types of desired results that may be sought, depending on the situation. These are protection for the child and punishment for the perpetrator. One or both of these may be pursued.

When the focus is on protection for the child, the case is heard in a child protection court. The name of this court varies by jurisdiction. It may be "juvenile court," "family court," etc. Whatever it is called, the desired results are a finding of maltreatment, and a court order for an appropriate case plan and related case management activities. When MBP has been confirmed as part of the maltreatment, an extremely important goal is for the judge to determine explicitly that MBP maltreatment has occurred, and to order an MBP-specific case plan and MBP-specific case management activities (see Chapters 9, 10, and 11). Without a specific finding by the child protective court that MBP has occurred, it is difficult to justify these MBP-specific elements.

When the focus is on punishment of the perpetrator, the case is heard in criminal court. The goals are a finding that the perpetrator is guilty of the charges, and an appropriate sentence.

Child maltreatment investigation is a specialized professional activity. Not all professionals, even in law enforcement and CPS, are well grounded in sound investigative activities and techniques. Investigation is not the same as clinical assessment. Well-trained investigators have specialized knowledge, skills, and sources of information. For example, they are familiar (as health care or social services professionals may not be) with reluctant or potentially deceptive witnesses, with chain-of-evidence procedures, and with gathering legally sound evidence for use in court. Professionals from other fields should not assume that their knowledge or skills are the same as those of professional investigators. Without meaning to do so, professionals who do not have sound investigative knowledge and skills may jeopardize the case. Protection of a potentially victimized child should take precedence over pride or professional rivalries.

MBP maltreatment investigations require even more specialized competencies than other maltreatment investigations. In addition to knowledge about MBP, these investigations require the skills to engage in activities such as interviewing and evaluating information from an MBP perspective. They also require the ability to understand and evaluate information about physical and mental health conditions/problems. False accusations and failure to confirm maltreatment are more likely when people without MBP knowledge and skills conduct the MBP investigation and confirmation/disconfirmation process.

Non-MBP child maltreatment investigations are planned and carried out much differently from those in which MBP is or comes to be suspected. If MBP is subsequently suspected in a case being investigated for another reason, the investigation needs to be replanned. Additional information needs to be gathered, additional individuals need to be interviewed and others reinterviewed. All information, old and new, must be reevaluated in light of the MBP suspicion.

The MBP definition presented in Chapter 1 is the foundation of the MBP investigation and confirmation/disconfirmation process.

> Munchausen by proxy is a dangerous form of maltreatment (abuse and/or neglect) in which caretakers deliberately and repeatedly exaggerate and/or fabricate and/or induce physical and/or psychological/behavioral symptoms and/or illness in others. The primary purpose of this behavior appears to be the gaining of some form of intangible gratification, such as attention, for the perpetrator.

As discussed in Chapter 5, there are two criteria for the confirmation of MBP:

1. Does proof exist, through direct and/or circumstantial evidence, that the suspected perpetrator has deliberately exaggerated and/or fabricated and/or induced a problem or problems in another (MBP-like behavior)?
2. Does the behavior constitute MBP maltreatment, or something else?

Throughout the investigation, involved professionals must focus on whether there is direct and/or circumstantial evidence that:

1. The suspected perpetrator has deliberately exaggerated and/or fabricated and/or induced physical and/or psychological problems in the suspected victim.
2. The primary purpose appears to be the attempt to fulfill an internal emotional need.

Answering these questions will require the gathering of considerable information. Even if the suspicion report indicates belief that MBP has been confirmed or that a perpetrator has been caught in the midst of induction, unless a thorough, correct investigation and confirmation/disconfirmation process has been accomplished this confirmation should be considered provisional until a full investigation is completed.

The "Questions for Suspected and Confirmed MBP Cases," introduced in Chapter 5 as Box 5.1, should be answered during the investigation. The purpose of these questions is to obtain information that can be used to address the criteria. The specific questions are, as already stated, only a general outline that will need to be modified for each case. They will usually need to be followed up with much more detailed information. Most of these questions should also be supplemented by the additional questions: "How do we know?" "What information do we have that may refute this information?" and "What additional information do we need to be sure?"

At its most basic, investigation is a research process. That is, an investigation involves some combination of observation, interviewing, collection of written records, activities unique to the particular kind of investigation, and appropriate evaluation of all information to arrive at a conclusion. MBP investigations typically require the gathering of extensive information from various sources. This includes information about the suspected/confirmed victim(s), suspected/confirmed perpetrator(s), other children presently or formerly in the suspected/confirmed perpetrator's (perpetrators') home, and sometimes others. Information must be gathered from all jurisdictions in which it is known or suspected that these individuals have lived. In identifying potential information sources, it is important to continually remember the MBP definition and perpetrator-consistent characteristics. Participants in the investigation should ask themselves, "Where else and from whom else might information be found that will help in confirming or disconfirming MBP?" Information must also be followed up if it might lead to the discovery that MBP maltreatment has *not* been perpetrated. For example, if the caregiver alleges that the child has a rare disease, information about this disease and whether the child has been adequately evaluated for it must be obtained. At all times, the goal of the investigation should be to find out the truth, not to prove a predetermined suspicion.

In suspected MBP cases, the information needed is very detailed. In the beginning of the investigation and confirmation/disconfirmation process, it is impossible to predict what will be important, and much information may be found in apparently inconsequential details. For example, in one case a nurse's note stating "mother said a sibling [of the suspected victim] died several years ago" led to the discovery that that baby had died as a result of the same problems as the current suspected victim.

Two major sources of information in the MBP investigation and confirmation/disconfirmation process will not be discussed in this chapter, as they are covered in other chapters. The initial suspicion report, discussed in Chapter 5, sets the stage for everything that will follow. Great care should be taken in ensuring that as much information as possible is obtained during the reporting conversation. Discussion of the initial MMT meeting, including a suggested agenda, appears in Chapter 7. As a result of each professional's sharing and comparing their experiences, significant information is obtained.

Written records, documents, interviews, and other methods are additional important sources of information. These will be discussed in this chapter.

WRITTEN RECORDS AND DOCUMENTS

The MBP investigation and confirmation/disconfirmation process requires that complete written records be obtained from a variety of sources. As already mentioned, not only should the suspected victim(s)' complete records be gathered, but also complete records of other children presently or formerly in the home of the suspected perpetrator(s). "Complete" records means from conception on, and means full records, not summaries. It means records relating to multiple areas of the children's lives, for example, school records even though the presenting problem may be medical. Records as far back as possible should also be obtained for the perpetrator(s) and sometimes others. Careful analysis of records that have accumulated over time often reveals patterns of deception or falsification throughout the suspected perpetrator's life, not just in association with the suspected victim(s)'s problems or alleged problems. Associations between the perpetrator's presence and the victim's problems or alleged problems, verification that purported "problems" do not exist, and other indicators that MBP is occurring or has occurred are especially important. Records can also reveal and help identify the harm suffered by the victim, numbers of hospitalizations or procedures, medications prescribed unnecessarily, days of school missed, and so on. Potential victim harm can also be identified.

Information in records often overlaps. For example, a record listed in a child's name may also contain information about parents, siblings, relatives, and others—and vice versa. As records are put together, a picture of the family (nuclear and extended) and situation grows. This picture may include alleged health problems, past suspicions/confirmations of MBP and/or factitious disorder/Munchausen syndrome, perpetrator-consistent characteristics, situational suspicion indicators, discrepancies and inconsistencies in information, past and present involved agencies and professionals, reported family history, and other potentially vital information. In some situations, records reveal a provable pattern consistent with MBP maltreatment that can justify the confirmation or provisional confirmation of MBP by or with the assistance of a credible MBP expert.

Records should be obtained directly from the original source to avoid the possibility of tampering. Examine records carefully when they are received, as they are often incomplete. Health care and other records may not include "face" or "cover sheets," information kept in other than the main record, "special records," etc. Often agencies send only summaries or portions that they believe are pertinent. Without complete records, critical information is likely to be missed.

Records will ordinarily not be supplied without legal authorization, usually a release of information signed by the person whose records are being requested or his or her legal custodian, a subpoena, or a court order. Until the child is safe, everything possible should be done to keep suspected perpetrators (or anyone who might tell them), from finding out about the suspicions. When a child comes into the custody of a child protection agency, the agency usually has the right to access information about the child, including records. The extent of this right varies by jurisdiction. If the child protective agency does not have the right to obtain needed records on its own authority, it may ask adults, such as the parents/custodians, to sign releases of information voluntarily. However, these requests may be denied. Then CPS must request that the court subpoena or order the release of the needed records.

Judges or other involved officials will probably not understand what MBP is and why the requested records are critical to MBP confirmation or disconfirmation. Such extensive records are not usually necessary in other kinds of child maltreatment investigations. To obtain the needed information, it will probably be necessary for an MBP expert consultant to provide education through testimony, reports, or affidavits.

Release-of-information forms are usually not as detailed as is necessary in MBP cases. Generally, the release-of-information form does not allow for personal contacts and conversations in addition to exchange of written material. A sample of a recommended, more complete, release-of-information form is shown in Box 6.1. Language from this sample form could also added to an existing form or used in a subpoena or motion for a court order.

Examples (not to be considered a complete list) of record sources that should be considered regarding individuals discussed earlier, and others as appropriate include:

- Hospitals (inpatient, outpatient) "clinic" and emergency departments
- Mental health facilities (inpatient and outpatient)
- Physicians, including psychiatrists and medical examiners
- Psychologists (including those associated with schools and health care facilities)
- Nurse practitioners and physician's assistants
- Pharmacies
- Disease-specific agencies and organizations (e.g., Easter Seals, March of Dimes, wish-granting agencies, etc.)
- Public health departments and public health/home care "visiting" nurses
- Emergency responders (911) ambulance/emergency organizations, fire departments, etc.
- Other nonphysician medical, mental health, pharmaceutical professionals, and facilities
- Law enforcement agencies
- Public and private educational programs (including day care, Head Start, preschools, elementary schools, middle/junior high schools, colleges, universities, and trade/vocational/adult educational schools)
- State and county child welfare agencies (child protective services, foster care, adoptions, etc.)
- State and county public assistance ("welfare") agencies including food stamps, financial benefits, Medicaid, training programs, parenting programs
- Federal programs such as Supplemental Security Income (SSI, which includes disabled children)
- Other social services agencies such as Women, Infants, and Children (WIC) supplemental food program, home visitor pro-

grams for infants, employment services, counseling agencies, adoption agencies, etc.
- Health and other insurance carriers (public and private). Insurance "runs" should be requested to obtain information about what care has been provided, where, and by whom
- Court records and transcripts
- Places of past and present employment
- Military facilities, including services and providers located there
- State and county vital records offices (for birth, death, and marriage certificates)
- Department of Motor Vehicles
- Voter registration records
- Libraries, especially medical libraries or collections

INTERVIEWS

Interviews have two major purposes. First, they are a source of new information. Second, they may clarify, augment, corroborate, or identify discrepancies in information already obtained. Individuals who have already been interviewed for other reasons than an MBP investigation must be reinterviewed from the MBP perspective. It may be necessary to interview people more than once during the MBP investigation and confirmation/disconfirmation process.

When MBP suspicion is reported or significant MBP-related events occur, a skilled investigative interviewer who has a solid understanding of MBP maltreatment and MBP perpetrator characteristics should go immediately to the scene (e.g., hospital, clinician's office, school, etc.) to personally assess the situation, obtain information, and take statements from involved professionals and staff while they are available and events are fresh in their minds. This person should also work with planning and coordinating other initial activities such as the initial MMT meeting and/or emergency meeting of available, involved professionals if there is no time to gather those to be included in the MMT. If the assigned investigator is inexperienced in MBP, an MBP expert consultant should participate directly and/or provide consultation. Remember that MBP perpetrators should be considered even more dangerous if/when they learn that they are suspected. Until the

BOX 6.1.
Authority to Release/Divulge Records
and Information

To: _____
_____
_____

Re: Full Name   Other Possible Names   Birth Date

_____
_____

You are hereby authorized and requested to release records and other written information and divulge information through personal contact and conversations to:

_____

This includes all information related to physical health, mental health, education, employment, social/family situation, or other information related to the above individuals. It should include ALL and COMPLETE records and information such as primary care records, consultations, nursing notes, social work/social services notes, initial and subsequent histories, face sheets, or other care provided, anything related to or impacting diagnoses, recommendations, treatment, or decision making. Professionals involved in the case are authorized to discuss this situation with others as necessary to investigation and case management activities.

The foregoing authority shall continue in force until revoked by me in writing. A copy of this authority shall carry the full force and effect of the original.

Signature: _____

Printed name: _____

Date: _____

victim and other potential victims are safe, nothing should be done that could tip off the suspected perpetrator.

Interviews must be planned carefully, even when the investigator is responding immediately to a report. Interviews should be conducted in person so that the investigator can observe body language and other nonverbal cues. Only as a last resort should they take place via telephone. Hold initial interviews with individuals by themselves. Family or group interviews are inappropriate as an initial investigative activity.

Careful consideration should be given to the time and place for the interview. Interview strategy must be planned so that those interviewed do not have a chance to compare stories or share what happened during their interviews. Nor should the interview be held in a place where others are likely to interrupt or try to become involved in the conversation.

Some people believe that it is advantageous to audiotape or videotape interviews. They argue that this will not only allow review of the information obtained, but may help answer later criticisms that the interviewer coerced, led, or misinterpreted the interviewee. Given the strong positions taken by many who do not believe that MBP occurs, as well as recent controversies over testimony by both children and adults in child sexual abuse cases, a video of a well-conducted, neutral interview may later prove very useful. However, taping may also allow specific attacks on interviewing methods should the case go to court. The local situation and interviewer preferences should be taken into account as this decision is made.

Audiotapes and videotapes should be transcribed promptly. Written documentation should be completed quickly after the interview to minimize the chance of forgetting or confusion with other data sources. Transcribers should be careful to include an accurate summary and exact quotations that appear significant. Interviewers testifying in court may be accused of misinterpreting what was said. The interviewer should review the main points at the end of the interview, ask if the subject has understood, and document the answer by having the subject sign and initial the documentation if possible. Written and other documentation such as tapes should be made a part of the official investigative file and kept in a place where tampering is not possible.

Who Should Be Interviewed

Anyone with potential information about the nuclear or extended family should be interviewed. This often includes the following:

1. Suspected/confirmed perpetrator(s), but only after victim safety is assured.
2. Suspected/confirmed victim(s), if old enough, but only after their safety has been assured. Some victims have said later that they had information to give but were never asked.
3. Suspected perpetrator's spouse/significant other(s), past and present, including child's father.
4. Day care or school staff.
5. Other individuals presently or formerly living or working in the home.
6. Present or former relatives, friends, neighbors.
7. Professionals or other staff mentioned in records or involved in producing records. (Such individuals often have much more information than they documented.)
8. Professionals or other staff not mentioned in records, but known to have had contact with the family.
9. Individuals who supposedly witnessed the alleged symptoms/ illness/behavior or relevant events.

Methods for Interviewing

Good investigative procedure dictates that initial interviews are conducted with the interviewee alone. This prevents one person from inhibiting or influencing the responses of others, and also prevents a unified front in which all participants tell the same story. When interviews have been done separately, the information obtained can be compared and discrepancies discovered. For example, if both parents are interviewed together (father is the suspected perpetrator and mother is not), the father's presence and power or the mother's loyalty may coerce the mother into agreeing that she has seen signs of genuine problems. Mother may deny that father has ever been alone with the child when the problems began. It is far more likely that the truth will emerge if each is interviewed by himself or herself.

Begin the interview with open-ended questions. These are questions that cannot be answered with "yes" or "no," or with a single fact such as a date. The open-ended question should be neutral, to avoid later assertions of bias. A good opening question is, "What do you think about (victim or perpetrator's) situation?" The answer will give the interviewer a good indication of what subjects understand about what has happened and what they know—or think they know. Another good open-ended question is, "I don't know much about (suspected perpetrator/spouse/victim/etc.). How would you describe what he or she is like?" This question will assist the investigator in obtaining a picture of the person in question. It will also assist in determining whether or not perpetrator-consistent characteristics may be present. Detailed examples should be requested: "Can you tell me about a time that she seemed to crave a lot of attention [repeating words used by the interviewee]?" "Can you give me examples of him or her 'lying'?" Questions such as these also help the interviewer to evaluate the reliability of the information that is being provided.

Information obtained about the suspected perpetrator can be compared with the list of MBP perpetrator-consistent characteristics. Information about the victim and siblings can be compared with the normal expectations for children of a given age. It is amazing how much information is revealed by answers to initial questions like these, and by body language. Particular attention should be given to the interviewee's spontaneous comments.

Later in the interview, open-ended questions can give way to more direct inquiries. These should not be limited to information about the suspected victim(s) and perpetrator(s). Information should be sought regarding others presently or formerly in the home, relatives, and others as relevant. This may reveal other potential sources of information, other possible victims, or even multigenerational MBP. Typical and useful questions include (but are certainly not limited to) those shown in Boxes 6.2 and 6.3. The questions in Box 6.2 are more likely to be useful with nonprofessionals, while those in Box 6.3 are more likely to be useful with professionals. Note that most are worded in a neutral way. Specific information is being sought, but the respondent is not being "led." The goal is to find out the truth, so information that disconfirms MBP is as important as information that confirms it. Until the investigation and confirmation/disconfirmation process is com-

BOX 6.2.
Some Suggested Questions
for MBP Investigation Interviews
(Use As Appropriate)

- How long have you known _____ (the suspected perpetrator, child, family member, etc.)?
- What was she or he like growing up?
- What is she or he interested in?
- What does she or he like to talk about?
- Why do you describe her or him that way? Can you give some examples?
- What kinds of problems has she or he had? How do you know?
- Has the child (have the children) ever had any problems? What kinds of problems? How do you know?
- Were you ever present when there was a problem? Tell me about it.
- What was done about the problem? By whom? How do you know? Tell me about it.
- Has anyone else in the family had problems? How do you know? Tell me about it.
- Who else is involved with the family? Who has been involved in the past?
- Who else is living in the home? Who has lived there in the past?
- Who else has taken care of the child(ren)?
- Are any agencies or organizations currently helping the family? Have any helped in the past?
- Can you think of anyone else who might be able to talk to me about the family?
- Does (suspected perpetrator) have any other children? Where are they? What is going on in their lives? Did they have any problems?
- Where else has the family lived?
- What day care providers or schools have family members attended?
- Have you ever been concerned about any family members or what was going on with the family? Why?

BOX 6.3.
Some Suggested Questions for MBP Investigation
Interviews with Professionals
(Use As Appropriate)

- What can you tell me about _____ (the kind of problem[s] the victim is supposed to have)? For each problem:

  How frequently have you worked with this problem? Do you have special expertise in this field?
  How does it usually present ("show up")?
  How common is it (overall); how common in a person of this age?
  How is it usually evaluated and diagnosed? Is there any test that can tell conclusively whether it is present?
  How is it usually treated?
  How has it been treated in this case? What have been the results of treatment?
  How dangerous is this condition?
  What is its usual outcome; how do most people respond to treatment?
  What are the common side effects of treatment?
  What other conditions can look similar to this problem?
  How dangerous are other conditions that look similar to this one?
  How frequently do people with this problem have emergencies/ need to call the ambulance/need to come to the hospital or emergency room, etc.?

- In this case, how much have you depended on reports from other persons? Who, and what did they say?
- What conditions have been included in the differential diagnosis (list of possible diagnoses) in this case? Have they been eliminated as possibilities? How was that done?
- Have problems in the environment (e.g., allergies, pollution, radon, other toxins and sensitivities, etc.) been considered as possibilities? Have they been ruled in or out? How?
- Are there any things about the problem in this situation that have puzzled you, or that seem different from the usual presentation of this problem?

pleted, conclusions should not be drawn and investigators should be wary about finding only what they expect to find.

Interview anyone who has reportedly seen the alleged problem or witnessed any medical or psychological/behavioral events. A primary concern is determining whether the witness was present at the onset of the alleged event. The following example shows how such a critical topic might be addressed. It also illustrates how the interviewer's expression and relationship-building techniques can be used to help the interviewee open up and recall specific details of an emotionally charged situation. When interviewing, the way questions are asked is often as important as the questions themselves.

Case 6.1

Cynthia Butler is suspected of having caused cyanosis—turning blue from lack of oxygen—in Jerry, a cousin for whom she babysits. She says that her uncle, Matt Robinson, witnessed one of Jerry's cyanotic episodes when he was visiting. The investigator conducted the interview alone with Mr. Robinson. After a brief "warm-up period" to build rapport, part of the interview might progress as follows:

INVESTIGATOR: Mr. Robinson, has anyone in the family ever had problems?

MR. ROBINSON: Oh yes, especially Jerry.

INVESTIGATOR: What kind of problems has Jerry had?

MR. ROBINSON: Oh, he turns blue all the time and can't breathe right.

INVESTIGATOR: How do you know that?

MR. ROBINSON: Well, Cindy told me about it lots of times.

INVESTIGATOR: Were you ever around when Jerry had a problem? [Investigator gives only as much information as necessary to ask the question.]

MR. ROBINSON: Yes, I was over at Cindy's house. It was just awful. I was scared to death. He turned blue and was having a bad time breathing.

INVESTIGATOR [very concerned and sympathetic]: That must have been frightening! Tell me what happened. [Mr. Robinson describes Jerry as pale and limp and gasping.]

INVESTIGATOR [puzzled]: How do you know that was cyanosis?

MR. ROBINSON: Well, Cindy told me to call the ambulance because he was having a cyanosis again. She knows all about things like that.

INVESTIGATOR [leaning forward, showing concern]: When did you first realize Jerry was having problems? [This question is asked very quickly as a technique to cause Mr. Robinson to answer quickly.]

MR. ROBINSON: Cindy came through his bedroom door with him and he was just lying in her arms. She yelled for me to call 911, and I just ran for the phone.

INVESTIGATOR: Have you ever seen anything like that in your life before?

MR. ROBINSON: No, and I hope I never do again. Cindy and I thought we had lost him.

From this interview, the investigator has learned that Mr. Robinson did not see the alleged cyanosis begin, and that Mr. Robinson thinks Jerry had cyanosis because Cynthia, the suspected perpetrator, told him it was cyanosis. The investigator has also learned that Mr. Robinson believes Cynthia has some kind of medical knowledge and will, at some point, want to find out more about this. For example, where did she get her knowledge? How does he know this?

As the investigator continues to focus on the alleged event in this case, appropriate questions include:

- What happened next?
- What did your niece do?
- How long had you been there before this problem started? What did you see and hear before the problem started?
- What was Cynthia doing in the bedroom with Jerry? How do you know?
- How long was she there before she came through the bedroom door with Jerry in her arms?
- Can you show me what he looked like when he was limp? Where did he look pale? Where did he look blue?
- What happened when the ambulance personnel arrived? What did Jerry look like then, and what did they say and do?
- How long afterward did you stay? What happened during that time?
- Who else was there before, during, or just after all this happened?
- What did Cynthia say about it? What did Jerry's parents say about it?
- Has anything like this ever happened to Jerry or Cynthia before? How do you know?

After asking questions about the specific event apparently witnessed by Mr. Robinson, the investigator should ask other open-ended and direct questions as already discussed, as well as questions suggested by the investigation so far. For example, the perpetrator may have stated that cyanosis "runs in Jerry's family." The investigator should ask Mr. Robinson what he meant when he indicated there were other problems in the family, what they are, how he knows, etc. (Note that the investigator did not ask whether cyanosis runs in the family. This would be a leading question, and might also limit the information that, potentially, Mr. Robinson could provide.) Alternatively, the investigator could use a list of conditions, including cyanosis, and ask if each runs in the family. Information should also be sought or followed up upon that might suggest other explanations than MBP for what has been heard or observed.

OTHER METHODS OF INFORMATION GATHERING

Diagnostic Separation

Separation of the suspected or confirmed victim from the care, custody, control, and influence of the suspected or confirmed perpetrator is an excellent confirmation/disconfirmation tool. It must, of course, be part of an appropriate, carefully made plan. Separation can be used as an information-gathering tool before MBP confirmation, and can also be useful after confirmation to validate and strengthen the case. Although separating a child from the parent is a very serious measure, it is justified by the seriousness of the situation. Separation also ensures victim safety, allows any needed medical and mental health care to be given to the victim, and reduces the danger that a potential legal or court case will be undermined.

Diagnostic separation may be accomplished either through an inpatient facility hospitalization or foster placement, depending on the case needs. Court intervention is almost always required. Whether placement is in the hospital or a foster home, if visitation by the suspected perpetrator is allowed, it must be strictly supervised. (Planning for placement and supervising visitation are discussed further in Chapters 9 and 10.) The suspected victim must be placed in a neutral, emotionally and physically uncontaminated environment in accordance with a carefully designed monitoring and evaluation process. Placement in the home of a relative or friend must be avoided, as it cannot guarantee impartial monitoring and evaluation or protection of the child or case.

Prior to placing the victim, or immediately after, obtain a specific description from the suspected perpetrator of the child's problem(s) and usual patterns. This will help in planning the minimum length for the separation. If the separation is shorter than the usual "problem-free" interval, the suspected perpetrator may later claim that the lack of problems during placement was not significant. Careful documentation of the suspected perpetrator's information will help to clarify whether the patterns and problems are occurring as reported.

The following list shows the purpose of diagnostic separation.

1. To discover whether the alleged problems are actually present. For example, the caregiver states that the child runs fevers. Can these be documented?
2. To discover whether the alleged problems are as serious as has been claimed. For example, the caregiver has stated that the child's fevers are over 105°. If fevers occur, are they as high as has been reported?
3. To discover whether problems occur spontaneously. For example, if the high fevers have been documented, do they occur out of association with the perpetrator?
4. To discover whether problems improve in the absence of the perpetrator. For example, the child might have a high fever on admission to the hospital, but it resolves and does not recur once the perpetrator does not have access to the child.

Diagnostic separation may help to exonerate a suspected perpetrator if the problem is real. The length of time required for diagnostic separation will depend on the nature of the problem(s) reported. Physicians and/or mental health professionals (as appropriate to the condition) should be involved in formulating the suspected victim's medical and/or mental health diagnostic, monitoring, and evaluation plan. Again, do nothing that will alert a suspected perpetrator before the suspected victim is safe.

Covert Electronic Surveillance

MBP perpetrators may be "caught in the act" by audiotape or videotape. Using these methods, statements made by a perpetrator, as well as actions, may be documented and compared with other information. For example, a perpetrator may induce behavior in the victim by commenting, "You have a lot of pain now, don't you?" Perpetrators may also make remarks to others, in person or on the phone, such as reporting that the child has had symptoms or is gravely ill, when this is not the case. Physiological recordings (e.g., patterns such as heartbeat and breathing) from medical monitors may also provide indications that problems are being induced or that equipment has been tampered with.

Covert video surveillance must be planned and carried out very carefully due to legal, ethical, and practical problems. One protocol reflecting British law can be found in Southall and Samuels (1996); protocols may also be obtained from institutions that have gained experience in this area. Leadership must be provided by a professional familiar with the use of electronic recording in MBP. The MMT, MBP expert, and legal counsel should be involved in considering video surveillance and in planning for it.

As already discussed in Chapter 3, many ethical issues are associated with electronic recording. Professionals must consider whether privacy of the possible perpetrator or others will be invaded, how consent is to be obtained for this procedure, and whether the risks inherent in recording are counterbalanced by the benefits expected. Covert recording, in which the child's custodian does not know about the presence of the recorder, raises significant ethical questions. It should not be undertaken without careful consideration of the issues. Legal counsel and the administration of the institution in which it takes place should be involved in decision making regarding covert recording.

If electronic monitoring is to be undertaken, and the legal and administrative hurdles have been cleared, there are still practical considerations to be worked out. The logistics for the equipment and its placement must be determined. Generally, cameras with sound recording capability are hidden in the room occupied by the victim. This should be a private room so that the confidentiality of other patients and family members is not compromised. There are differences of opinion about the aiming of the camera. Some professionals believe that the camera should be focused only on the bed where the child/victim sleeps. This is suggested to reduce violations of privacy when the suspected perpetrator or others, for example, change clothes in the room. However, if the suspected perpetrator removes the child/victim from the bed, subsequent actions will not be visible. The suspected perpetrator might also prepare injections, draw blood, or take other actions out of view of the camera, which would provide evidence if recorded. For example, cases have been documented in which incriminating actions occurred in the bathroom. Alternatively, the camera may be focused on as much of the area as possible. This placement maximizes evidence but potentially raises more ethical issues. A means of immediate communication with medical personnel may also be used to signal the need for intervention, and this should also be tested before the video surveillance begins.

Law enforcement and audiovisual technicians should be involved in arranging and understanding the equipment. Once it is in place, there should be sufficient testing to assure that the equipment is working in the way that is desired. For example, lighting of the room should be adequate, sound levels should be adequate, and the overall function should be tried and adjusted until clear recordings are produced. Recordings should be in a format that can be readily used by those who will need to see them at other locations. Use of nonstandard equipment, or the lack of technology to easily make usable copies of the full recording, could compromise the confirmation/disconfirmation process as well as court proceedings and other legal activity. Technology problems have caused cases to be stalled for months.

A sufficient supply of tapes or other recording media should be available. Recording should be continuous, and tapes should not be reused because "nothing has happened." Full recordings will be required for the confirmation/disconfirmation process and potentially later if the case goes to court.

Appropriate staff (e.g., law enforcement, CPS, security, or health care professionals) should observe the room at all times while recording is taking place. Provision must be made for adequate staffing and for coverage during breaks. Staff must be in a position to intervene at any time if the child is in danger. In one case, a child almost died while being filmed but not observed.

Observers must be trained in MBP basics, and given detailed case information and specific instructions for monitoring and logging. Observers, or a technician who is also present, must know how to operate and troubleshoot the equipment. Observers should receive guidelines in advance about when and how they are to intervene. These should be based on the suspected victim's problems and the hypothesized method(s) used to create them. However, observers should also be prepared that the unexpected may happen, related to MBP, to genuine problems, or to something else. For example, non-

MBP physical abuse has been documented in cases being recorded for suspicion of MBP (Southall et al., 1997). The goal is to obtain definitive evidence of maltreatment, if it is occurring, without subjecting the suspected victim to serious injury. This may be difficult, and calls for a good deal of discretion on the part of the observer.

Covert electronic monitoring can be highly effective in confirming the presence of MBP-like behavior, but does not prove that the behavior constitutes MBP. Professionals should also understand that a lack of findings using electronic monitoring does not disprove MBP. All case information must be taken into account.

As useful—and dramatic—as covert monitoring can be, it is simply one technique of many. At present, the majority of genuine MBP cases appear to be confirmed through solid circumstantial evidence. All investigative "eggs" should not be put in one "basket." Other information still needs to be gathered and evaluated. Good decision making about the case and good case planning will come from the full investigative process, and not from any single technique.

Polygraphs

"Lie detectors" are controversial, and are sufficiently imprecise that courts will usually not admit their results. These machines measure physiological responses to the anxiety generally associated with deception. False results may be obtained from people who are unusually nervous, as well as from people who can lie without anxiety. Some MBP perpetrators are likely to be in the latter category. Sometimes lie detectors are used strategically as an investigative tool, particularly with witnesses or perpetrators who believe the machines to be accurate. The threat of a polygraphic examination may be used, along with other inducements, to persuade a reluctant person to speak. Such uses are situation specific and controversial.

Mental Health Evaluations

As part of an investigation, or for other reasons, mental health professionals are often asked to evaluate a suspected perpetrator through interview(s) and psychological testing "to determine the presence or absence of MBP." This is a mistake, based on the assumption that MBP is a mental disorder. No mental health test or evaluation can determine whether MBP has been perpetrated, although some findings may suggest that it is more or less likely. (That is, they may confirm or refute some suspicion indicators.) Mental health evaluations of MBP perpetrators often report "normal" results. Such findings do not mean that MBP has not occurred.

A mental health evaluation performed by a professional who has credible MBP education and experience and is part of an MBP investigation and confirmation/disconfirmation process may, however, be valuable in other ways. For example, the mental health professional may be able to elicit information that can be compared against other case information. Even if apparently cooperative, however, the suspected perpetrator may or may not be giving accurate information. Mental health evaluations can also be useful to gather additional information. They may be able to determine the presence and extent of coexisting mental illness or personal concerns, comment on the subject's capacity for empathy, need for attention, or other perpetrator-consistent characteristics. This can be very helpful to the investigation or future therapy. As has already been discussed in Chapter 1, it is not useful to consider MBP a mental illness that someone "has."

Mental health professionals may be able to answer questions about the implications of mental illness or psychological damage in both perpetrators and victims. They can assist the team on a collegial basis if there are unresolved interpersonal issues, or if questions arise about mental health reports. They cannot say whether the suspected perpetrator is the "kind of person" who would perpetrate MBP.

Additional Information

As the investigation proceeds, information will be obtained that adds to the context of the situation. This information may support suspicions of MBP, or it may suggest additional possibilities and lines of inquiry. All such information should be noted and followed up as thoroughly as possible.

Chapter 7

Information Evaluation, Information Organization, and the Confirmation/Disconfirmation Decision

INFORMATION EVALUATION

Decisions will be made based on information that has been gathered, so it must be reviewed for completeness and evaluated for quality and relevance. The four major criteria for evaluating information are:

- Is it credible? Why or why not?
- Is it useful for confirming/disconfirming MBP? Why or why not?
- Is it useful for other case activities or decisions? Why or why not?
- If necessary, can it be used in court? Why or why not?

Each time questions are asked and data are reviewed, an additional question should be asked: Why or why not? This question is very useful in focusing on further tasks to be accomplished and on the justification for decisions.

The information gathered must always be considered as a whole, and especially from the standpoint of consistency. Organizing information, as discussed in the next section, will help to identify inconsistencies. If inconsistencies are found, there should be an attempt to find the reasons for them and resolve the discrepancies through seeking additional information. In cases of MBP, some inconsistencies will be related specifically to the exaggeration, fabrication, or induction behavior, and there will probably be others in the life of the suspected perpetrator. In cases that initially appear to be MBP, but are not, other explanations for the inconsistency will be found. Still other inconsistencies will occur because various information sources are used, interpretations of events differ, and memories are faulty. None of this will be clear when the information is initially received. For example, suppose that most informants claim a specific incident occurred at County Medical Center. The victim's aunt is "sure" that it occurred at St. Luke's. It will be important to obtain information both from County Medical Center and from St. Luke's. Do not simply assume that the aunt is mistaken. The aunt may be mistaken, but additional incidents involving the family and St. Luke's may be discovered. Alternatively, the aunt may be the only person who remembers the incident correctly or who was actually there. Other family members may have heard only a garbled version. However, exploration at County Medical Center may reveal additional incidents involving the family. When all possible information is gathered, organized, and evaluated, patterns of exaggeration, fabrication, and induction, if present, should stand out clearly.

Is the information credible? Why or why not?

Information comes from a variety of sources, written and verbal. It may appear to be factual, but a closer look may show that it includes items that are not true or that demand further verification. Even "official records" frequently contain honest mistakes, "hearsay," and "falsehoods disguised as truth"—seemingly true statements that are not true, for example, those that record the informant's statements as fact. Professionals generally believe and document what they are told by parents, relatives, and others. Spouses/partners, relatives, and friends may be repeating what the suspected MBP perpetrator has told them. This "history" may be reviewed by other professionals and repeated in various kinds of other records. When MBP is suspected, what is *said* (which may be true or false) must be separated from what has been verified and is therefore known to be true. MBP investigators must constantly ask themselves where information originated or might have originated, whether it has been verified, and how it can be verified if its truth is not established.

The source and method of obtaining information should be considered and documented along with its content. Was information obtained directly from the original source? If not, there is a possibility that it has been distorted in some way. Was the source qualified to form the conclusion that was made? Was the source objective? Information is often mistakenly "documented" in records as if it were truth. The following examples illustrate this.

> Example 1: (Excerpt from a child protective services initial report): *On April 8, Telephone Intake received a report from psychologist Amy Sandivar indicating suspicion of sexual abuse.* Betsy (age eight) is multiply handicapped and has many medical problems. Recently she has become belligerent and aggressive, complains of pain in her genital area, plays sex games with her dolls, and does not want to visit her father on weekends. *Dr. Sandivar scheduled an appointment to see the child for the first time next week (April 14, 3:30 p.m.).*
>
> Example 2: (Excerpt from a certified medical record provided by a hospital): *This is the fifth admission for Benjamin at this facility.* He has continued to have seizures at home, *and arrived in status epilepticus* [a state of prolonged seizures]. The older brother has a history of seizure disorder and breathing problems.

In both examples, only the italicized material can be considered beyond suspicion. The information about the children's symptoms and behaviors outside the hospital, and the information about the older brother in Example 2 were based on someone's report. If these are genuine cases of MBP, the reporter was probably the perpetrator, but could also have been someone to whom the perpetrator gave this information. The writers should have identified the sources of their information by using terms such as "according to mother" or "according to father" rather than writing down unverified history as if it were fact. (This is a good general practice, not just in cases of suspected MBP.) People investigating MBP cases should continually ask themselves questions such as, "Do we know where this information originated? If not, where did it likely originate? Is the source reliable?" The suspected perpetrator and anyone who could have received the information from the suspected perpetrator—no matter how well-intentioned—cannot initially be considered reliable sources of information.

Any material is questionable if suspected perpetrators or those close to them *might* have initiated or had access to it. Even people regarded as "trustworthy" have sometimes removed, added to, or changed information because they believed what perpetrators told them. Suspected perpetrators frequently offer to "help" by obtaining or hand carrying information, but this should not be allowed under any circumstances. Records must be obtained in such a way that tampering cannot occur.

Is the information relevant for confirming/disconfirming MBP? Why or why not?

Information is relevant if it is pertinent to possible MBP exaggeration, fabrication, or induction, or to alternative explanations for the problem, especially if patterns of attention seeking or deception are found. Early in the case, however, conclusions about relevance should not be drawn too quickly. It is better to accumulate information and later decide that it is not relevant than to overlook something potentially important.

Is the information relevant for other case activities or decisions? Why or why not?

During the MBP investigation and confirmation/disconfirmation process, other issues besides MBP may surface or be addressed. Some of a perpetrator's actions may constitute non-MBP child maltreatment or other illegal or harmful behavior. Other information may help with decisions about siblings, placement, prognosis, etc.

If necessary, is the information potential court evidence? Why or why not?

Suspected and/or confirmed MBP cases almost always require court action. Although investigators should not assume that MBP will be confirmed or that the case will go to court, they should be aware of these possibilities and think strategically. Some information will be of a type and quality that can be used in court. As information accumulates, the investigators and MMT should consider what may be useful in court and identify potential witnesses. If information appears important but is not presently usable in court, action may be indicated. For example, "hearsay" evidence (i.e., that which comes from a third party) is ordinarily not admissible in court. Knowledge of a fact by hearsay can lead the investigator to search for another source resulting in evidence that can be used in court.

ORGANIZING INFORMATION

A review of as much information as can possibly be gathered is key to the determination of whether MBP has or has not occurred. MBP maltreatment should not be confirmed based on one event. Even if the event constitutes MBP-like behavior, much more is involved. The *pattern* of events is crucial. For example, any caretaker may occasionally be mistaken about symptoms or details. If a review of all records shows no more than this, then MBP would not be confirmed. More typically, however, cases later determined to be MBP show dozens of inconsistencies and falsifications involving the perpetrator as well as the victim, and strong associations between the presence or influence of the caretaker and the presence of problems. These patterns become clear only when a careful analysis of information is undertaken.

A large amount of information from a variety of sources is usually accumulated during the typical MBP investigation and confirmation/disconfirmation process. Some information will be relevant to determining the presence or absence of MBP and some will not. Merely reviewing the stacks of records and interview information without organizing them in a meaningful way will not contribute to thorough and correct MBP investigation, decision making, MBP determination, court preparation and presentation, and later case planning. Relevant information must be identified and organized.

As the case progresses, it is essential to keep track of many activities and to officially document that they have taken place, including:

1. who is to be interviewed, when, by whom, and the status of the interview (i.e., completed or pending);
2. what records need to be collected, when they are requested, and when they are received;
3. who needs basic MBP education and when this is provided;

4. who are potential witnesses should the case go to court; and
5. important dates in the case process (i.e., meeting dates, report deadlines, upcoming interviews, court hearings if the case goes to court, etc.).

Unless a system is developed and followed, important information and ideas will be forgotten. Lists should be developed for potential information sources, persons in need of education, potential witnesses, and tasks to be accomplished. However, gathering information by itself is not enough. It is only the first step in a process that (hopefully) leads to confident decision making. A good decision about the presence or absence of MBP can be made only when information is organized and competently analyzed.

The importance of well-organized data in MBP cases cannot be overstated. Significant amounts of time can be wasted if people "think" they can remember an event, statement, or source, but cannot find documentation for it and compare it to other information. Without careful information organization, patterns will not be detected. In court, witnesses are expected to speak authoritatively and back up their statements by references to specific documents and statements. If they cannot do this quickly and competently, they lose credibility.

A suggested method of information organization consists of five steps:

- Separate information into sources.
- Assign each information source an identifying name and number. Make a list of the sources and numbers.
- Number the pages within each source.
- Develop categories for information.
- Place information (exact quotations from the source) and potential witnesses in each relevant category.

1. *Separate information into sources.* Example: St. Luke's Clinic, Dr. William Green, Martin Luther King Elementary School, etc.
2. *Assign each information source an identifying name and number.* The ordering of these is arbitrary. Example: the hospital is given #1, the pediatrician is given #2, the school is given #3, the

person reporting the case is given #4. Be sure to keep a list of what number is assigned to each source.

3. *Number the pages within each source.* This allows specific information to be coded and easily found again when needed. For example 2-14 would mean source 2, page 14.

4. *Develop categories for information.* The number and type of categories will depend on the case. Additional categories can be added at any time or categories can be subdivided or collapsed as needed. Frequently used categories are shown in Box 7.1.

5. *Place information (exact quotations from the source) in each relevant category.* As relevant or potentially relevant information is identified, direct quotations (with quotation marks and specific source number and page number clearly identified) and names of potential witnesses should be placed into the appropriate category or categories. Some information will need to be placed into more than one category. Comments or paraphrasing should not include quotation marks, so that actual quotes can be differentiated easily. The system should be kept simple, followed consistently, and communicated to anyone who will be analyzing information.

Case 7.1

Ms. Doyle, a neighbor, was interviewed by CPS worker Vicki Adams on September 13, 2002. She was eventually coded as Source 4. On page 10 of the interview transcription, Ms. Doyle stated, "Their mom, Monica, says they're all sickly in that house. She's always going to the doctor herself, and taking them to the doctor too. None of them look sickly to me. Jennifer's more on the quiet side, but I see Sam running around all the time."

Vicki Adams also interviewed Dr. Cromwell, the pediatrician. He was coded as Source 2. On page 6 of the interview transcription, he stated, "I never saw anything wrong with those kids, except for normal colds and flu. Oh, Sam broke his arm one time playing soccer, but Jennifer is a healthy little girl."

This material was coded and organized on work sheets. Two examples are shown in Box 7.2. The same material was also placed on other work sheets for Sam (Jennifer's brother) and for inconsistencies in the case. As additional information was obtained, it was added to each appropriate work sheet.

As cases become more complex, it can also be useful to construct a time line that includes significant dates and relevant information. This should be done in chronological order, earliest to latest, with

---

BOX 7.1.
Some Possible Categories and Subcategories
for Organizing Information

- Each suspected perpetrator
- Each suspected victim
- Each child not currently considered a victim who was presently or formerly in home or born to suspected perpetrator (even if deceased, not living with perpetrator, or now an adult)
- Spouse/parent/significant other (past or present) not suspected of MBP
- Other close relatives of suspected victim
- Inconsistencies
- Past or current suspicion or confirmation of MBP in nuclear or extended family, or in children cared for by suspected perpetrator
- Past or current suspicion or confirmation of factitious disorder/ Munchausen syndrome in suspected perpetrator or nuclear/ extended family
- Other suspected or confirmed maltreatment (linked to or separate from MBP)
- Suspected or confirmed exaggeration of events
- Suspected or confirmed fabrication of events
- Suspected or confirmed inducing of events
- Professionals involved in case including role and contact information
- Nonprofessionals involved in case including role and contact information
- Credible information that refutes the idea of MBP and/or supports other possible sources for the problem(s)
- Comments, e.g., things that need to be followed up on, ideas, etc.

---

appropriate coding for sources, categories, and page numbers. This can show, for example, how problems moved from one child to another, how patterns developed over time or were random, or how the perpetrator consistently exaggerated and/or fabricated and/or induced in many facets of life.

The full task of correctly and thoroughly completing the MBP maltreatment category analysis is extremely time-consuming, whether it is accomplished by hand or by computer, particularly since the same information often must be included on several work sheets. Using a

---

BOX 7.2.
Sample Work Sheets for Monica and Jennifer

Category: Monica (mother)

Source	Information
4-10	From interview of Margaret Doyle by Vicki Adams, 9/13/02. "Their mom says they're all sickly in that house. She's always going to the doctor herself, and taking them to the doctor too. None of them look sickly to me."

Category: Jennifer (child, suspected victim)

Source	Information
4-10	From interview of Margaret Doyle by Vicki Adams, 9/13/02. "Their mom says they're all sickly in that house. She's always going to the doctor herself, and taking them to the doctor too. None of them look sickly to me. Jennifer's more on the quiet side.
2-6	From interview of Wm. Cromwell, MD, by Vicki Adams, 9/9/02. "I never saw anything wrong with those kids, except for normal colds and flu. Jennifer is a healthy little girl."

---

simple "sort program" (available in word processing software) enables the task to be accomplished much more quickly than if done by hand. It also requires careful thought and some experience to recognize subtle manifestations of MBP behavior. Thus, the task of organizing and analyzing information is often performed by an MBP expert consultant. If done well, it will ultimately produce information that will assist in identifying any existing MBP patterns as well as potential witnesses and other evidence. Alternatively, it will suggest other possibilities if MBP does not appear to be occurring. Categorization will provide a list of comments and a "to-do list," keep track of potential witnesses, and be invaluable if court preparation is necessary. Nothing else will contribute so positively to a grasp of case information.

THE MBP CONFIRMATION/DISCONFIRMATION
DECISION AND THE FUNCTIONING OF THE MMT

MBP investigations may have at least five possible outcomes:

- MBP confirmed and perpetrator(s) determined
- Other maltreatment (with or without MBP) confirmed and perpetrator(s) determined
- Other maltreatment (with or without MBP) confirmed but perpetrator(s) not determined
- Not enough information to make a confirmation/disconfirmation decision
- No maltreatment confirmed after a thorough investigation and confirmation/disconfirmation process

MBP Confirmed

To confirm MBP maltreatment, there must be proof (usually through circumstantial evidence) that one or more problems have been deliberately exaggerated and/or fabricated and/or induced in the victim. There must also be sufficient information to conclude that the situation constitutes MBP maltreatment rather than something else. For example, if there is clear induction of problems for the primary purpose of external gain, or a primary intent to torture or kill, this may be non-MBP child maltreatment.

If MBP is confirmed, the behavior must be labeled as MBP as part of the confirmation process, so an appropriate case plan, including elements unique to MBP, can be legally justified. Otherwise, short- and long-term victim protection is unlikely.

Other Maltreatment (With or Without MBP) Confirmed

Confirmed MBP will manifest as physical abuse, emotional abuse, neglect, sexual abuse, or a combination. Alternatively, a case that was initially suspected as MBP may turn out to constitute non-MBP maltreatment. Even though the focus is determining the presence or absence of MBP, do not lose sight of other forms of harm that may be occurring. If these are found, they should be dealt with according to established protocols.

Not Enough Information

In some cases, there is insufficient information to conclude that MBP or other forms of child maltreatment are occurring. For example, a court may have refused to order the release of information about a suspected perpetrator. The MMT should do all within its power to brainstorm approaches to information gathering that may discern whether maltreatment is occurring.

Maltreatment (MBP or Other) Is Disconfirmed

Sometimes the result of a thorough and appropriate investigation is a consensus that no maltreatment has occurred. For example, a rare disease may have been confirmed as the cause of the child's problems. Disconfirmation is a positive finding. Time spent on the investigation should not be regarded as wasted; the process has worked to uncover the truth. Members of the MMT have also gained knowledge and experience during the course of the investigation.

The Identity of the Perpetrator May Be Determined

Often there are suspicions of the perpetrator's identity at the time that possible MBP is first considered. All possibilities must be considered during the investigative process. Statistically, birth mothers are the most common perpetrators, but other caregivers have also been identified. As more reports of MBP are received, more categories of perpetrators will emerge.

As the investigation proceeds, if the case is genuine MBP, a pattern usually emerges of one person being associated with the problem(s). Most important, if patterns of deception and opportunity emerge, they usually center around one person. When this occurs, involved professionals can feel more confident in determining that a single person is the likely perpetrator, and further action can be taken.

The Identity of the Perpetrator May Remain Undetermined

Sometimes the perpetrator of MBP or other child maltreatment cannot be determined. For example, in one instance an infant died of a skull fracture. Circumstantial evidence suggested that both parents were home alone with the infant at the time that the fracture must have occurred. Both parents denied hitting the baby, and denied any knowledge of how the injury occurred. They did not change their stories during police interrogation or court action, and were ultimately jailed for medical neglect—failure to seek medical assistance for an injured child.

Every effort should be made to identify the perpetrator. Without such identification, it becomes very difficult to adequately protect the identified victim, and even more difficult to know whether siblings are in danger. Realistically, however, there may be some instances in which this determination cannot be made.

Deciding whether MBP has occurred is a serious and complex task. But if the investigation and information organization process have been conducted correctly and thoroughly, the task can be accomplished. Working through the Questions for Suspected and Confirmed MBP Cases (Box 5.1) and deciding what information is sound and what conclusions can be agreed upon will help with the confirmation/disconfirmation process. These questions must be answered fully in order to validate and continue to validate the initial MBP confirmation/diagnosis and prepare for court and related activities. When questions cannot be answered, further investigation and brainstorming may be necessary. In some circumstances, information will not be available in spite of everyone's best efforts. This may limit the conclusions that can be reached and further action that can be taken.

Sometimes there are differences of opinion over whether MBP should be confirmed. Often this occurs when one or more professionals lack an understanding of MBP basics and/or case information. It may also occur when one or more professionals, in spite of information, find it impossible to give up their own views of the situation, or to accept that this form of abuse occurs and may have occurred on their "home turf." Ultimately, whatever the opinion and recommendations of the MBP expert consultant and MMT, the legally appointed child protective agency must make the final decision of whether to take action and/or make recommendations to the court.

THE WORK OF THE MMT:
INITIAL AND SUBSEQUENT MEETINGS

The multiagency-multidisciplinary team (MMT), which is composed of key professionals involved in the specific case, provides ideas, expertise, and a "sounding board" to those involved in the investigation and confirmation/disconfirmation process as well as post-confirmation case activities and decision making. The presence of the MMT also allows for the building of a consensus among those involved in the case. Reasons for utilizing an MMT were discussed in Chapter 4. The old clichés of "many heads are wiser than one" and "many hands make light(er) work" are never more true than in the labyrinth of an MBP case, when it is terribly easy for anyone, no matter how skilled, to miss important observations and information and to be led astray by a perpetrator and/or their own feelings. To ensure proper decision making and recommendations during the investigation and confirmation/disconfirmation process, and for short- and long-term victim protection, case planning, and case management, the MMT must meet throughout the life of the case.

As has been stated repeatedly, MBP perpetrators are accomplished deceivers. They usually have plausible-sounding reasons for their behavior and look like good caregivers. They are often adept at perceiving someone's vulnerabilities and "pushing their buttons." For example, if someone believes that parents are always good and that the "system" is destructive, the perpetrator may claim to have been entrapped by the "system." The MMT helps those involved in the investigation and case process to remain objective and to recognize deception and manipulation.

On the other hand, innocent persons may be falsely accused if professionals jump to conclusions or use incorrect methods. Either type of error—failure to confirm actual maltreatment or false accusation—can be extremely damaging to victims, accused, and accusers. The active involvement of a multiagency-multidisciplinary group of professionals who work through all possibilities together, will reduce these dangers and increase the probability that a thorough and correct investigation and confirmation/disconfirmation process will be conducted. If MBP is later confirmed, this process will also reveal weak spots in the case that must be overcome for successful victim protection and perpetrator prosecution.

The first meeting of the MMT should be called as soon as a report has been received involving MBP suspicion. The reporter (if a professional), another concerned professional, or the child protection agency can request and organize the initial MMT meeting. Ultimately, however, because CPS is the legally mandated child protection agency, it should ensure that the meeting takes place and that all known/appropriate professionals are requested to attend. This is a meeting for professionals only, for the purposes of discussion and planning, and should not include perpetrator or suspected perpetrator, family, or friends. Since present or future court action may be involved, minutes of MMT meetings should be taken carefully. These minutes should show process as well as decisions and include attendance, methods of decision making, and reasons for decisions. They can be used later to establish the credibility of the professionals involved, the alternative plans that were considered, and the care that went into planning.

The first meeting should include all known professionals who have been involved with the family, so that all possible information can be gathered. Those who are no longer active with the family may not be needed after the first meeting. Appropriate professionals might include CPS staff, law enforcement officers, community agency staff, school personnel, emergency responders, and health care providers. Professionals who have not previously been involved with the family, but who will need to be part of the case, should also be asked to attend. The person inviting others to attend the meeting should explain the situation, the urgency, the need for attendance, and the meeting's structure and purposes. A typical agenda for the initial MMT meeting is shown in Box 7.3. If the child is currently hospitalized in a physical or mental health care facility, a hospital social worker can help in identifying and contacting appropriate physical or mental health staff and other facility personnel as well as arranging meeting space if needed. Hospital personnel may include representatives from social services, risk management, nursing, security, administration, and others. Should someone resist attending the meeting, a gentle nudge may help. For example, the person coordinating the meeting could explain the need for the person's information and expertise: "I understand how busy you must be, Detective Jones. But this may be a life-threatening situation and we need to have an officer at the meeting. I have to document those who attend, and the names of anyone who can't be there and why they said they couldn't attend. Are you sure you can't attend—or what should I write in my official record?" Often such a statement will change the professional's mind. There should be no hesitation about "pushing" people to attend. An inclusive, well-functioning MMT is vital. It is the key to success in attempting to protect a child.

BOX 7.3.
MMT Initial Meeting Agenda

I. Sign in and introductions.
II. Review the MBP definition and terminology:
  A. Remind participants to include the words "by proxy" when referring to MBP so that MBP maltreatment and factitious disorder/Munchausen syndrome will be clearly distinguished.
  B. Review perpetrator-consistent characteristics (Box 2.1), situational suspicion indicators, criteria for confirming or disconfirming MBP, and the "Questions for Suspected and Confirmed MBP Cases" (Box 5.1).
III. Review purposes of meeting:
  A. To share and clarify presently known information.
  B. To formulate strategy and come to consensus regarding future case activities and recommendations.
  C. To clarify involved facility/agency/organization roles, procedures, expectations, and next steps.
IV. Review presently known case history and information (physical, mental health, social, educational, etc.) The "Questions for Suspected and Confirmed MBP Cases" (Box 5.1) can be used to structure this discussion.
  A. Each person should share his or her knowledge and the bases for it.
  B. Raise questions, concerns, inconsistencies, etc. Clarify where possible and identify unresolved areas.
V. Discuss and strategize, make recommendations and decisions. Document each and include rationale.
  Typical topics include:
  A. Does the team agree at this time that this case involves MBP? On what basis? Why or why not?
  B. If MBP is not confirmed, does the team remain suspicious that MBP is involved? Why or why not?
  C. What other information is needed? What investigative activities will need to be accomplished? How will they be done? Who will take responsibility? By when?
  D. Regardless of MBP confirmation status, does the MMT believe that the victim is at high risk or in immediate danger? Why or why not?

(continued)

(*Box 7.3, continued*)

  E. Does the team recommend that the suspected/confirmed victim(s) be separated from the suspected/confirmed perpetrator's care, custody, control, and influence and placed in a neutral, carefully monitored environment? Is this primarily for safety and/or as a diagnostic confirmation/disconfirmation tool? Are any strategies other than seeking protective custody likely to ensure protection? Why or why not?
  F. If a decision is made to take or seek protective custody, what action will be taken, who will take it, and how will the situation be evaluated/monitored? Will any special characteristics or competencies be required in the foster home? See Chapters 8 and 9.
  G. If there are other children in the victim's home, does the MMT recommend that any action be taken to remove or request removal of them from the home? Why or why not?
VI. Review recommendations and decisions, what is to happen next, who is to do what, and in what time frame. Decide when/where the next MMT meeting will take place. Ensure that meeting documentation is accurate.
VII. Adjourn

The meeting chairperson should be designated in advance, and should have demonstrated leadership skills in chairing meetings. Someone involved in the meeting must have verified, extensive MBP knowledge and experience. An MBP expert consultant could participate by telephone conference call or video teleconference if time or budget do not allow for physical attendance. The chairperson should prepare and ensure distribution of the agenda and selected MBP educational handouts prior to the meeting if possible. Otherwise, this material should be available at the beginning of the meeting. To ensure that everyone will be working from a common background, educational handouts should be provided to all participants, even those who have had prior training or insist that they have sufficient MBP knowledge. A competent and responsible recorder should also be designated, preferably in advance, to keep minutes of the meeting.

All participants should personally sign an attendance sheet, indicating their name, position, agency/organization, mailing address, telephone number, fax number, and e-mail address. The attendance sheet should also indicate any individuals participating via electronic technology, with documentation as to who is "signing in" for them. Notation should be made of any individuals who arrive after the meeting begins or leave before the meeting ends, including exact times. Notations should also be made of the times that various topics are discussed. This is important documentation, and can potentially be used in court as proof of who was involved in recommendations and decision making at a given meeting.

The chairperson should ensure that all participants receive basic MBP training prior to their participation in formulating strategy, recommendations, or decisions. It is counterproductive and potentially dangerous to discuss and make decisions regarding MBP cases without a foundation of correct knowledge. If time does not allow for full training before or during the meeting, training should be scheduled as quickly as possible after the meeting. Time must be allocated at the beginning of the meeting, even in emergencies, for a review of basic definitions, MBP perpetrator-consistent characteristics, situational suspicion indicators, and criteria for confirming MBP. As the meeting progresses, participants will be asked to share their relevant experiences and impressions. Allowing them to speak in the order of their involvement is one system that lends coherence to these sometimes confusing recitals. It also may curb the desire of any professionals to assume that their voice or perspective should dominate. As recommendations and decisions are made, the chairperson should read them back to the group, formally asking how many agree. Both agreement and disagreement should be documented, with reasons recorded.

The initial MMT meeting is likely to be a lengthy process, as there is a great deal to be accomplished. Facilities should be available and participants should be prepared to spend at least three to four hours. Conducting this first meeting correctly, however, will save time in the long run. By the end of this meeting, all professionals involved in the case, and particularly the child protective services investigator responsible for the case, should have a clear understanding and acceptance of the investigative "game plan."

*Case 7.1. MBP Investigation and Confirmation/Disconfirmation
with the MMT*

Monica Stewart, age three, had numerous hospitalizations and emergency room visits for hypoglycemic (low blood sugar) episodes. The cause of these was a mystery. The mother, Mrs. Stewart, insisted that Monica was a "brittle" (i.e., hard-to-control) diabetic, but glucose tolerance tests in the hospital were normal. Nevertheless, within a few days of hospital discharge, Monica always returned with another hypoglycemic episode.

A pediatric resident (physician in training), Dr. Randolph, reported the case to CPS as possible MBP because he was ordered to do so by his chief resident, Dr. Bridgeport. Susan Masters, a CPS investigator, was assigned to the case. Susan had previously received MBP basic education. When she discussed the case with her supervisor, it was agreed that the first investigative activity would be the convening of an MMT within twenty-four hours and that the supervisor would seek approval for the funding of an MBP expert consultant. Funding was obtained and Yvonne Black, a recognized MBP expert consultant, was contracted.

Susan contacted the following persons and requested their presence at the initial MMT meeting: Dr. Randolph, Dr. Bridgeport, the hospital social worker, the nurse manager from the young children's ward, and the hospital's risk manager. A public health nurse, Brenda Paxton, was invited to the meeting because, Susan discovered, she had been to the home on many occasions to provide health guidance for Mrs. Stewart's elderly parents, who lived with Mrs. Stewart. A police officer from the city's juvenile division was also invited.

Dr. Randolph initially resisted attending the meeting because he "was not sure it was fair to accuse a concerned parent without proof." However, Susan explained that MBP was only a possibility at this stage, and that Mrs. Stewart was not being accused. Susan also explained that the initial MMT meeting was the first step in an objective MBP investigation and confirmation-disconfirmation process. Susan explained that Dr. Randolph's input was very important to the meeting. Dr. Randolph agreed to attend.

Before the first MMT meeting, Susan sent all MMT members a meeting agenda, basic MBP training material prepared by Yvonne Black, and a journal article about MBP presenting as factitious diabetes. Susan discussed case details with Yvonne, faxed available records to her, and arranged for her to participate by telephone conference call at the initial MMT meeting and to present condensed, basic MBP training prior to case discussion.

At the MMT meeting, after the training, the group reviewed what they knew about the family and the facts in the case. Dr. Randolph stated that the hypoglycemia was genuine, proved on many occasions by laboratory tests conducted when the mother was not present. The nurse manager of the pediatric unit stated that Monica frequently had hypoglycemic symptoms on the ward, but she had never thought about whether these might coincide with Mrs. Stewart's visits. She promised to ask her nurses for their observations. The hospital social worker described the many times that Mrs. Stewart had come to her office to talk, in heartrending terms, about her own illnesses and the difficulties of living with a child "who could die at any moment." The home care nurse remained silent, only commenting that she did not know why she was invited since her field was geriatrics and she did not provide any care to Monica. She knew nothing of Monica's problems, except that Mrs. Stewart frequently said the child was in the hospital.

Susan described how she would like to proceed in her investigation. The agency had granted permission for Yvonne to provide consultation and technical assistance, to review further records, and to assist in interviewing and reinterviewing various individuals. Dr. Randolph agreed to assist Yvonne with any questions she might have after reviewing the medical information. It was decided that the records review and the information from the nurses on the young children's ward would be crucial in the team's decisions about next steps. Susan planned to interview other hospital personnel, and stated that she would have liked to interview the teacher at Monica's preschool, but this woman was described as a friend of Mrs. Stewart's and was likely to "tip her off" if a CPS investigator came to talk about Monica. She had tried to interview Mrs. Stewart's personal physician, but he refused to talk with her without a signed release of information from Mrs. Stewart. It was agreed that the team would meet again as soon as Yvonne completed the initial records review.

At the next team meeting, Yvonne was present in person. She had completed preliminary MBP category analysis work sheets from information she had reviewed thus far. A sample from the work sheet focusing on inconsistencies is shown in Box 7.4. The hospital record is source #1. The private pediatrician's record is source #2. The preschool's health record is source #3.

Another chart also showed that when Mrs. Stewart did not visit, Monica was free of symptoms. Yvonne stated that even though the investigation was not complete, she and Susan believed that this was very likely a case of MBP and that Monica and possibly her half brother were in need of protection. She asked the MMT for their input and reactions to this data.

Members of the MMT found Yvonne's data persuasive. However, Dr. Randolph was reluctant to "accuse such a nice woman" because the hypoglycemic episodes were genuine. Yvonne asked, "What could produce sudden and severe hypoglycemia in a young child?" Dr. Randolph stated that injections of insulin could do this. The public health nurse then revealed that Mrs. Stewart's father had insulin-dependent diabetes, so needles and insulin were easily available in the home.

This information led the team to wonder whether Mrs. Stewart might be using some of her father's insulin and syringes to inject Monica. The plan was developed that, at Monica's next visit with Dr. Randolph, she would be examined carefully for injection sites and asked outside her mother's presence what was the cause of those marks. When this plan was followed, Dr. Randolph's examination revealed puncture marks in the webs of her fingers, and Monica told him "Mommy gives me shots."

At the following MMT meeting, the team reviewed the facts uncovered by their investigation, using the "Questions for Suspected and Confirmed MBP

BOX 7.4.
Inconsistencies in the Stewart Case

Source	Information
1-242	(Lab slip from the medical chart, test done 11/10/01): "Normal results on glucose tolerance test."
2-3	Note from office record maintained by private pediatrician Dr. David Gamble, visit on 12/1/01: "Mother states previous pediatrician confirmed hypoglycemia via glucose tolerance test at hospital lab. Plan: repeat test."
1-243	(Lab slip from the medical chart, test done 12/2/01): "Normal results on glucose tolerance test." No indications on lab slip of any problems during test.
3-1	Health record, Rainbow Preschool, note dated 12/14/01: "Mother states that Monica has had several blood tests at the hospital that show she suffers from hypoglycemia."
2-4	Note from office record maintained by private pediatrician Dr. David Gamble, visit on 12/20/01: "Discussed with Mrs. S. that results of glucose tolerance test are normal. She stated that technician did not appear to know how to perform test, and that many errors and problems occurred. She does not trust results and asks that test be repeated on an emergency basis."
1-244	(Lab slip from the medical chart, test done 12/21/01): "Normal results on glucose tolerance test."

Cases" (Box 5.1) format. Some of these questions and answers are shown as follows.

4. *When was MBP maltreatment first suspected in this case? By whom? What specific reasons led to the suspicion?*

Dr. Bridgeport first suspected MBP because of Monica's frequent emergency department visits and the mother's insistence that she was a "brittle diabetic," contrasted with her normal glucose tolerance tests in the hospital. He could think of no other reason for this paradox besides some form of child maltreatment.

5. *If MBP was confirmed or is suspected:*

- *Who is believed to have perpetrated the maltreatment? Why? Who else was considered?* Mrs. Stewart is now considered to be the perpetrator because of Monica's statement that her mother gives her shots at home. This statement is supported by puncture marks in the webs of her fingers, and by the association between Mrs. Stewart's visits to Monica in the hospital and Monica's development of hypoglycemia. No other possible perpetrators were considered in this case. Other perpetrators and other possible causes of the situation would have been considered if Dr. Randolph's examination had not revealed puncture marks or if Monica had given a different cause for the puncture marks.
- *Who is believed to be the victim? What other children are in the home or under the care of the perpetrator?* Monica Stewart is believed to be the victim. Monica's half brother, Douglas, age five, is also in the home. It is not known whether he might be or have been in the past a victim of any form of maltreatment.
- *What specific physical and/or psychological-behavioral problems is the victim having that are believed to have been caused by the perpetrator? What specific examples support belief that the perpetrator has caused the problems? What specific examples refute this belief? What documentation is available? Are there other problems that do not appear to have been caused by the perpetrator?* Monica's frequent episodes of hypoglycemia are believed to have been caused by the perpetrator. Monica's statements, and the temporal association between Mrs. Stewart's hospital visits and Monica's development of hypoglycemia, support this. However, puncture marks can be nonspecific, and Monica is only three years old. It is possible that she is lying, misunderstood Dr. Randolph's questions, or was "led" in her answers. Further investigation needs to be done to determine if lab tests can show whether Monica has been given insulin, and perhaps what type she might have been given. This should be compared with the insulin known to be in the home. From time to time, Monica does have colds and other childhood illnesses that are not believed to have been caused by the perpetrator.
- *Does it appear that the method of creating these problems was exaggeration and/or fabrication and/or induction? Why? What documentation is available?* Based on Monica's statements, and the laboratory tests that have shown her hypoglycemic episodes to be genuine, it is believed that they are induced. In talking with others, Mrs. Stewart has also been very dramatic about the extent of Monica's illness, exaggerating the severity of her symptoms.
- *What form(s) of maltreatment, as defined in the jurisdiction, does the MBP appear to constitute? (For example, physical abuse, sexual abuse, emotional abuse, medical neglect, etc.) Why?* In

this jurisdiction, "physical abuse" includes "providing the minor with dangerous drugs, medications, or controlled substances" except when these are "part of treatment for illness . . ." Thus, the MBP appears to constitute physical abuse. It could also be considered emotional abuse, because of the ordeal to which Monica had been subjected through the mother's injections that caused unnecessary diet and activity limitations, frightening symptoms, and multiple hospitalizations. In some jurisdictions, this behavior would also constitute medical neglect, since the mother was not providing appropriate health care to Monica.

- *What MBP perpetrator-consistent characteristics have been identified? What documentation is available for these? What alternative explanations appear reasonable, and what documentation is available for those?* Mrs. Stewart has spoken to nurse Mike Takaki, the hospital social worker, and some of the ward nurses in a very dramatic manner about her own personal problems and her feelings about Monica's illness. All of these hospital personnel have been asked to write statements about their contacts with Mrs. Stewart, and some observations of her "dramatic tendencies" already are present in Monica's medical record. Other interview information obtained and documented by Yvonne suggested that Mrs. Stewart sought attention in many facets of her life, and was seen by friends and professionals as often exaggerating her "stories." Perhaps these behaviors are unrelated to Monica's illness, or are an appropriate response to a difficult life situation that includes a very sick child. Until the team is more sure about whether Mrs. Stewart is inducing symptoms, it will be impossible to know whether this is the case.

- *What physical and/or psychological-behavioral interventions (office visits, hospitalizations, medications, surgeries, etc.) has the victim been subjected to unnecessarily because of the perpetrator's exaggeration and/or fabrication and/or induction behavior? What harm has occurred because of these? What harm might have occurred?* Monica had been in the Emergency Department twenty-seven times, with twenty-two hospital admissions because of hypoglycemic symptoms. Generally on arrival at the hospital she was unconscious or close to unconscious. She had at least 120 physician visits for monitoring of blood sugar or as follow-up to hospitalizations. During each episode of hypoglycemia she received injected medicines. Blood tests were done in the emergency room, hospital, and in conjunction with physician visits. As a "diabetic," Monica was also placed on a restrictive diet and limited in her active play. Monica suffered frightening losses of consciousness, pain, separation from her family, and restrictions of her normal activities. Insulin is a dangerous drug. Harm that Monica could have sustained (but did not) includes death, coma, brain damage, seizures, and the development of allergies to insulin that could have caused skin damage or limited her ability to use insulin if needed in the future.

* *What other possibilities besides MBP have been considered? Which have been excluded, and why?* Drs. Randolph and Bridgeport initially considered Monica's hypoglycemia to be genuine, and treated it accordingly. However, Monica's lab tests in the hospital (when Mrs. Stewart was not present) suggested that she did not have diabetes. The physicians considered whether Monica might be in an early stage of developing diabetes, and thus her laboratory tests might be inconsistent, but could never find evidence of hypoglycemia except when she was in the emergency room or in association with Mrs. Stewart's visits while she was hospitalized. They considered whether she might truly have the "brittle diabetes" that Mrs. Stewart described, but never found the high blood sugar readings they would have expected with the disease. The physicians presented Monica's case to an experienced endocrinologist (diabetes specialist) who wondered whether Monica might have a tumor of the pancreas. However, an ultrasound of her pancreas was normal.

After these questions were reviewed, the team was asked how they felt about the criteria for confirmation/disconfirmation: Was there proof, through direct and/or circumstantial evidence, that the suspected perpetrator had deliberately exaggerated and/or fabricated and/or induced a problem or problems in another (MBP-like behavior)? Did the behavior constitute MBP maltreatment or something else?

The team felt that they had both direct and circumstantial evidence that Mrs. Stewart was inducing hypoglycemic episodes in Monica through injections of insulin. Monica's statement, the presence of needle marks, and the laboratory evidence of nonhuman insulin in her body provided direct evidence. Circumstantial evidence included (among other things) the presence of insulin and needles in the home, the frequent association between Mrs. Stewart's visits to the hospital and Monica's symptoms, and insulin in the home of the same type as had been identified in Monica's body.

After concluding that MBP-like behavior was occurring, the team turned to the question of whether this was a case of MBP or something else. Mrs. Stewart did not appear to have any mental illness that would cause her to be confused about reality or about Monica's symptoms. It did not appear that she was simply an overanxious/overprotective mother. Nor did it appear that she was trying to kill Monica (i.e., attempted murder); a larger dose of insulin, or a delay in seeking help, could easily have accomplished this if it had been Mrs. Stewart's goal. Diabetes education provided by Brenda Paxton had stressed the calculation of insulin doses and the dangers of overdose.

No information was found to suggest that Mrs. Stewart profited in any material sense from Monica's illness; in fact, the family was thousands of dollars in debt from medical bills. So this did not appear to be a case of "malingering by proxy" or fraud. (Even if there were some material gain, if this was not a primary motivation it would not invalidate a finding of MBP.)

- *Where is the victim now? What has been done so far to ensure the victim's safety? What plan has been created to continue to monitor and evaluate the victim?* Monica was hospitalized immediately after the clinic visit at which she reported that "Mommy gives me shots." Yvonne worked with the team to build an appropriate plan for her close supervision, and for management of Mrs. Stewart's visits. (See Part III for discussion of these issues.)

6. *Has MBP maltreatment been disconfirmed by any individual, team, etc.? If so, who? How can they be reached? What are the specific reasons for the disconfirmation? What are their qualifications in relation to MBP?* No other individual or group is known to have considered MBP in this case.

   By using the "Questions for Suspected and Confirmed MBP" and the criteria, and by coming to agreement on each piece of this complicated case, the team felt that they were completing a process that was orderly and fair. The questions structured their discussion, pointing out what they knew at this point and what they did not know. As a result of reviewing the case in this way, the MMT was able to confirm that, in their opinion, MBP was occurring. They also had a number of insights. These included:

- For the first time, the team realized that Monica's half brother, Douglas, might also need protection. They decided to begin a confirmation/disconfirmation process focusing on him.
- The importance of "diagnostic separation"—removing Monica from Mrs. Stewart's care and influence as a means of testing whether her symptoms were genuine—became clearer. The team realized that it would help to resolve alternative explanations for Monica's symptoms, and that it would increase Monica's safety. They agreed that placement of Monica in a foster home would be the next appropriate step.

A summary statement reflecting the team's agreement that MBP should be confirmed was prepared by Susan Masters and signed by all members of the MMT. It was used by CPS to gain emergency protective custody of Monica.

This is a reasonably straightforward case in which the MMT was able to come to an agreement and confirm MBP. Many other case situations will be more complex, uncertain, lengthy, and contentious. This case illustrates, however, the importance of assembling as many people as possible who can contribute ideas. Without the team process, including both Susan and Yvonne, it is likely that Dr. Randolph would have remained resistant to considering MBP. Without the structure provided by the questions, this complicated and emotional discussion might well have gotten off track, failed to consider important elements, or failed to come to specific conclusions. If that had happened, it is very likely that Monica would have continued to receive dangerous and unnecessary insulin injections that could, if the mother had miscalculated, easily have killed her.

PART III:
CASE PLANNING
AND CASE MANAGEMENT
IN CONFIRMED MBP

Chapter 8

Essential Elements in Case Planning and Case Management When MBP Has Been Confirmed

The desired outcome when MBP has been confirmed is protection of the victim. This generally requires that CPS place the victim in a protected setting, most often foster care. Court action is usually necessary as a part of the process to initiate or continue placement and establish a court-ordered case plan. As was noted in Chapter 4, there are four essential elements in case planning and case management. If they are followed, cases are far more likely to be "won" in court. Case management and the tasks of ongoing risk assessment, planning, placement, visitation supervision, etc., are also more likely to be managed appropriately if these essential elements are used. These elements were discussed in Chapter 4, but their application after MBP confirmation is slightly different:

- basic MBP and continuing education;
- ongoing participation of the case-specific multiagency-multi-disciplinary team (MMT);
- an MBP expert who will continue to provide consultation and technical assistance, and who will serve as an expert witness in court proceedings; and
- a competent, correctly MBP-educated attorney who is willing to prepare thoroughly for court and related activities, and to work as a team member with the MBP expert and others.

THE ESSENTIAL ELEMENTS
FOLLOWING CONFIRMATION

MBP Basic and Continuing Education

The importance of basic MBP education was discussed in Chapter 4. After a suspected MBP case has been confirmed, new professionals may become involved in the case and/or the MMT. For example, the child protective agency may assign an out-of-home placement worker once the victim is placed in a foster home. Before they participate in case decision making, these new professionals must receive basic MBP education and detailed case information.

Throughout the life of a case, which may extend for years, it is also common for personnel to change. New people will join the MMT, and they will require training. Continuing members who have received basic MBP education may need "refreshers" from time to time, and should also be kept up-to-date on new developments in the field. If people do not understand MBP, or if their understanding is not complete and current, they will not be able to protect the victim and make appropriate recommendations. Education can be done by the MBP expert, or by someone else who has sufficient, correct, and up-to-date information. The need for education must be met promptly and thoroughly as long as the case is active.

Ongoing Participation of the Case-Specific Multiagency-Multidisciplinary Team (MMT)

The composition, functioning, and advantages of the MMT were described in Chapter 4. The use of the MMT does not end when MBP is confirmed. The MMT should be used as long as the child protective agency is involved. The MMT should meet at least monthly to share and compare detailed case information about the perpetrator, victim(s), others who are involved, and the case as a whole. In MBP cases it is virtually impossible for any professional, including the involved therapist, to form recommendations regarding the perpetrator's progress (or lack thereof) in isolation from other case-involved professionals. Major decisions should not be made nor should the case be closed without the input of the MMT. Especially when crucial decisions are to be made, such as decisions about reunification of the victim with the perpetrator, the MMT should either have a member with advanced and current knowledge of MBP, or access to an MBP expert. If possible, the MBP expert originally involved in the case should be consulted. Also, if possible, at least one person on the MMT should have been involved in the case when MBP was first confirmed.

The MBP Expert

When MBP maltreatment is confirmed, the MBP expert will continue to have a vital role. In addition to providing general consultation and detailed case planning and management recommendations, the expert should complete or assist in the completion of the initial victim risk assessment. The expert's role also includes assisting the attorney in preparation for court and related activities. This will include providing additional education, consultation, and technical assistance. The MBP expert may also function as the expert witness in court hearings or trials. Activities related to the attorney and to court proceedings are discussed in Chapter 11.

A Competent, Correctly Educated Attorney Who Is Willing to Prepare Thoroughly for Court and Related Activities and to Work As a Team Member with the MBP Expert and Others

No matter how solid the MBP confirmation and recommendations, the attorney who has responsibility for preparing and presenting the case is the key to successful court-related activities. Court cases that include allegations of MBP are complex. Thus, the attorney must be competent. But this, by itself, is not enough. If there is to be a successful outcome, the attorney assigned to an MBP case must be open to learning and working in partnership with other members of the MMT and especially with the MBP expert. Attorneys and others who may become part of the court case must receive correct MBP education about MBP basics and issues specifically related to their role. They must understand MBP well enough to explain it to others independently and through the presentation of testimony. They must be able to appreciate their contribution to the welfare of the victim(s), and to advocate effectively for MBP-specific requests that will be made of the court. Cases can be lost if attorneys deny the need for

MBP education or put it off until just before the hearing when it can only be done in a hurried or incomplete fashion.

Attorney participation and preparation must begin early and continue throughout the case process. As with other professionals, the attorney's involvement and time commitment may far exceed what is required for other kinds of maltreatment cases. Although most attorneys are dedicated and willing to learn and prepare in the best possible manner, a few have refused to become properly educated about MBP or to prepare to the extent required for MBP case success. If an attorney does not have the time, interest, or ability to give to the case, it is imperative that the problem be corrected. The stakes are too high to continue with such an attorney.

SUMMARY OF THE FORMULA FOR MBP CASE SUCCESS:
A CASE EXAMPLE

The working of elements will be reviewed, continuing the case example of Annie Martin from Chapter 4.

Case 4.1, continued
(Summary: Annie Martin, age twelve, was referred to the juvenile court by her elementary school due to truancy concerns. Mrs. Martin stated that Annie's frequent absences were due to health problems, but these could not be verified. Mrs. Martin also alleged that Annie had Tourette's syndrome and Prader-Willi syndrome. Jackie Lam, Annie's guardian ad litem, was the first to hear about MBP. She obtained medical records and engaged an MBP expert, Mr. Johnson. At his suggestion, an MMT was formed. Based on their sharing of information, as well as additional information provided by the CPS investigator, MBP was confirmed.)

The next step was for the child protective agency to seek authority to place Annie in a foster home. This placement would not only protect Annie from potential abuse, but would also serve as a "diagnostic separation." That is, it would test whether her problems resolved or improved when Mrs. Martin no longer had access to her (as was expected if Mrs. Martin was involved in their creation). At this point the newly assigned CPS attorney, Carolyn Cabonilla, joined the MMT. She received basic MBP education from Mr. Johnson, and seemed very eager to understand her role and the contribution she could make to Annie's safety.

The MMT's detailed summary of its findings and conclusions was presented to the court by the CPS worker as part of the agency's petition for temporary custody. During the hearing, Mr. Johnson provided basic education about MBP and its dangers, linking this information to the facts of the case. In both instances, Ms. Cabonilla and Mr. Johnson helped the witnesses to prepare their testimony; through questions Ms. Cabonilla guided the presentation to the court. The court granted the petition.

Mr. Johnson, Ms. Lam, and the CPS investigator were present when Annie was removed from Mrs. Martin's care. In temporary placement with an exemplary and experienced foster family, Annie was initially confused and lonely, but soon began to adjust. Under the care of her pediatrician and a new psychologist, her medications were tapered off. She showed no evidence of seizures, bizarre movements, or inappropriate speech. She needed only a metered dose inhaler ("puffer") to control occasional wheezing. As the dose of steroids came down, her appetite (enthusiastic but not pathological) normalized. The foster mother sparked an interest in healthy food choices to control her weight. Annie sometimes complained of being "too tired" in the mornings, but the foster mother made it clear that this was no reason to miss school.

By the time the case came to court again for the full evidentiary hearing, Annie was thriving in the foster home. She was no longer taking any oral medication, and she could monitor her wheezing and use her inhaler appropriately. There was no evidence of tics or verbal outbursts at home or in school. In the opinion of the foster mother and psychologist, she was a normal but shy and self-conscious twelve-year-old. She showed some harm from the MBP maltreatment: probable bone damage and growth retardation from long use of steroids, poor educational achievement and social skills from being out of school and away from her peer group, nightmares about her life at home (no content related to abuse by her father), and confused sadness whenever she received a phone call from her mother. (All contact was carefully planned and managed in adherence to the visitation guidelines discussed in Chapter 10. In-person visitation was not allowed and phone calls were carefully monitored on both ends.)

During the evidentiary hearing, Mr. Johnson again served as the MBP expert witness. In his testimony, he answered questions he and Ms. Cabonilla had carefully prepared. He provided more extensive MBP education to the court, related the education to the case, and gave his opinion and the rationale that supported it. He also presented MBP-specific detailed case recommendations. The judge ruled that MBP maltreatment had occurred and had manifested as physical and emotional abuse. The judge awarded continued custody to the child protective agency. In the "dispositional" phase of this hearing, CPS requested an order for the recommendations Mr. Johnson had made. The judge approved these recommendations and included them in the court order

Several important events followed the court hearing. First, Mr. Martin and his new wife returned to the community, following notification by Mrs. Martin that "the state had kidnapped Annie." They met with representatives of CPS, Ms. Lam, and Mr. Johnson. Mr. Martin did not comment directly on the MBP, but said that Mrs. Martin's "hypochondria" was a major factor in the divorce. Mr. Martin and his wife said they would welcome Annie into their home. Mr. Martin adamantly denied that he had ever abused her. After a thorough MBP-specific relative assessment (as discussed in Chapter 10), and with the concurrence of the MMT, the child protective placed Annie in the home of her father. On follow-up six months later, Annie remained off oral medication, had no signs of illness, and had missed no days of school.

Mrs. Martin continued to insist that she had done nothing wrong. She had brief interactions with several lawyers, but broke these off when they would not challenge the court's findings. Contrary to the court-ordered case plan and offers of financial assistance, she discontinued psychotherapy when her insurance benefits ran out. Six months after Annie had moved to her father's home, Mrs. Martin called a suicide and crisis line to report that she had taken "every pill in the house," including Annie's leftovers. By the time police arrived, she was dead.

Case Discussion

1. *MBP basic and continuing education:* During this phase of the case, the members of the MMT and the child protective agency needed further education related to managing the case. The attorney, now newly involved in the case, needed basic MBP education.

2. *The case-specific, multiagency-multidisciplinary team (MMT):* The concurrence of the MMT with the expert's opinion and recommendations was a key factor in convincing the court that temporary custody should be awarded to the state, and later in making the decision that placement should be awarded to the father.

3. *The MBP expert:* Mr. Johnson continued to provide information, training, and suggestions following the confirmation of MBP. As an expert witness in the evidentiary hearing, he provided basic education to the court, related theory and information to the case, and rendered opinion. Later he provided detailed case recommendations. This resulted first in foster placement, and later in a court order designed to protect Annie in the long-term. He also advised the MMT as they considered whether Annie should live with her father.

4. *An MBP-educated attorney who is willing to prepare thoroughly for court and related activities, and to work as a team member with the MBP expert and others:* Ms. Cabonilla prepared for, negotiated, and presented the case competently. She participated in the MMT, including its educational sessions. She worked closely with Mr. Johnson in preparing for court and related activities, and on questions that allowed him to present his case clearly and convincingly. She was very willing to learn as well as to contribute.

This case resulted in a good outcome for Annie because the essential elements facilitated a thorough understanding of the situation and teamwork in investigation, court action, and case planning. Each participant in the case had an important role. Two participants, however, deserve special commendation. Ms. Lam's conscientious work as guardian *ad litem* went far beyond what is usually done in this role. She even obtained funds to pay the MBP expert. She remained in contact with Annie and continued to telephone after she was placed in her father's home.

The school nurse's alertness led to concerns, and thus to the truancy petition. Although this case was about far more than truancy, the petition was the means through which Annie's problems were addressed. School personnel had wrestled with the question of referring Annie to court for truancy. It was an unusual step for this elementary school. Preparing the petition took time at the end of a busy school year, and the school district had not always been satisfied with the results of court referrals. Mrs. Martin was furious when told of the referral, and threatened to "report" the principal to the school board. The principal and school nurse worried that they would appear cruel if Annie were truly dying. In the end, they asked themselves a simple question: Would they rather explain to a judge and their own consciences why they took action, or why they did not?

Chapter 9

Initial Postconfirmation Victim
and Case Protection

As shown in the following list, four general tasks must be accomplished when MBP maltreatment is confirmed.

- Risk must be formally assessed.
- The safety of the victim and the integrity of the case must be ensured.
- The victim must be removed from the care, custody, control, and influence of the perpetrator and placed in an approptirate setting.
- The perpetrator must be confronted with case decisions and actions.

INITIAL TASK 1: RISK ASSESSMENT

Although assessing potential risk should be a focus of investigative activity from the time MBP is first suspected, and risk issues may appear obvious, formal risk assessment should occur immediately upon MBP confirmation or provisional confirmation. The first priority must be to protect the victim. Plans for the victim's safety must be individualized, building on knowledge of risks in the specific case. Justification for removal or requests for removal of the victim(s) from the home and restriction of contact—both of which are normally essential for protecting the victim(s) and the case—are developed through the process of risk assessment. Periodic risk assessment is also a major method of measuring case progress over time, functioning as a method of case evaluation.

The concept of risk assessment is familiar in child protection. Many agencies use risk assessment tools that are based on known or hypothesized factors that increase or decrease risk to children. Risk assessment tools developed for other forms of maltreatment, however, are rarely, if ever, appropriate for MBP cases. Their use will result in a false sense of safety because they are based on situations and factors that are irrelevant to MBP. For example, they may contain elements such as "cooperation," "perpetrator/victim dynamics," past CPS involvement, perceived parenting skills, household cleanliness, etc. These are misleading when determining risk in MBP cases. Unless investigators are skilled and knowledgeable regarding MBP, they may take at face value what appears to be true on the surface—for example, a loving relationship, cooperation with the agency, the perpetrator's apparent concern for the child's health, appearance of the house, the ability of the family to support the child financially, the perpetrator's education or ability to say the "right" thing.

The following should be kept in mind when assessing risk to victims of MBP:

1. Risk is not diminished because the perpetrator knows of the suspicions, has been accused, has been caught in the act, or has admitted to the perpetration. Risk to the victim increases under any of these conditions. As already discussed, perpetrators may continue or escalate the MBP maltreatment in an attempt to "prove" that the victim truly has problems. They may also flee or attempt to flee with the victim.
2. Cases that appear to be "only" exaggeration or fabrication should not be perceived to be less dangerous than those cases in which induction has occurred. Serious short- and long-term suffering and even fatalities have occurred with these methods of perpetration. The Sylvia Grant case illustrates this.

Case 9.1

Sylvia Grant, a fifteen-year-old girl, was admitted to the hospital based on her mother's report that she had severe rheumatoid arthritis. She routinely took twenty-two different daily medications, including high doses of steroids and narcotics for pain. Sylvia's mother gave her other drugs on an "as-needed" basis. Ms. Grant said that she had been told Sylvia "did not have long to live," and Sylvia had already taken two trips funded by a wish-granting organization for seriously ill children. She had attended school only ten days in her life.

Sylvia Grant lived for fifteen years as a "dying child." MBP maltreatment began when her mother fabricated her "problem" by falsely presenting symptoms, diagnosis, and treatment recommendations on what appeared to be doctor's letterhead stationery, created by Ms. Grant. At that time, the case involved "only fabrication." It might not have been taken seriously by CPS. Yet, as a result of the fabrication, Sylvia endured fifteen years of physical, emotional, and educational maltreatment as well as medical neglect (that is, failure to provide the care she *should* have received) because of her mother's fabrication. Through the years, Ms. Grant's continuing fabrications and the resulting medications caused extreme harm to Sylvia's body. The treating physician stated that had the MBP maltreatment not been identified, Sylvia would have been dead within six months.

The MBP risk assessment work sheet (appendix to this chapter) should be used from the time of confirmation or provisional confirmation through the entire case. It should be used on an ongoing basis along with the case plan to evaluate progress toward risk reduction. "Unknown" answers suggest a need for further information. The first risk assessment work sheet(s) should be completed when MBP is confirmed or provisionally confirmed. Along with correct MBP education and specific case details, the work sheet can be used to justify removing the victim or requesting authority to remove the victim from the control of the perpetrator. It can also be used during the initial court hearing (sometimes called the "probable cause hearing"), which is almost always held within a few days after the child has been removed.

A risk assessment work sheet should be completed for each victim, suspected victim, possible victim, or potential victim immediately upon confirmation or provisional confirmation of MBP. (Remember that even though one child has been confirmed as an MBP victim, others may also be victims or at risk of becoming victims.) The presence of each potential risk category should be assessed. The team or individual making the risk assessment should then consider whether this category increases risk *in this specific case.* Whatever the answer in the "Risk Increased?" column, the team or individual should be ready to answer, "Why or why not?" For some categories, information will be unknown. Efforts should be made to find out this information. Occasionally, items may not be applicable to the case at hand. Additional sheets should be added to give details of answers or to provide documentation. The risk assessment work sheet should also be used in combination with the recommended case plan components presented in the appendix to Chapter 10.

The specific elements of risk identified in the work sheet are as follows.

1. *MBP maltreatment confirmed, provisionally confirmed, or suspected for person assessed on this work sheet.* This is the starting point for use of the sheet. Regardless of how other questions are answered, a yes here means that the case should be considered at high risk.

2. *Does the person assessed on this work sheet have any special risk characteristics?* This category assesses the victim's vulnerability to the manipulations of the perpetrator. Victims identified so far in the literature or through experience are disproportionately infants and young children, and their inability to "tell" makes them vulnerable. So the victim's age may constitute a special risk characteristic. However, just because a child is old enough to "tell" does not mean that the child is emotionally able to tell or recognizes the manipulation and deception.

Other characteristics may also make a child more vulnerable to manipulation by a perpetrator. Conditions such as mental retardation or physical disability diminish a victim's awareness, credibility, or capacity to evaluate and respond to situations. A child who is very shy or emotionally very close to the perpetrator may not have the capacity to speak up effectively, so this could increase risk. Individual situations may also present other factors that would work against detection of problems.

3. *Is MBP maltreatment confirmed, provisionally confirmed, or suspected for any other person presently or formerly under the perpetrator's care?* If information exists to suggest that MBP perpetration may have extended beyond one child, there is even more reason to fear that the behavior is persistent and ingrained. The assessment of risk to a specific actual or potential victim cannot be done without knowledge of the full context. This item also serves as a reminder that the investigation should not be limited to the identified victim(s). If the possibility of other past and present victims was not considered prior to confirmation or provisional confirmation, it should be done at this point. Any future children born to or in contact with the perpetrator must also be considered at risk.

4. *Has anyone else under the care of the perpetrator died in a manner that was suspicious or never adequately explained?* (See Chapter 5 for a more extended discussion of this as a Suspicion Indicator.) A

history of death(s) among children exposed to the perpetrator, even if these were not identified at the time as suspicious, may suggest that MBP and/or other maltreatment was perpetrated in the past. If this was not considered prior to confirmation or provisional confirmation, it should be addressed at this point. Such a history may also suggest that the perpetrator is capable of using highly dangerous methods, and was not deterred from MBP even by the death of a child.

5. *Has anyone else under the care of the perpetrator experienced unexplained problems?* As with unexplained deaths, the presence of unexplained problems may suggest that MBP and/or other maltreatment has occurred more extensively than has been recognized, and this suggests increased risk. Again, if this was not considered prior to confirmation or provisional confirmation, it should be addressed at this time.

6. *Has there been any other suspicion of MBP maltreatment within the nuclear or extended family?* The investigation may also reveal patterns that raise suspicion of MBP associated with other family members. For example, sometimes the current perpetrator was herself or himself a victim of MBP as a child. Such multigenerational MBP may suggest an even poorer chance that the perpetrator can make significant change in her or his own life.

7. *Have case plan components 1, 3, 4, 5, 6, 7, 8, 9, 10 under Box 10.3 Part A been successfully completed and are 2 and 11 currently occurring?* Attach detailed status of each component. These case plan components are discussed in detail in Chapter 10. They specify gains that a perpetrator must have made in order to be considered safe with a child. These gains include a sincere admission to the pattern of MBP behavior and its impact on the victim(s), and insight into why the behavior occurred and how it can be prevented in the future. The perpetrator should also have cooperated fully and sincerely with CPS in the disclosure of information, in therapy (item 2), and in all other case plan elements (item 11). An attachment to the risk assessment work sheet should provide information about the status of each component of the case plan.

8. *Have case plan components 1 and 3 under Part B in Chapter 10 Appendix been successfully completed and is 2 currently occurring?* Attach detailed status of each component. These case plan components are also discussed in detail in Chapter 10. Components specify that victims and potential victims will have completed a mental health

evaluation to determine their treatment needs (if any), their physical and mental health care is coordinated by one "point of contact" who understands MBP, and that those providing care to the victim (e.g., foster parents) have received education about MBP and information about the case. An attachment to the risk assessment work sheet should provide information about the status of each component of the case plan.

9. *Have case plan components 1, 2, 3, 4, 5, 6, 7 under Part C in Chapter 10 Appendix been successfully completed and is 8 currently occurring?* Attach detailed status of each component. These case plan components are also discussed in detail in Chapter 10. Components specify that any adults having close and consistent contact with the victim(s) understand and believe in the occurrence of the MBP, understand the perpetrator's motivation(s), understand the effect on the victim, and are cooperating with the child protective plan.

If the victim is ultimately to be safe with his or her family of origin, those close to the perpetrator must understand what MBP is, how it occurred, and how serious it is. Without understanding what MBP is, they cannot monitor what is going on with the child. Without understanding how serious MBP is, they will not be motivated to report recurrence of problems, including apparently minor ones. Such reporting is an important safeguard for the victim and other potential victims in the perpetrator's care. This understanding of MBP begins with basic MBP education. An attachment to the risk assessment work sheet should provide information about the status of each component of the case plan.

10. *Is the case being managed as described in Part D of the Appendix to Chapter 10?* Attach detailed status of each component. As discussed in Chapter 10, this part of the case plan speaks to the involvement of the MMT, involvement of a credible MBP expert, selection and role of appropriate therapists for the perpetrator and/or victim(s), appropriate safeguards for any contact between perpetrator and victim(s), and issues affecting placement. This is the agency's portion of the case plan. An attachment to the risk assessment work sheet should provide information about the status of each component of the case plan.

11. *Does the perpetrator continue to say that the exaggerated and/or fabricated and/or induced problem(s) are/were real?* For risk to be reduced, the perpetrator should consistently state that the prob-

lem(s) never existed, or never existed as reported. The MMT can be particularly useful in determining whether the perpetrator is telling different stories to different people. Ultimately, the perpetrator must honestly and sincerely acknowledge that the pattern of MBP perpetration has occurred. A grudging or manipulative agreement, a statement to some people but not others, or the admission of isolated incidents is not enough.

12. *Has the perpetrator been diagnosed with or is the perpetrator suspected of having factitious disorder/Munchausen syndrome?* If the perpetrator exaggerates and/or fabricates and/or induces illness in herself or himself, the problems associated with the case are compounded. A longer time in therapy will probably be required for perpetrators to gain insight into their behavior and bring it under control—if they are ever able to do so. In speaking of the interaction of factitious disorder and factitious disorder by proxy, Ostfeld and Feldman (1996a, p. 84) state, "Because each disorder is a risk factor for the other, the diagnosis may lead to recognition of the other; the mysterious crises in a mother's health may suddenly become understandable when her FDP behavior is detected."

13. *Does the perpetrator have other problems (physical and/or psychological-behavioral/ mental health) that could affect case progress?* As already mentioned, mental health evaluations of MBP perpetrators may be "normal." But if a mental health diagnosis is identified, the task of helping the perpetrator to make meaningful change is even more complex. This is true even if the perpetrator cooperates with treatment. The responsiveness of the mental condition to treatment, and the thought dynamics associated with that condition, will be an important part of therapy and case planning. For example, many perpetrators are depressed, and this illness is often quite responsive to medication and therapy. If the depression contributed to the MBP perpetration, then the risk of recurrence may be less when there is adequate treatment. On the other hand, "personality disorders" are difficult to change and far more resistant to treatment. If the personality disorder contributed to MBP perpetration, then its existence may suggest a poorer prognosis. This does not mean, however, that the mental health problem is the *cause* of the MBP perpetration, or that when specific diagnoses are dealt with the risk of further MBP maltreatment to the victim will be gone.

By the same token, the perpetrator may have or claim to have other problems, such as physical challenges, which also influence risk. For example, the perpetrator might have a physical limitation that makes it difficult to attend therapy or fulfill other elements of the case plan. In such a situation, case progress would clearly be affected and the lack of progress would mean that the victim continues to be at risk.

14. *Does the person evaluated on this work sheet have genuine physical and/or psychological/behavioral/mental health problems that could make monitoring of the case difficult?* If the victim continues to have genuine problems, whether physical or nonphysical, this increases the difficulty of monitoring the situation. For example, suppose a victim has genuine mild asthma, which the perpetrator exaggerated. If the victim returns to the care of the perpetrator, the agency staff and medical personnel will have to make difficult judgments. Are the symptoms being reported real? Are they exaggerated? Has perpetration (whether exaggeration, fabrication, or induction) begun again? Particularly when the problem involves subjective judgments (e.g., complaints of pain), it will be hard for anyone to know what is true and what is false. Thus the presence of these "confounding" true conditions increases the risk to the victim.

15. *Are there any external barriers that might be problematic to case progress?* This criterion requires the assessor to consider the external (e.g., situational, environmental) factors that may affect the perpetrator's and family's ability to receive the help that they need. Availability of transportation, ability to pay for help, insurance coverage, and similar factors are important in allowing people to get assistance. For example, a perpetrator with an unreliable car, living in an area without public transportation, is at a disadvantage in obtaining therapy even if motivated to receive it. Whether friends, relatives, and other helpers are supportive or unsupportive can also influence the case. For example, the availability of a brother to transport the perpetrator might allow services to be received. If the perpetrator has long since "worn out his or her welcome" with the brother, risk to the victim is increased because it is less likely that the perpetrator will receive help.

Factors in the child welfare/mental health systems may also help or hinder adequate services to families. For example, in some areas, community mental health centers are available and well staffed with qualified professionals. In other areas, they are not. Some involved or potentially involved agencies, professionals, and communities are willing to be educated about MBP and receive consultation; others resist. In some areas, there are good relationships among agencies, health care providers, and law enforcement. Such circumstances are part of the resource network within which the perpetrator is to receive treatment. When the environment that should provide help is inadequate, this increases risk to the victim.

16. *Other risk factors and information:* Every case is different. This space on the work sheet is provided for additional information that may be pertinent (such as explanation of some of the risk factors) and for describing other risk conditions that may be part of the situation but are not provided for in the checklist. For example, a perpetrator who is a citizen of a foreign country, and whose passport includes his or her children, would be at high risk of taking the victim(s) beyond the reach of any American court or agency. Such a situation would constitute an additional risk not covered by the categories on the form.

17. *Risk summary statement:* The risk assessment ends with a risk summary. This is a synthesis of the MMT's assessment of the risk in the situation. It should contain the MMT's overall conclusions about the degree of risk and its sources. This summary statement can be useful in court petitions or testimony, in communicating to other professionals as the case plan is executed, and in providing a baseline for future actions and assessments of risk.

18. *Date and signatures:* The risk assessment ends with the date it was prepared and the signature, title, and agency affiliation of the person preparing it. The signatures and agencies of those who have reviewed the information and concur should also be added. If this is done, the risk assessment becomes even stronger for legal or planning purposes.

When prepared carefully and used in conjunction with the case plan, this risk assessment work sheet can be a powerful tool in protecting the victim throughout the life of the case. A case example, with a risk assessment work sheet, follows.

Case 9.1, continued
    When Sylvia Grant was admitted to the hospital, her care was assigned to Dr. Murphy, who had not treated her before. His physical examination showed that she was very weak and had wasted muscles. She moved only with difficulty, guarding her joints. Dr. Murphy was extremely concerned

about the number and types of her medications. He contacted physicians identified by the mother as having taken care of Sylvia previously, but could find none who had ever said that she was terminally ill. Several doctors said that when they had suggested reducing some medications, Sylvia and Ms. Grant had not returned for follow-up. None of the physicians was aware of the number of other health care professionals who had been or were treating Sylvia, or of the number and kinds of medications Sylvia had been taking.

Dr. Murphy was familiar with MBP. He made a report of MBP suspicion to CPS, and an initial MMT meeting was convened two hours later. The MMT strongly concurred that secret video and audio surveillance should be conducted. Sylvia was moved to the special hospital room equipped for this purpose. This could be done without a court order since the hospital's standard consent for admission, signed by Ms. Grant, included a provision that that anyone could be audio- and videotaped within the facility as a diagnostic procedure. Videotapes revealed Ms. Grant telling Sylvia that she "knew" Sylvia was in unbearable pain, even though Sylvia was exhibiting no signs of pain. Ms. Grant encouraged Sylvia to request more drugs from the nurses and to tell them how much pain she was in. Ms. Grant was deliberately fabricating the pain and inducing pain-related behavior (e.g., Sylvia telling staff that she was in unbearable pain and needed medication, when this was not true). Ms. Grant also made telephone calls to Sylvia's grandparents in which she said that Dr. Murphy had predicted that Sylvia would be "crippled for life." Dr. Murphy had said nothing that could be interpreted this way, and so this was another instance of fabrication.

Based on the videotape and other information that had been obtained, and with the strong recommendation of the MMT, a provisional MBP confirmation was made. (It was considered provisional because, at the time, information was still being gathered.) A protective order was successfully obtained through family court. The order placed Sylvia in the temporary custody of CPS and denied physical or verbal contact with Sylvia to anyone except specifically identified professionals. Dr. Murphy immediately began weaning Sylvia off the medications.

Over the next few weeks the MMT continued to meet, and a full investigation followed. It was discovered that when Sylvia was an infant, just after her parents separated, Ms. Grant created letterhead stationery and wrote a memorandum apparently from a pediatrician. This stated that Sylvia had severe arthritis and recommended aggressive treatment. Ms. Grant took the letter to a pediatrician in a city to which she and Sylvia had just moved. She told the new physician that the former doctor had died in a fire and that all of Sylvia's records had been destroyed. The new physician accepted the letter and began to treat Sylvia accordingly. Thus, Sylvia's fabricated history began. It was compounded, with the assistance of unsuspecting health care professionals, for the next fifteen years as each new professional accepted the "diagnosis" and apparent ongoing symptoms unquestioningly. Based on a thorough investigation and confirmation/disconfirmation process, MBP was fully confirmed.

Dr. Murphy later stated his belief that, without intervention, Sylvia would have been dead within six months due to the kind and variety of medications she was receiving. Instead, six months later, Sylvia was off all her medications and attending school daily. It was determined that she did not have—and had never had—arthritis.

The risk assessment work sheet for Sylvia Grant (appendix to this chapter) was done at the time of the provisional confirmation, and before Ms. Grant was confronted. Throughout the life of the case, these answers will change.

INITIAL TASK 2: PROTECTING THE VICTIM AND THE CASE

MBP victims should not remain with or have anything but the most strictly supervised contact with perpetrators, or with anyone who might be influenced by the perpetrator. This statement may be harsh, but experience validates it. Appropriate protective custody is the only effective means of protecting the victim and keeping the court case free of "tainting." Perpetrators are even more dangerous when they realize they are suspected, and may continue—or escalate—perpetration in an attempt to "prove" the victim's problems even if CPS or others are monitoring closely. The risk that they will take the child and flee is also particularly high. Even if the perpetrator appears to take responsibility for his or her actions, there are too many uncertainties in the situation to predict what the perpetrator will do. This is true even if the other parent, relatives, etc., are in the home and promise to supervise the situation. Even daily contact by a monitoring agency cannot ensure the victim's safety.

Nor can safety be ensured if the victim is in the hospital but remains accessible to the perpetrator. Exaggeration, fabrication, and induction of problems occur frequently in hospitals. Even constant supervision by hospital staff in the room is not necessarily sufficient to guarantee the victim's safety. For example, one parent concealed pills in her mouth, and pushed them into the child's mouth during a kiss. Perpetrators are skilled manipulators and deceivers. Hospitals are designed to deliver health care, and hospital personnel are largely health care professionals. Neither the institution's design nor the professionals' training equips them for the kind of intense surveillance and protection of patients that is required in MBP cases. Hospitals will do all they can to protect children, but without legal authority they cannot limit parents' access or prevent legal guardians from removing a child. Preventive action should be taken so that the hospital, police, and/or child protective agency are not required to deal with a crisis.

It is also not safe for the *case* if perpetrators or those who might be influenced by them continue to have contact with victims. Separating the victim through protective custody and appropriate out-of-home placement is the only way to safeguard the case from potential contamination by the perpetrator. If the perpetrator has contact with the victim and successfully fabricates or induces without being detected, it will appear that the child really does have the symptoms. Fabrication or induction can happen indirectly through verbal or physical cues and through other people, as well as directly. One of the most powerful means of confirming, continuing to confirm, or refuting the presence of MBP is through separating the victim and suspected or confirmed perpetrator. Insuring the integrity of this process is of the utmost importance if both victim and case are to be protected.

Case 9.1, continued

For example, consider again the case of Sylvia, presented earlier in the chapter. Suppose that Sylvia was placed in foster care. The primary purpose of this placement is, of course, to protect Sylvia from her mother. But an important secondary purpose of the placement is to continue to evaluate Sylvia's health status, including whether Sylvia needs her medications. The MMT's belief is that Sylvia does not have rheumatoid arthritis. However, they acknowledge that there is a chance they could be wrong.

Suppose that, while in placement and off her medications, Sylvia only became sicker. This would lead all professionals involved in the case to consider whether a mistake had been made. Testing for medical disorders would probably begin again. It might well be decided that MBP was not occurring. Sylvia would probably be returned to her mother—as ought to happen if maltreatment is not occurring.

Now suppose that Sylvia was in placement, but was able to receive telephone calls or letters from her mother, or others who were sympathetic to her mother. It would be very easy for someone to "cue" Sylvia to complain about pain. There might be subtle reminders of how lonely the mother was without Sylvia, and how "you know how to come home if you really want to." If Sylvia's joints then began to "hurt" again, it would look as though she has a true medical illness. The integrity of the case would not have been protected. Because of that, Sylvia herself would not have been protected from further maltreatment.

Relatives, friends, or neighbors may also attempt to exaggerate, fabricate, or induce to help the perpetrator. Their actions may be deliberate or unwitting. They may be sincere in their belief that the perpetrator has done nothing wrong and is being unfairly accused by the "authorities." If they have access to the victim or knowledge of where the victim is, they may give messages (personally or via telephone), medications, or gifts, etc. Because these may be dangerous to the victim and/or "taint" the case, separation from the perpetrator must also include these people.

INITIAL TASK 3: REMOVING THE VICTIM FROM THE CARE, CUSTODY, CONTROL, AND INFLUENCE OF THE PERPETRATOR; PLACEMENT IN AN APPROPRIATE SETTING

Ideally, children should be taken into protective custody, pending full investigation, as soon as MBP is seriously suspected. Realistically, however, placement at the time of first suspicion is often impossible. Judges are usually reluctant to remove a child without strong indication that maltreatment has occurred and/or that probable cause exists to believe the child is at substantial risk. Even so, the MMT should request removal (and document the request) if they feel that the situation justifies it. Removal should certainly occur if MBP is confirmed.

Protective authority in MBP cases is obtained through the same statutory processes as with other forms of child maltreatment. Steps to take the victim into protective custody vary according to the jurisdiction. In some cases, CPS or law enforcement may have the right to make the decision themselves and take the child into protective custody. In other jurisdictions, a judge or other designated court official must grant a request for the child to be taken into custody.

If removal of the child involves a judge, other court official, or the police, the person(s) requesting protective authority must be ready to explain the specifics of the situation. They must provide education about MBP and the dangers of continued contact, give convincing reasons why removal is necessary, and provide recommendations and rationale if a court order is necessary.

Access to the victim and other children who have been taken into custody must be limited to specifically identified CPS staff, law enforcement officers, and health care providers. As already discussed, there should be no visitation or contact with the perpetrator, other parent, relatives, or anyone else except involved and specifically identified professionals. If, in spite of recommendations, contact must occur during this initial period, the guidelines described in Chapter 10 must be followed.

As a general rule, protective custody will be taken or sought without notifying the perpetrator or others likely to inform the perpetrator. Once the child is safe, the parent should be confronted with the suspicions and the action that has been taken. If there are other children in the home, they should be included in the removal action. Even if removal of other children is not possible under local guidelines, or if authority to remove is not granted, carefully document that the appropriate official attempts were made and why removal was not possible. All children in the home should be considered at high risk, even if they do not appear to be maltreated. MBP perpetrators may victimize children serially (one child at a time) or concurrently (several children at the same time). When the first identified victim is removed, other children in the home are at increased risk. Special attention is warranted if the perpetrator is pregnant or becomes pregnant during case supervision, as the new baby will be at risk of MBP maltreatment.

Managing Removal and Placement in an Appropriate Setting

If the victim is in the hospital when protective authority is received, appropriate hospital staff (often the social worker or nurse responsible for the child) should be notified as quickly as possible. The hospital representative can then notify the attending physician, hospital security, and the appropriate hospital unit. An entry should be made in the medical chart, and perhaps a cautionary sticker or note should be placed on the front of the chart, if hospital policy allows. The following steps will increase safety in the hospital after protective custody is taken:

- Ensure receipt of the protective custody order by the appropriate hospital representative.
- Place the child in a different room under an assumed name.

- Consider perpetrator safety.
- Consider staff safety and well-being.
- Inform the child about the placement if old enough to understand.

1. *Official documentation of protective custody should be immediately faxed or delivered to the appropriate hospital representative.* This representative should ensure placement of copies as appropriate in the child's medical chart, with the hospital's legal or risk management department, etc., as required by hospital policy. Involved or potentially involved hospital staff should be notified of the situation, where the documentation is located, and what to do in case of an emergency. The child protective agency should also provide any other necessary instructions at this time.

2. *The child should be placed in a different room under an assumed name (most hospitals have a procedure for this) and should be placed on "no information" status.* Only authorized persons should be allowed to receive information about the victim. This means that, even if someone discovers the assumed name, he or she cannot call the hospital's patient information service to learn about the child's condition or room assignment. A password is a good precaution to allow only authorized persons to receive the information they need; MBP perpetrators could impersonate child protective or other personnel.

3. *Perpetrator safety should also be considered by the MMT or other planning group.* Perpetrators frequently are or appear to be depressed. When they learn that the child has been taken into CPS custody, they may develop or present with apparent mental and/or physical health problems. They may threaten or hint at suicide—saying, for example, "I can't live without my child." It is impossible to know whether such talk represents a true desire to die, an exaggeration, an idle threat, or a plan to make an attention-getting gesture. Although it can be difficult to sympathize with perpetrators, they may be in genuine distress. As much as possible, their welfare should be protected. Liability is also reduced if mental and physical health consultation is offered to perpetrators. The perpetrator's statements and the response of involved professionals should be documented. Even if perpetrators do not report mental health symptoms or make self-destructive state-

ments, they should be offered the opportunity to talk with a mental health professional. This offer and the perpetrator's response should be documented.

4. *Staff safety and well-being should also be considered.* If it is possible that someone may attempt to retaliate against the personnel associated with the placement, security or the police should be contacted. Staff who are closely involved in the case or who have been close to the perpetrator may wish to consider whether their home address is known or publicly listed. They may need to alert their family members, building security, or doorman, etc.

The whole process of taking custody and confronting the perpetrator may be difficult or upsetting for hospital staff. They may have believed in the perpetrator and feel betrayed; they may still believe in her or his innocence. MBP education, debriefing, or even counseling may be necessary to staff who are upset about the situation and need to understand it better. If well-informed about MBP and not enmeshed with the perpetrator, the hospital social worker probably can offer or coordinate this assistance. It would also be an appropriate role for a consultant psychiatrist or psychologist familiar with MBP who is able to work collegially with hospital staff.

5. *If the child is old enough to understand language, he or she should be informed about the placement.* A trusted person should explain that the caregiver must be gone for a while, or give another reason that will make sense to the child. If the child is older, a full and more truthful explanation may be appropriate.

If the child is not in the hospital when protective authority is received, removal from the perpetrator's custody requires careful planning. The goal is to minimize risk to all participants, to pave the way for the later confrontation interview, and to minimize the chance of a "scene" that may involve parents, friends, relatives, neighbors, etc. The removal can be accomplished best in a neutral setting. One might think that this would be more frightening to the child, since children often fear being taken where parents will be unable to find them. However, it may be less traumatic than forcible removal from the arms of a parent who is or appears to be hysterical. If the child attends school or day care, removal can occur there. A general explanation for the action and the choice of site should be given, in keeping with rules of confidentiality.

If there is no naturally occurring neutral setting, someone can ask the parent to bring the child to the CPS office, clinic, or hospital. A minimum of information should be given about the purpose of this contact. Perpetrators should not be told that the purpose of the visit is to remove the child from their custody. Nor should they be asked to bring the child's belongings.

If the child must be removed from the home itself, this should be planned to minimize the chance of a "scene." The contact should be kept short and there should be no attempt to argue. Court documents can be presented and the decision and next steps stated. Involved professionals should move briskly and convey a need for quick action—"we need to leave now." The perpetrator should not be given time to pack a suitcase or engage in other delaying activities. If the child is on medications, they should be requested for possible use as evidence. A new supply should be obtained for the child's use, however, and medications from home should not be used because of the risk of tampering. The child's belongings can be brought when the perpetrator and CPS staff member meet together to discuss what has happened (the confrontation interview). This confrontation interview should be held as quickly as possible so that the family understands what has happened and why.

The victim must be placed initially in a neutral environment for protection, observation, and monitoring. Whether the child remains in the hospital or is placed in a foster home depends on the case specifics. A monitoring and evaluation plan should be developed. The attending physician, lead mental health professional in a psychological/behavioral case, and MBP consultant should be involved in and integral to the formation of this plan. Depending on the circumstances, the child may remain hospitalized, placed in another medical or mental health inpatient setting, placed in a foster home, or moved from one setting to another. A neutral environment cannot be accomplished when the child is placed with the nonoffending spouse or relatives. Consideration of placement with the nonabusive parent, friends, neighbors, or relatives requires specialized activities beyond those appropriate with other kinds of child maltreatment (see Chapter 10). It may be appropriate as a long-term plan, but not in the initial case stages. People with emotional ties to the perpetrator or victim rarely believe or understand the maltreatment that has taken place, and are subject to the perpetrator's manipulations. No matter how sincere they may seem, they cannot be relied upon, at least early in the case, to protect the victim and follow instructions.

When their health allows, MBP victims should be placed initially in an agency foster home. The foster placement must be carefully selected not only with regard to care and protection of the child, but of the case as well. The foster parents should be considered as key potential court witnesses, able to testify regarding the victim's condition and behavior while in their care. In an MBP case, foster parents are usually much more involved than in other kinds of child maltreatment. Foster home selection, activities, and guidelines include the following:

> • At least initially, use foster parents who have a proven track record of cooperation with the agency and careful adherence to guidelines and instructions.
> • The foster parents should have the knowledge and skills necessary to care for the victim.
> • The foster parents should be good observers and capable of providing clear written and verbal documentation and communication.
> • Prior to the victim's placement in the foster home, the foster parents should receive at least basic MBP education and detailed case information.
> • The foster parents should receive specific instructions for child care and monitoring activities.
> • There should be absolutely no contact between the victim, foster family, and perpetrator, nonoffending parent, relatives, or friends. The whereabouts of the foster home should not be divulged.

1. *The foster parents should have the knowledge and skills necessary to care for the victim.* In MBP cases, the knowledge and skills necessary to care for child victims often go beyond those normally expected of foster parents. For example, detailed observation and logging of the victim's behavior and health are necessary. Ability to follow medical regimens or learn to use medical equipment may be required. When the victim is first placed, it is impossible to know the extent of the problem(s). They may fall anywhere on a continuum between nonexistent to every bit as serious as the perpetrator has claimed. The MMT has acted on its best assessment of the child's

problems, but there is always the possibility that they are wrong. The agency and foster family need to be prepared for the possibility, even if remote, that the child's problems are more serious than has been estimated. Therefore, a plan needs to be developed prior to placement for all case participants to understand how to assess and respond to any problems the child has been alleged or seems to have. The foster parents need to understand their part in this plan thoroughly.

2. *Foster parents should have a proven track record of cooperation with the agency and careful adherence to the guidelines and instructions given to them.* Compliance with required observation, logging, health care, court orders, and agency instructions must be ensured.

3. *Foster parents should be good observers and capable of providing clear written and verbal documentation and communication.* Their observations, writing, and testimony may be needed in court or as a basis for court actions.

4. *Prior to the victim's placement in the foster home, the foster parents should receive at least basic MBP education and detailed case information.* This should include at least the definition of MBP, an explanation of what it is and why it is dangerous child maltreatment, and perpetrator-consistent characteristics. This information should be communicated clearly and in person, not simply through handouts or articles. Detailed information should be given about the case, the perpetrator, and how or why it is believed that MBP maltreatment has been perpetrated. This information forms the basis for the foster parents' understanding of why the guidelines and instructions they are given are so important. With this understanding, they will be more likely to comply and to deal correctly with unexpected situations.

5. *The foster parents should receive specific instructions for child care and monitoring activities.* This would include such things as administering and logging medications, administering and logging treatments, special diet restrictions, and permissible activities. Each case is different and will require different instructions. A daily running record (log) should be kept and include:

- the child's general condition (activity level, emotions, etc.);
- the presence or absence of problems (especially the problems reported by the perpetrator), and whether these are observed by the foster parent, observed by others, or reported by the victim;

- medications taken, particularly those being tapered or those given at the request of the victim; and
- "critical" or "key" incidents that may reflect on the presence or absence of problems, the victim's state of mind, or how the ex-aggeration/ fabrication/ induction was accomplished. For exam-ple, in the case of Sylvia it would be important for the foster parent to note if she complained of pain primarily when she was homesick and talking about her mother.

These data can show trends such as the disappearance of problems, the lack of necessity for medications, etc. In paying attention to symp-toms and logging, however, foster parents should be "matter-of-fact" and "low-key" to avoid reinforcing the child's symptoms through at-tention.

6. *There should be absolutely no contact between the victim, foster family, and perpetrator, nonoffending parent, relatives, or friends, at least in the early stages of the case.* Whereabouts of the foster home should not be disclosed. If the perpetrator and/or others on her or his "side" know where the child is placed, attempts may be made to manipulate the victim and foster family, harass them, raise false alle-gations, or even remove the child. Efforts by any of these people to contact the foster parents should be immediately documented and re-ported to the child protective agency. The foster parents should not be asked to transport the child to visits or anywhere else that they might encounter the perpetrator or victim's family.

INITIAL TASK 4: THE POSTCONFIRMATION/ CONFRONTATION INTERVIEW

Once MBP maltreatment has been confirmed or provisionally con-firmed and the protective action is in place for the victim (and poten-tial victims if possible), a confrontation interview with the perpetra-tor must take place immediately. This quick action is a matter of justice, is legally necessary, and may reduce the possibility of the per-petrator involving others in the deception. The purpose of the con-frontation interview is to discuss the MBP allegations, inform the perpetrator that the child is now in protective custody, and explain what official activities will follow. In addition, this may be the last or only time that an interview with the perpetrator will be possible. (She or he is likely to obtain an attorney, who will probably advise not talking to the authorities.) Therefore, it is important to make the most of the opportunity that this interview provides to obtain as much information as possible.

General Recommendations

The confrontation interview should be planned strategically. Recommendations and planning for the confrontation interview include:

- Ensure victim safety before the confrontation interview.
- Attempt to ensure other children in home are safe, and document this.
- Plan the interview carefully.
- Use a neutral setting with complete privacy, freedom from interruption, and security available.
- Interview the perpetrator by himself or herself.
- Keep the number of people attending to a minimum, but include: the CPS investigator, the key physical or mental health professional who agrees with the confirmation/provisional confirmation the professional who confirmed/provisionally confirmed MBP, the hospital social worker or another hospital representative if the victim is hospitalized, the MBP maltreatment expert, and law enforcement if involved and they wish to attend.
- Know what the next steps will be and how they will be handled.
- Plan how to get the perpetrator to the confrontation interview alone.
- Plan who will attend the interview, and what the role of each person will be. Decide who will chair the interview. Finalize the sequence of activities.
- Plan what information might be obtained from the perpetrator before informing her or him about the MBP confirmation.
- Plan what will be said to inform the perpetrator about the MBP confirmation.
- Plan what will be said to inform the perpetrator that the child has been taken into protective custody.
- Have mental health assistance present or on standby (for immediate needs only).
- Discuss what to expect from the suspected perpetrator's behavior during confrontation; consider the suspected perpetrator's welfare and safety.

- Obtain agreement that, after confrontation, the suspected perpetrator will not be allowed to "say good-bye."
- Plan how to ensure that the perpetrator leaves the property promptly after the end of the interview.

The confrontation interview should take place in a neutral setting that offers complete privacy, freedom from interruption, and the availability of security. In accordance with good investigative practice, the perpetrator should be interviewed alone. If the interview is conducted in the hospital, the session should take place away from patients and visitors. If conducted outside the hospital, the setting should be businesslike. The CPS office may be used. A physician's or mental health professional's office is usually less satisfactory because of close quarters and the presence of other people, but may sometimes be necessary because of the professional's schedule.

When the perpetrator is asked to attend the interview, only a general reason for the meeting should be conveyed; e.g., "to clarify some issues regarding your child's condition." A strategy should be developed so that the suspected perpetrator comes to the interview by herself or himself. When alone, the suspected perpetrator may give different answers than she or he would give in front of others. If present, others may also try to answer questions or take over the discussion. Part of the investigation is a comparison of the perpetrator's statements with other information. If the perpetrator is present when others are interviewed, it may influence their comments. This can occur because of either verbal or nonverbal interactions.

The number of other persons attending should be kept to a minimum, depending on the situation. The child/victim should not be present. Participants in the confrontation are detailed in the list at the beginning of this section.

Law enforcement may or may not want to attend. If law enforcement chooses to interview the suspected perpetrator separately, this should be done after the confrontation. The police may or may not be planning to arrest the suspected perpetrator. Even if they wish to interview separately or arrest, law enforcement should be given an opportunity to participate in the confrontation interview.

A mental health professional should be available for crisis intervention or consultation as needed regarding general and immediate mental health issues. For example, the perpetrator may become, or may appear to become, extremely depressed and agitated, stating, "I can't live another day without my child." A mental status evaluation and determination as to whether the perpetrator should be involuntarily transported to a mental health facility would need to be discussed, and acted upon as needed. The presence of the mental health professional increases safety for the suspected perpetrator, and reduces potential liability for the agency/facility holding the interview. This mental health professional will not necessarily have ongoing clinical responsibility for the perpetrator. Unless the mental health professional has received basic MBP education and has served as part of the MMT to date he or she should not become involved in the case itself.

Security should be available outside the interview room. The perpetrator may become agitated or even violent. Security may also be necessary to escort the perpetrator off the premises at the end of the interview.

Those planning or participating in the confrontation interview should think strategically. They should know how the confrontation interview relates to the overall safety plan for the victim(s), and to building and protecting the case against the perpetrator. They should know what the next steps will be following the confrontation—usually further legal action and (if the legal action is successful) long-term case planning, care, and treatment for the victim(s).

Steps in the Confrontation Interview

The interview should begin with a general introduction of persons present and the general purpose of the meeting. Typically, the person chairing the session might say, "we are here to discuss your child's situation." The following steps have been shown to work well:

- Introduce the people present.
- State a *general* purpose for the interview, e.g., "to discuss your child's situation."
- Review the "history" of the problem.
- Ask the perpetrator questions to gain additional information, as planned in advance.

- Inform the perpetrator that MBP has been confirmed. Do not argue.
- Inform the perpetrator that the victim(s) is/are in protective custody, and provide information and documentation.
- Express concern for the perpetrator and offer assistance. Involve a mental health professional if necessary.
- Do not allow a "good-bye" between the perpetrator and victim(s).
- Escort the perpetrator to transportation and ensure that she or he leaves the property.

1. *Depending on the victim's problems, the physician, mental health professional, or MBP expert gives a review of the victim's past situation ("history").* This may be framed around the idea that the child's problems have been complicated and confusing. This first phase of the interview is a good time to ask the suspected perpetrator a variety of questions. The purpose of these questions may be to gain new information, to check previous information, or to assess consistency of the story over time. The person who has presented the review of the history should ask these questions, and inquire if any of the other professionals have any additional questions. Some questions that might be used are:

- Are there any providers not mentioned who have had substantive contact with the child?
- Has the child undergone any procedures not mentioned?
- Does the perpetrator have anything to add in the way of ideas about the cause of the problem, or the things that have made it better or worse, even if these ideas are different from those that have been considered so far?
- What does the perpetrator believe would help the child at this point?
- What are the perpetrator's and family's attitudes toward the problem? How have they adapted to the presence of the problem?

Questioning should be done early in the interview because, once the suspected perpetrator is told about the suspicions, she or he may cease giving information. Questioning can, of course, occur at any point in the interview. The most important questions, however, should be asked at the beginning.

2. *The previous questioning leads to the conclusion that MBP or MBP-like behavior has occurred, and the reasons for this conclusion.* MBP as a term may or may not be used. The speaker might say that "it seems that you want _____ to have problems," or may simply describe the suspected perpetrator's behaviors. The presentation should be succinct, careful, and reasonable.

3. *The CPS investigator then explains that the child has been taken into protective custody.* Information should be given about what to expect while the child is in placement (e.g., upcoming court hearings, contact with the child as discussed in Chapter 10, etc.), and the next steps in the process. Any legally required documents should be provided. The perpetrator can be told that additional information will be gathered during the time the child is in placement, and that it is possible that the separation may produce information that is valuable to the perpetrator.

4. *Although the focus has been on the victim, the meeting should close with an expression of concern for the suspected perpetrator.* The interviewer can recognize with the perpetrator that this is a very upsetting charge. The suspected perpetrator should be asked how she or he is feeling, how she or he is going to get home, where her or his spouse/partner is and how that person is likely to feel about the situation, whether she or he would like to talk to a mental health professional, etc. These questions and the perpetrator's responses should be carefully documented. This part of the interview should not be prolonged, however, and the focus at the end of the meeting should be getting the perpetrator on her or his way. The perpetrator should be escorted to her or his car (or other means of transportation) to ensure that she or he has left the property.

Suspected perpetrators often ask to see the victim "one last time," to "say good-bye" before separation or placement. This is not advisable. It offers another opportunity for problem creation and attention getting through "grandstanding"—manipulation of the victim, hospital personnel, or bystanders. The suspected perpetrator may offer promises, but cannot be trusted to keep them. If the suspected perpetrator has belongings (e.g., a purse) with the child, or there is another reason to return to the child's room, someone else should take care of this. The perpetrator should not be left alone until it is certain she or he is off the premises. Security or law enforcement, if available, may be involved if there is concern that departure will not be quiet and prompt.

The confrontation interview may take a short period of time, or may last several hours, depending on how much each speaker has to say and to what extent the suspected perpetrator wishes to respond. During the confrontation interview, the suspected perpetrator will almost always continue to exhibit perpetrator-consistent characteristics. The perpetrator may attempt to argue with the conclusions/decisions, and may make dire predictions of the "harm" that will result from this "terrible mistake." It will be useless to counter these assertions or try to convince the perpetrator of the suspicions or that placement is necessary. The perpetrator's explanations or pleas will not make a difference in what has been decided and done. However, those present will want to hear what the perpetrator has to say. The perpetrator's state of mind, receptiveness to help, or future strategies might be revealed by statements such as, "Without him I have nothing to live for" (suggests possible suicide risk), or, "I know why you're doing this—you're frustrated because you can't find out what's wrong!" (suggests that the perpetrator remains closed to insight/help, and may use this assertion later in court as a defense tactic).

The suspected perpetrator may be very emotional (crying, angry), or may show little emotion. One set of emotions may be shown in the interview room, but an entirely different set may be shown outside when the perpetrator is caught off guard or is unaware of being observed. For example, the perpetrator may be crying and appear to be upset. She or he asks to go to the rest room. After a few minutes, the social worker goes to the rest room and finds the perpetrator laughing and talking animatedly on a cell phone. Any of these emotions may be genuine or feigned. The suspected perpetrator's behavior may be calculated; it is very possible that she or he anticipated the confrontation and planned responses.

If the perpetrator has a history of factitious disorder/Munchausen syndrome, or a pattern of creating dramatic events, these may occur during the confrontation interview. For example, a suspected perpetrator with a pattern of "hysterical" fainting may do this during the confrontation or while being escorted off the premises. Knowledge of the perpetrator's patterns will allow the team to plan responses to such situations. For example, a physician could check the perpetrator briefly after she or he has fainted, rather than sending her or him to the emergency room, which would delay departure, gain sympathy and attention, and increase the risk that she or he might discover something about the victim's whereabouts.

Perpetrators almost always deny the MBP perpetration. Admissions, if made at all, usually concern only what they have been caught doing, and usually include justifications. They may answer questions with questions and attempt to steer the conversation off the subject, or make statements that no one can prove or disprove. It may be difficult to resist this manipulation. Seemingly plausible reasons for behavior will probably be given. The suspected perpetrator may appear so believable that interviewers find themselves wondering if a mistake has been made. Preparation, reliance on the team and process, and a clear sense of what is to be accomplished will help the interviewers stay on track. The professionals involved in the confrontation will need time afterward to discuss, debrief, and engage in planning for the next steps.

Confronting an MBP perpetrator is a difficult task. It can be emotionally draining. But with preparation and teamwork, this essential and inevitable step can be accomplished successfully.

APPENDIX:
MUNCHAUSEN BY PROXY RISK ASSESSMENT
WORK SHEET

Sample Work Sheet

Note: This work sheet should be completed when MBP maltreatment has been confirmed or provisionally confirmed. A work sheet should be completed for each victim or potential victim. Attach additional sheets to give details of answers. This work sheet should be used in combination with the case plan components document.

Date prepared: _____

Name of person assessed on this work sheet:

_____

Date of birth: _____

MBP maltreatment is (circle one):   confirmed   provisionally confirmed

                                      suspected   not suspected at present

Confirmed/Provisionally Confirmed Perpetrator:

Name _____

Relationship of perpetrator to the person assessed on this work sheet:

_____

	RISK FACTOR	Present? (circle)	Risk Increased? (circle)	UNK. or N/A (circle)*
1.	MBP maltreatment confirmed, provisionally confirmed, or suspected for person assessed on this work sheet.	Yes No	Yes No	Unk. N/A
2.	Does the person assessed on this work sheet have any special risk characteristics?	Yes No	Yes No	Unk. N/A

3.	Is MBP maltreatment confirmed, provisionally confirmed, or suspected for any other person presently or formerly under the suspected perpetrator's care?	Yes No	Yes No	Unk. N/A
4.	Has anyone else under the care of the perpetrator died in a manner that was suspicious or never adequately explained?	Yes No	Yes No	Unk. N/A
5.	Has anyone else under the care of the perpetrator experienced unexplained problems?	Yes No	Yes No	Unk. N/A
6.	Has there been any other suspicion of MBP maltreatment within the nuclear or extended family?	Yes No	Yes No	Unk N/A
7.	Have case plan components 1,3,4,5,6,7,8,9,10 under Ch. 10 Appendix Part A, MBP Perpetrator been successfully completed and are 2 and 11 currently occurring? Attach detailed status of each component.	Yes No	Yes No	Unk. N/A
8.	Have case plan components 1 and 3 under Ch. 10 Appendix Part B, Victims and Potential Victims been successfully completed and is 2 currently occurring? Attach detailed status of each component.	Yes No	Yes No	Unk. N/A
9.	Have case plan components 1,2,3,4,5,6,7 under Ch. 10 Appendix Part C, Non-Offending Spouse/Other Adults been successfully completed and is 8 currently occurring? Attach detailed status of each component.	Yes No	Yes No	Unk. N/A
10.	Is case being managed as described in Ch. 10 Appendix Part D, Case Management? Attach detailed status of each component.	Yes No	Yes No	Unk. N/A

11.	Does the perpetrator continue to say that the exaggerated and/or fabricated and/or induced problems are/were real?	Yes No	Yes No	Unk. N/A
12.	Has the perpetrator been diagnosed with or is the perpetrator suspected of having factitious disorder/Munchausen syndrome?	Yes No	Yes No	Unk. N/A
13.	Does the perpetrator have other problems (physical and/or psychological/behavioral/mental health) that could affect case progress?	Yes No	Yes No	Unk. N/A
14.	Does the person evaluated on this work sheet have genuine physical and/or psychological/behavioral/mental health problems that could make monitoring of the case difficult?	Yes No	Yes No	Unk. N/A
15.	Are there any external barriers that might be problematic to case progress?	Yes No	Yes No	Unk. N/A

*Unk. = unknown; N/A = not applicable

Other Risk Factors and Information:

_____
_____
_____
_____
_____

Risk Summary Statement:

_____
_____
_____
_____
_____

Prepared by: _____

Title: _____

Agency: _____

Concurring:

Signature   Agency

_____   _____

_____   _____

_____   _____

_____   _____

_____   _____

BP Risk Assessment Work Sheet for Sylvia Grant

Note: This work sheet should be completed when MBP maltreatment has been confirmed or provisionally confirmed. A work sheet should be completed for each victim or potential victim. Attach additional sheets to give details of answers. This work sheet should be used in combination with the case plan components document.

Date prepared:_____1/17/02_____

Name of person assessed on this work sheet: __Sylvia Grant_____

Date of birth: _____4/28/88_____

MBP maltreatment is (circle one):confirmed (provisionally confirmed)

                                  suspected   not suspected at present

Confirmed/Provisionally Confirmed Perpetrator:

Name <u>Lilah Grant</u>

Relationship of perpetrator to the person assessed on this work sheet:

_____mother____

	RISK FACTOR	Present? (circle)	Risk Increased? (circle)	UNK. or N/A (circle)*
1.	MBP maltreatment confirmed, provisionally confirmed, or suspected for person assessed on this work sheet.	**Yes** No	**Yes** No	Unk. N/A
2.	Does the person assessed on this work sheet have any special risk characteristics?	**Yes** No	**Yes** No	Unk. N/A
3.	Is MBP maltreatment confirmed, provisionally confirmed, or suspected for any other person presently or formerly under the suspected perpetrator's care?	Yes **No**	Yes **No**	Unk. N/A
4.	Has anyone else under the care of the perpetrator died in a manner that was suspicious or never adequately explained?	Yes **No**	Yes **No**	Unk. N/A
5.	Has anyone else under the care of the perpetrator experienced unexplained problems?	Yes **No**	Yes **No**	Unk. N/A

6.	Has there been any other suspicion of MBP maltreatment within the nuclear or extended family?	Yes No	Yes No	(Unk.) N/A
7.	Have case plan components 1,3,4,5,6,7,8,9,10 under Ch. 10 Appendix Part A, MBP Perpetrator been successfully completed and are 2 and 11 currently occurring? Attach detailed status of each component.	Yes (No)	(Yes) No	Unk. N/A
8.	Have case plan components 1 and 3 under Ch. 10 Appendix Part B, Victims and Potential Victims been successfully completed and is 2 currently occurring? Attach detailed status of each component.	Yes (No)	(Yes) No	Unk. N/A
9.	Have case plan components 1,2,3,4,5,6,7 under Ch. 10 Appendix Part C, Non-Offending Spouse/Other Adults been successfully completed and is 8 currently occurring? Attach detailed status of each component.	Yes (No)	(Yes) No	Unk. N/A
10.	Is case being managed as described in Ch. 10 Appendix Part D, Case Management? Attach detailed status of each component.	Yes No	Yes No	Unk. (N/A)
11.	Does the perpetrator continue to say that the exaggerated and/or fabricated and/or induced problems are/were real?	(Yes) No	(Yes) No	Unk. N/A
12.	Has the perpetrator been diagnosed with or is the perpetrator suspected of having factitious disorder/Munchausen syndrome?	Yes No	Yes No	(Unk.) N/A
13.	Does the perpetrator have other problems (physical and/or psychological/behavioral/mental health) that could affect case progress?	Yes No	Yes No	(Unk.) N/A
14.	Does the person evaluated on this work sheet have genuine physical and/or psychological/behavioral/mental health problems that could make monitoring of the case difficult?	(Yes) No	(Yes) No	Unk. N/A

15.	Are there any external barriers that might be problematic to case progress?	Yes No	Yes No	Unk. N/A

*Unk. = unknown; N/A = not applicable

Other Risk Factors and Information:

Case is "provisionally" confirmed and perpetrator is "provisionally identified" only because information is still being gathered. Further information is needed in order to confirm that the behavior is MBP and not just "MBP-like."

Comments on risk factors:

#1 Physical abuse, emotional abuse, medical neglect, and educational neglect caused by deliberate fabrication of medical symptoms and deliberate "coaching" confirmed by video/audiotape on 12/6/2001 and supported by other information (physician and hospital records, telephone discussions by Dr. Murphy with other providers, etc.).

#2 Even though Sylvia is a teenager, she is still extremely vulnerable to manipulation by her mother. She appears very immature and dependent on her mother. She is isolated from peers and other family members.

#6, 12, 13, 15 Information still pending.

#7-11 Perpetrator has not been confronted, and case plan has not been formulated.

Risk Summary Statement:

This is an extremely high-risk case. Munchausen by proxy (MBP) maltreatment has been provisionally confirmed with Sylvia Grant as victim and her mother, Lilah Grant, as perpetrator. Physical abuse, emotional abuse, and medical neglect have been confirmed. Ms. Grant has deliberately fabricated physical problems and induced related behavior in Sylvia. This has resulted in very serious consequences to Sylvia's physical and emotional health, including physical debilitation and severe medication side effects which are life threatening. The danger is likely to remain for the foreseeable future.

Prepared by:	William Wright	AND	Lani Kamakele
Title:	CPS Investigator III		MBP Maltreatment Expert Consultant
Agency:	Central Valley Department of Human Services		

Concurring:

Signature	Agency
L. C. Murphy, MD	Attending Pediatrician
Jane A. Peterson, RN	Clinical Nurse Specialist, Child Abuse Team, Central Valley Hospital
Robert J. Brown, MSW	Medical Social Worker, Pediatrics, Central Valley Hospital
Rowlene Phillips	Principal, Central Valley High School
Victoria Ortiz	Risk Managment Department, Central Valley Hopsital

Attachments: Comments, MMT minutes, Central Valley School Attendance Report, Central Valley Hospital medical records (excerpts).

Chapter 10

MBP Case Planning
and Management

MBP cases do not end with the evidentiary court hearing. If there has been a finding of MBP child maltreatment, CPS and other involved agencies will enter a long-term process with victim(s), siblings, if any, perpetrator, and others. Throughout this process, the essential elements for MBP case success continue to be important. Those essential elements, which were discussed in Chapter 4, are correct MBP education; continued information gathering and evaluation; advice from the MMT; the MBP expert; and a competent, MBP-educated attorney.

Child protective agencies and/or courts are required to develop a case plan when child maltreatment is determined. The initial plan must be completed within a specified period, and is usually presented at a dispositional court hearing. At this hearing, the judge listens to both sides' recommendations and arguments, and then makes decisions. The case plan must be in agreement with and responsive to the findings of fact in the evidentiary hearing (the hearing at which information was presented to the judge and the judge decided—"found"— the facts of the case). For example, if CPS made an allegation of physical abuse that was confirmed by the court, the case plan then would have to address and attempt to solve the conditions that led to the physical abuse.

Thus, if MBP has been confirmed it is vital that this is included in the court's findings of facts. Otherwise, there will be no justification for including MBP-related elements in the case plan. If such elements are included without such a finding, they can be challenged.

CASE PLANNING IN CHILD PROTECTION
AND MBP CASES

Because every case of confirmed child maltreatment requires a case plan to guide child protective activities and expectations, case planning is a common activity for child welfare personnel. Good case plans are individualized and reflect the child protective agency's thinking about the risks to the child, the causes of the risks, and the best ways to resolve the risks so that the child can be protected. Elements should be included in a case plan because they are needed—that is, because they reflect assessed risks—not because they are commonly used or part of a "boilerplate." For example, many abusive or neglectful parents are referred to parenting classes to learn about such issues as child discipline. This is appropriate if it has been determined that they do not know or use good parenting skills. MBP perpetrators should not automatically be referred to parenting classes unless problems have been identified with their parenting skills. This would only give them an opportunity to demonstrate compliance in a meaningless way, since it would not contribute to the resolution of identified risks. A perpetrator could later say that the victim should be returned to her or his custody because the perpetrator cooperated with the case plan.

Case planning in today's child welfare practice means working within a time limit toward a permanency goal for the victim(s) and siblings if they have also been brought into state custody. Attempts may be made to reunify the victim and sibling(s) with the perpetrator, or it may be decided early on that a different permanency plan will need to be recommended and court approved.

The child welfare agency pursues four general goals during the case planning and management process:

* ensuring the safety of the victim(s) and any siblings(s);
* providing appropriate case services to the child victims and siblings if in placement;
* determining the permanency goal and time line; and
* planning for the future.

Each will be discussed in detail later in this chapter.

Cases do not remain static, and case plans and actions may be changed. Throughout the case planning and management process, the focus should be on the child/victim's long-term safety and welfare. One way to assess this is to consider the original risks that brought the child to the attention of CPS. The risk assessment work sheet in Chapter 9 is useful for ongoing reassessment. Have those risks resolved because the parents have successfully completed elements of the case plan? If so, then it may be time to consider contact or increased contact between the parent(s) and child(ren). If the risk conditions have remained the same or gotten worse, then it may be necessary to extend placement or consider other permanency options. Thus, accurate initial and continuing risk assessment and accurate continued monitoring of the case situation are vital to the case planning and management process. Evaluation of case plan progress should be made at regular meetings (for example, every month to six weeks) of involved case professionals, including the involved therapist(s), as will be discussed later in this chapter. If the MBP risk assessment work sheet is used each time the case is reviewed, the agency will have ongoing documentation of progress, or lack of progress, with each risk factor.

MBP perpetrators are not likely to change quickly. True change, if it occurs at all, requires a great deal of time and effort. Until it is accomplished, perpetrators may seem appropriate and cooperative, but are likely to continue deception, manipulation, and use of the child(ren) and situation to meet their own emotional needs. Even if they admit to perpetration, they are likely to claim that it is in the past now. They will probably not admit to the pattern and extent of maltreatment. They may claim to have undergone a religious conversion or to have changed their lives in other significant ways. These statements may be true, but the situation as a whole must be evaluated appropriately before they are believed. Because change is slow and unpredictable, MBP cases should be followed on a long-term basis. It is dangerous for the welfare of the victim, present siblings, and any potential future siblings for CPS to withdraw from or close a case too quickly.

Some MBP cases will need to remain open over many years. There will be times of activity, such as during court hearings or crises, and times when only periodic review and updating is necessary. Eventually, some MMT members will retire, move away, or otherwise become unable to serve. They will have to be replaced, and when this is done it will be necessary to educate new members about MBP and about the specific case. The case should be considered as an ongoing investigation, with information checked and not taken at face value. Case planning and casework will continue to be much more time-consuming in MBP cases than in other maltreatment cases. Communication among professionals, making arrangements for the MMT to meet, and continued information gathering and evaluation are time-consuming tasks. Workers as well as their supervisors must continue to allocate sufficient time to their MBP cases if they expect to provide adequate services and ensure victim and sibling safety.

Although perpetrators may not have access to the child, they are likely to continue to use their victims as objects to meet their own emotional needs. Perpetrators have been known to contact the press and make allegations about various people involved in the case; for example, a perpetrator may allege that the physician made the child protective referral because of an inability to diagnose the illness. They may ally themselves with support groups for persons who feel victimized by child protective agencies. They may engage crusading attorneys who file multiple motions and lawsuits. They may write letters to politicians or bring charges before state licensure and professional review boards. These tactics are further reason for continued involvement of the MMT.

A single professional, working alone, may find it impossible to determine progress, or lack thereof, toward victim risk reduction. If necessary, members of the MMT will be available to support one another through such processes, to keep one another from being "sucked in" by continued deception, or to testify honestly to their colleague's good faith and competence.

The appendix to this chapter shows recommended elements for case plans in confirmed MBP, to be used as appropriate. As each of the four goals for case planning is discussed, relevant case plan elements are repeated for convenience.

CASE PLANNING GOAL 1: ENSURING THE SAFETY OF THE VICTIM(S) AND SIBLING(S)

The goal of ensuring victim and sibling safety is usually accomplished by placement in a neutral, agency foster home, with foster parents who exhibit skill, compassion, and appropriate judgment about problems. Guidelines for immediate placement were discussed in Chapter 9, and continue to be valid throughout the life of the case. Ensuring the integrity of the case through appropriate placement also continues to be an important part of protecting them as long as the court is involved or additional legal action *could* be brought. Perpetrators can and do appeal decisions or sue persons and agencies involved in removing the child from their care.

Once CPS has protective authority, the agency is responsible for the safety of the child. Regardless of where the child is placed, long-term supervision of the placement is essential. Victims and potential victims must continue under the "agency umbrella" of close monitoring until it is safe for them to return home or until another permanency goal has been established for them. In practice, this means that agency supervision often continues for years.

Case plan recommendations for foster placement include the following:*

> B3. MBP basic education and detailed case histories will be personally shared with all adults with whom victims or potential victims are placed.
> D9. Foster parents will be considered part of the MMT.
> D10. Foster parents will have no contact with the perpetrator, non-perpetrating spouse, other adults in the home, or other friends and relatives of the family. If such contact occurs, it will be limited to necessary formal discussion. The location of the foster home will not be divulged. Transportation to/from any visits will be performed by the agency responsible for the case.

As described in Chapter 9, placement in an agency foster home makes it easier to protect the victim(s) and less likely that the case can be tainted. The criteria from Chapter 9 for selecting foster parents, for educating them about MBP and the case, and for clear instructions and logging remain throughout the life of the case. Should any change in foster parents occur, the new foster parents also need instruction about MBP, case-specific details, and the expectations of the agency. This is true whether the child protective agency is using its "own" agency or one under the supervision of another agency.

---

*Letter/number references in boxes refer to elements listed in the appendix to this chapter.

Foster parents should be considered full participating members of the MMT. This will provide them with ongoing education about MBP and the case. In addition, foster parents can also make a significant contribution to the team's understanding of the case through their observations of the child(ren)'s progress and reports of information that the child(ren) have shared with them.

The agency responsible for the case should also take steps to protect the foster family. Information about the victim's location should be withheld not only from the perpetrator, but also from relatives and friends. The primary purpose of this is to diminish the possibility of contact with and manipulation of the child(ren) in placement, and potential harassment and manipulation of the foster family. The foster family should have no contact with the perpetrator, other adults in the home, or friends and relatives of the child(ren)'s family. For example, agency staff should manage transportation for visits. If contacts cannot be avoided or occur accidentally (for example, during a court hearing), the foster parents should be instructed to keep interaction minimal and businesslike. Because of the danger of manipulation by the perpetrator, the foster family should not attempt to reach out to the child(ren)'s family or to befriend them.

Placement with Relatives and Friends

D8. Placement with relatives or friends of the family is potentially dangerous in MBP cases and will be allowed only after a specialized process (over and above what is normally done in approving relatives) and recommendation from the MMT, including the agency responsible for the case.

Occasionally, relatives or friends *do* understand what has happened and believe that the perpetrator is the cause of the problems. For example, they may have been the first to raise suspicions, perhaps acting out of a sincere concern for children with whom they have a meaningful relationship. Even in this situation, initial placement should not be with relatives and friends. Generally, there is not time to assess them and their situation. They might still be ambivalent. They might give in to pressure or clever manipulation by the perpetrator or the nonoffending spouse.

Alternatively, CPS may be required by court or policy to look for and assess relatives as resources for out-of-home placement, even if they believe it inadvisable. In this situation, or if relatives/friends *appear* to be appropriate for consideration, the placement should be considered high risk and a more thorough, detailed, and MBP-specific screening process should be undertaken. This process is described as follows. The perpetrator's family of origin is particularly questionable for placement, as they may have contributed to or shared the perpetrator's problems. Perhaps the perpetrator is not typical of his or her family, but did develop personality and behaviors within this family context.

Throughout contacts with relatives and friends, for whatever purpose, information gathering about the case should continue. Information obtained during the investigation, although sufficient for confirmation, is often insufficient for a full understanding of what has happened, its extent, the perpetrator's motives, etc. This is not unique to MBP. Thus contacts with potential caretakers should be used to gain more information about the perpetrator, the family, the victim, and the victim's purported problems, and especially unanswered questions. For example, perhaps the perpetrator has stated that seizures run in the family. In accordance with good investigative procedure, general questions should be asked prior to specific questions. The investigator should ask, "Do you know of any physical or mental health problems that any family members have had?" After the response, the interviewer should name several physical and mental health problems, including seizures. Each positive response should be followed with a probe such as, "How do you know?" or "Who told you about that?" In addition to providing case information, the interviewees' answers will suggest the extent to which they believe the perpetrator, or are making excuses for the perpetrator, etc. As with other information obtained in the case, statements should be evaluated, compared with other sources to detect inconsistencies, and documented in the case record and data summary.

Child welfare agencies ordinarily have procedures for assessing potential caretakers related to the victim(s). These procedures may include references, collateral contacts, law enforcement screenings, and corroboration of information. These activities should be conducted in an MBP case, but from an MBP point of view. For example, information obtained from the relatives should be carefully corrobo-

rated and not taken at face value. In addition to usual evaluation activities, a specialized MBP evaluation should be conducted, as shown in
Box 10.1 and detailed in the text following. Two professionals should
be involved in the process, one to lead the sessions and the other to assist in observing and documenting. The latter should not interrupt or
interject questions or information; the lead professional should, at
least before the end of the conversation, ask the other if he or she has
any questions to ask. If more than one home is being considered, this
process should be completed separately for each.

Step 1: Initial Relative Interviews

Relatives who wish to be considered for child placement should
first be interviewed separately (even couples) without allowing them
to talk with one another between interviews. More information and
more clues to information will be uncovered in this way.

One of the first questions to be asked could be: "So much has been
going on. What do you think of what has been happening?" The inter-

---

Box 10.1.
Specialized Evaluation of Relatives
as Potential Caretakers of MBP Victims

1. Initial information-gathering interviews (all adults in the home
   interviewed separately)
2. Provision of basic MBP education (all adults in the home together)
3. Overnight time interval for adults to think about/discuss situation
4. Second relative interviews (all adults in the home, interviewed
   separately)
5. Provision of detailed case information related to basic MBP
   education followed by discussion (all adults in the home together)
6. Decision or recommendation made by CPS with consultation
   from MMT

If more than one relative's home is being considered, a separate
process must be completed for each. Assessment should not be
done as a group process.

viewee should be allowed to talk while the interviewers listen and observe body language. No attempt should be made to argue, teach, or try to change the person's feelings and beliefs, as the purpose of this interview is to obtain information. No case information or case discussion should be part of this interview; the focus should be on the interviewee's statements about the situation. Both interviewers should be alert for material which indicates that the interviewee questions the existence of MBP in this case, any thoughts that the perpetrator should be "given another chance," or any ambivalence about the placement of the child(ren).

The next question might be: "How do you think (spouse/partner/other adult relatives in home) feels about the situation? Why do you think she or he feels that way?" Follow-up questions should be asked to clarify or to obtain more information. This, of course, can be compared with information obtained in the interview with the other person. Discrepancies—for example, the wife appears to believe in the MBP, but the husband says she still believes the perpetrator is innocent—should be taken very seriously.

At this stage, information about the case should still not be given. The focus remains on obtaining verbal and nonverbal information about the relatives' attitudes toward the case. Notice any indication that the relatives do not believe that the maltreatment has occurred or that the perpetrator poses a potential danger to the child.

After these lines of questioning have been followed, the interviewer should use the opportunity to obtain the interviewee's perspective on any other issues that may be helpful to the investigation or to decision making about placement. This material may contribute to the evaluation of the interviewee, but its primary purpose is to contribute to the case as a whole. Answers provided by the interviewee should not be taken at face value, but should be compared to other information in the case.

Step 2: Provision of Basic MBP Education

Immediately after completion of Step 1, the relatives under consideration for placement should receive basic MBP education together. This step has two purposes: (1) to provide information about MBP basics, and (2) to observe the verbal and physical reactions of the adult family members to the MBP education. This will complement information already learned about them in Step 1. The interviewer should carefully provide and explain the definition of MBP, suspicion indicators, perpetrator-consistent characteristics, and situational suspicion indicators. The interviewer should emphasize how dangerous MBP maltreatment is, both in the short and long term, and how deceptive and manipulative perpetrators can be. However, case information should still not be given. Although general information is being provided, a major focus of this step is on continuing to observe the relatives' reactions and ability to integrate the facts they are being given. For example, the relatives may identify some of the perpetrator's behavior as they hear about the perpetrator-consistent characteristics. Alternatively, when told about the dangers of MBP perpetration, the relatives may continue to deny that the confirmed perpetrator "could ever have hurt her own children." Again, if there is any indication that relatives do not believe the maltreatment occurred or that the perpetrator poses a potential danger to the child, placement with them cannot be considered.

Step 3: Overnight Time Interval

After their separate interviews and the educational session, the relatives should have time to talk overnight. The process and conversations that follow may stimulate some change in their apparent or real attitude toward the case or toward serving as foster parents. This time interval also allows the interviewers to think and talk about their impressions and consider any additional lines of questioning that may be necessary.

Step 4: Second Relative Interviews

This step should occur the day after Steps 1 and 2. Again, separate interviews should take place, without the interviewees having an opportunity to talk to one another between their interviews. Questions to be asked include, "What do you think now about the situation based on what we discussed yesterday?" "How do you think your spouse/partner/other household adult feels now?" "Why do you think he or she feels that way?" During this step, the interviewer should ask any necessary follow-up or additional investigative questions, including those suggested by information received the day before.

Step 5: Provision of Detailed Case Information Related to Basic MBP Education, Followed by Discussion

The primary purpose of this session is to link the previously discussed MBP education with what has happened in this particular case and, again, to take note of what is expressed verbally and nonverbally by the relatives. Legal authority to release information (signed release forms of information by a parent or authority given by the court) must be in place prior to this session so that detailed case information can be shared. All adults in the home should be present at this session.

Special care should be taken to link the MBP basics with the case. Other information to be discussed includes the victim(s)' suffering through the MBP maltreatment and consequent physical or mental treatment needs, the risk if MBP continues or resumes, and the special activities and guidelines necessary to keep the victim(s) safe. If the interviewers have any concerns or issues, for example, about apparent inconsistencies, these need to be discussed at this time. The relatives should be encouraged to ask questions, make comments, provide other information, etc. As all adults in the home are interacting together during this session, there is a good opportunity for interviewers to observe dynamics and clarify statements that may have been made by one about another.

Step 6: Decision or Recommendation Based on Total Assessment

After a careful review of all information received, the child welfare agency will come to a decision about the suitability of the relative(s) in question as caretaker(s) for the child(ren). The input of the MMT can be very useful in making this decision, and can add weight to the agency's recommendations or decisions. The interviewers should consider carefully whether they have seen any clues which suggest that the prospective caretakers doubt that the maltreatment took place, believe that the children would be safe with the mother/perpetrator, or do not seem to understand the need for agency guidelines. If any reason exists to suspect that the relative(s) will not follow agency guidelines, they should not be considered for placement.

Court orders that place victims with friends or relatives should include language requiring notification to CPS if the caretaking family plans to move, and court permission for a move out of the jurisdiction. (Such stipulations will not, of course, be necessary for agency foster homes, as they must consult with CPS on all moves.) Monitoring by the child welfare agency should also be included in the court order. Placement with relatives who have completed a screening and educational process does not eliminate the need for long-term supervision. Similar language should be included in the caretaking family's agreement with CPS if there is not a court order. The perpetrator should also be ordered to report to the court and/or CPS if he or she assumes care for another child or moves. Female perpetrators must report pregnancy or giving birth.

The process becomes even more complicated if out-of-state relatives are considered. Normally, when interstate placement evaluation and decision making is done, a request is sent through official channels from one state to another. The receiving state generally conducts the prospective relative placement evaluation. An important consideration in MBP cases is whether the receiving state is likely to understand MBP case details and to supervise and manage the placement as well as could be accomplished within the original jurisdiction.

In considering whether to accept responsibility for the case, the receiving state must understand the increased time and complexity involved in overseeing this kind of relative placement and potential related activities. These include coordinating with the sending state agency, supervising visitation, working with the perpetrator should she or he move to the jurisdiction, etc. Both initiating and receiving states must be clear about expectations and agreements before final approval of the placement and transfer of the child to the relative(s)' home.

If the decision is made to proceed with the evaluation of out-of-state relatives as possible caretakers, the requesting agency must organize and perform the specialized MBP portion of the evaluation. The receiving agency should be given basic MBP education and detailed case information so that its personnel can conduct their monitoring activities from an MBP perspective. The MBP expert consultant should work with both jurisdictions.

Case Planning Goal 1: Ensuring the Safety of the Victim(s) and Sibling(s) Through Supervision of Contact

In MBP cases, the victim(s) should have contact with the perpetrator, relatives, friends, and even siblings only with the strictest of guidelines and supervision. This applies to anyone who may engage in MBP or related behavior, or convey harmful information in either direction.

In order to provide the most neutral environment possible in which to evaluate the child away from even subtle parental influence, contact is not recommended during the investigation and confirmation-disconfirmation process. Day (1998a) also believes that visitation should not occur during the early stages of perpetrator therapy because the perpetrator may feel driven to reabuse the victim. However, often the issue of early contact will be brought up in court. CPS should be assertive in giving reasons for believing contact is inadvisable. The MMT and MBP expert may be effective in reinforcing these reasons.

If contact does occur, whether early in the case or after confirmation, it must be extremely closely supervised. The case plan recommendations in the appendix to this chapter (repeated in Box 10.2) should be followed. They apply to siblings as well as to the victim(s) and to anyone other than case-involved professionals. They protect the case as well as the child(ren).

Contact between family members and children in placement should serve the needs of the children. Needs of the parents, other relatives, and friends of the family are secondary. Although a child has been maltreated, experience and psychological theory suggest that the child may need a relationship with the parent. The primary mission of the child welfare agency is protection of the child(ren), and the purpose of allowing visitation is to sustain the victim's well-being. Although the perpetrator or other relatives may claim to be suffering, as adults they have more resources to withstand the separation. The perpetrator, in particular, does not have an independent right to visit the child if there is reason to believe that further maltreatment is likely. This understanding lays the foundation for all other rules affecting visitation.

Contact should occur in a setting over which the agency has control. It is inadvisable for the visit to occur on the perpetrator's "turf," or in a public place. In either circumstance, the perpetrator is at an advantage and may harm the child, flee, manipulate behavior, give secret messages, etc. Pleasant surroundings should be chosen in the hospital, agency, or a site specifically designed for child-parent visitation. Security should be available.

Box 10.2.
MBP Case Plan Recommendations for Contact
with MBP Victims/Siblings in Placement

Note: Contact should not occur prior to confirmation unless ordered by the court. Contact may be inadvisable during the early stages of a perpetrator's therapy.

D4. Unsupervised contact with anyone will not take place unless the Case Plan Elements in Parts A and C (See Appendix) have been satisfied. Unsupervised contact will also not take place until it has been approved by the MMT, including the agency responsible for the case.

D5. Supervised visitation, if necessary to meet the needs of the child, will take place under the following conditions:

A. Visitation will take place in a controlled setting (e.g., not in the home).

B. Visitation will be supervised by a staff member of the agency responsible for the case. This person will have personally received basic MBP education and detailed case information as well as specific instructions for monitoring and logging.

C. The visitation supervisor will remain in the room where the visitation is occurring at all times, with attention directed only toward supervision.

D. No activities may occur during the visitation that the supervisor cannot hear or see.

E. Anything brought to the visit must either be left outside the visitation area or be searched.

F. No food, drink, medications, gum, candy, or anything else that can be ingested will be allowed during visitation unless absolutely necessary. If they must be provided, they must be prepared by an agency staff member using material supplied by the agency responsible for the case, and given to the child by the visitation supervisor at least several feet away from the visitor(s).

G. No discussion of the case, health care issues, or related subjects will be allowed during the visitation.

H. Prior to each visit, visitors will sign an agreement indicating their understanding of these rules.

D6. Telephone contact will be allowed only under the following conditions:

A. Telephone contact will be monitored from both ends of the conversation by a staff member of the agency responsible for the case who has personally received basic MBP education and detailed case information as well as specific instructions for monitoring and logging.

B. No discussion of the case, health care issues, or related subjects will be allowed during the telephone contact.

C. Individuals approved for telephone contact will sign an agreement indicating their understanding of these rules.

D7. Contact by mail will be allowed only under the following conditions:

A. Mail will be directed to the child(ren) in care of the agency responsible for the case.

B. Letters and packages will be opened and inspected by an agency staff member who has personally received basic MBP education and detailed case information.

C. Letters and packages will be sent to the child(ren) only if they are believed to be beneficial.

D. No discussion of the case, health care issues, or related subjects will be allowed in letters.

E. No gifts of food, drink, medications, gum, candy, or anything else that can be ingested will be allowed.

F. Individuals approved for mail contact will sign an agreement indicating their understanding of these rules.

Visitation should be supervised by a competent person, preferably a staff member of the child welfare agency, who has received MBP education and understands the case. In some agencies or hospitals, one-on-one supervision is routinely done by poorly trained and inattentive paraprofessionals who know little about the situation they are watching and perhaps contribute little more than physical presence. This is inappropriate in MBP cases, as interactions may be subtle and very close observation and detailed logging is required. A professional with a security or investigative background, if available, makes a good observer. The observer should have a clear understanding of the methods that have been used previously to exaggerate, fabricate, or induce, and what to do if problems occur. The observer should recognize that the perpetrator is fully capable of changing the forms of exaggeration, fabrication, and/or induction. If visitation supervisors do not believe what they have been told, they are not appropriate for the task.

Whatever occurs during the visit should be carefully logged. This log will be of great value if the child has problems during or following the visit. The log should also be used to carefully evaluate behavior and conversation that occurs during and following the visit. Even while the observer is in the room, subtle verbal or behavioral cues might be given. For example, a perpetrator's inflection when asking, "How are you?" might cue a child that she is "supposed" to be in pain. Some previously used cues may be known from case information. Others may only be revealed through analysis of the log.

The visitation supervisor must be able to see and hear everything that occurs during the visit. This means that the observer must be in the same room with the perpetrator and victim, not observing them through a one-way mirror or via video camera (although audio/videotaping in addition to supervision of the visit can be valuable). This is the only way to keep the perpetrator in the line of sight at all times, and to be able to respond immediately if inappropriate events occur. If more than one visitor is present (and this should be discouraged), more than one visitation supervisor may be needed. All conversations must be audible and in English unless the visitation supervisor is fluent in the language spoken or an interpreter employed by the agency is available. Visitors should not discuss the case or issues related to the condition(s) that are the focus of MBP during the visit. If these subjects are raised during the visit by the child(ren), the visiting adult(s) or supervisor must change the subject. No passing of notes or other forms of communication that the visitation supervisor cannot see or hear should be allowed.

The visitation supervisor must not engage in activities such as receiving or making telephone calls, going to the rest room, reading a book, watching TV, talking to someone else, etc. The perpetrator could engage in or cause inappropriate behavior during even a brief lapse of attention.

Any objects brought to the visit, including apparently unrelated objects such as purses and packages, should be inspected before they are allowed into the visitation room. Gifts should be limited because they may pose a subtle danger to the child. For example, a perpetrator might bring a book about a sick child or animal. This might be a subtle reminder that the child is "supposed" to be sick. Lavish gifts may even have the character of "bribes" or attempts to "buy" the child.

The purpose of the visit is contact between the familiar people and the victim; gifts may distract from this.

No food, drink, or medication should be brought into the visit because of the dangers of contamination. If the child must ingest anything—for example, it is time for prescribed medications or a bottle—these should be prepared and given by an agency staff member using materials that have not been in contact with the visitor.

Similar contact rules apply to telephone conversations, which must be preplanned so that monitoring occurs at both ends. Telephone conversation supervisors, like visitation supervisors, must have received basic MBP education, be familiar with the details of the case and past methods of perpetration, and have received monitoring instructions.

If the perpetrator or other adults wish to contact the child(ren) by mail, the mail must be directed to the child welfare agency. Otherwise, the location of the foster home would be revealed. Letters and packages must be read and inspected by a competent staff member who has received basic MBP education and is familiar with the details of the case. Nothing that can "cue" the child or that can be ingested should be allowed. The burden is on the perpetrator and other adults to plan time for this process and the subsequent delivery to the child(ren) of approved materials. Special occasions (holidays, birthdays) should not be used as an excuse to rush the process. These rules, and any additional conditions that the agency believes necessary because of the specific circumstances of the case, should be explained to potential visitors well in advance of the visit, telephone call, or mail contact. Those who wish to be in touch with the child(ren) should be required to sign a form verifying their understanding of the rules and willingness to comply. Contact should not be allowed unless this form has been signed.

CASE PLANNING GOAL 2: PROVISION OF APPROPRIATE CASE SERVICES

B1. Victims and potential victims will undergo a mental health evaluation to determine if mental health intervention is presently needed.

B2. Physical and mental health needs of victims and potential victims will be coordinated through one professional who has

personally received MBP education and detailed case information, believes that the MBP maltreatment has taken place,
is not challenging the MBP confirmation, and who has been
approved by the agency responsible for the case.

A major goal following confirmation is the victim's recovery, to the extent possible, from any damage that has occurred as a result of the MBP maltreatment. The experience of being in the more normal environment of a foster home, where the problem is not a major focus of attention and where physical or mental health instructions are followed correctly, often allows the child(ren) to make significant progress. Beginning or returning to regular school/preschool attendance, participation in family and neighborhood activities, and development of new skills and interests may result from the placement and lead to a mentally and physically healthier and happier lifestyle.

Health care while in placement may include tapering/discontinuing unnecessary medications, discontinuing unnecessary treatments, medical or surgical repair or reversal of physical damage, or procedures and treatments to compensate for damage that is irreparable. An initial mental health evaluation and follow-up treatment as necessary should also be arranged for the victim and other children involved in the case. Infant mental health professionals are available in many areas, but if a child is considered too young for evaluation early in placement, this should be done if needed when the child is older. Some issues that may need to be dealt with in psychotherapy include: a persistent self-image as "sickly"; guilt over having "told on" the perpetrator or failing to meet the perpetrator's needs; guilt over having failed to protect other siblings from maltreatment; or an inability to separate illness from love. Children will also need to make sense of the maltreatment in a way that allows them to feel that it was not their fault and that they are worthy of love and care. If they will not be returning home, they will need to deal with this issue (Jones, Byrne, and Newbould, 2000). Some victims may exhibit symptoms suggesting that they are beginning to develop factitious disorder/Munchausen syndrome, malingering, etc. This should be addressed in therapy to prevent future problems.

The healing process is facilitated if a member of the MMT coordinates all physical and mental health treatment that the victim(s) and siblings will receive. A pediatrician or family practitioner could assume this role, but it could also be performed by a nurse or social worker. The treatment coordinator, however, must have received basic MBP education and detailed case information, must believe the MBP confirmation, and must be willing to participate as a member of the ongoing MMT. As questions arise about treatment, the MMT will also have a wider range of expertise than any individual and will be a valuable resource for decision making.

Mental and physical problems may emerge well after a child has been removed from the care, custody, control, and influence of the perpetrator. Thus, it is important that the history of MBP victims and siblings accompany them wherever they are placed. For example, one child was repeatedly suffocated by his mother during infancy. More than two years later, the foster mother noticed him repeatedly suffocating his foster sister's dolls. It is impossible to know whether this behavior represented a memory or whether he was acting out what he had heard people say. However, it needed to be addressed and he was referred for therapy. If the victim(s) and siblings are returned to the care of the perpetrator, either permanently or temporarily, the role of care coordinator will continue to be important. The perpetrator cannot be allowed again to be the common link among specialists or the primary provider of information about the child(ren)'s illness. Nor can the perpetrator be allowed to select new care providers. These precautions will not guarantee that the perpetrator refrains from former behavior, but the presence and activity of the care coordinator will make relapeses more difficult and more likely to be discovered. Agency supervision also must continue long term.

CASE PLANNING GOALS 3 AND 4: DETERMINING THE PERMANENCY GOAL, TIME LINE, AND FUTURE PLANNING

Recent legislation requires that a decision must be made, often within a matter of months, as to the long-term goal for a child in state custody. This is a reaction to the many children over the years who have remained in foster care for inappropriately long periods, or who

have become "lost" in a system of multiple placements. Possible permanency goals include reunification with the family of origin, long-
term foster care or relative placement, or legal termination of parental
rights with the hope of adoption.

Factors specific to the case determine the appropriate permanency
goal. These include the kind of maltreatment, extent of damage, resources in the extended family, and potential for the perpetrator to
change within a reasonable length of time. All of these will affect
planning. In some situations, the maltreatment will have been so severe and the likelihood of the perpetrator to change in a reasonable
length of time so low that termination of parental rights will be pursued from the beginning. In other situations, the perpetrator will be
given a chance to work toward reunification with the child. But MBP
cases must always be considered high risk for reperpetration. In a follow-up study Davis et al. (1998, pp. 220-221) concluded:

> Even in the cases of Munchausen syndrome by proxy without
> physical harm [in which the victims were] allowed [to return]
> home, 17 percent were reabused in a two-year follow-up pe-
> riod. . . . The ongoing morbidity, further abuse of index cases
> and harm to siblings all demand a very cautious approach in
> child protection. Reintroductions to the home should be consid-
> ered only if the circumstances are especially favorable.

Similarly, Jones, Byrne, and Newbould (2000, p. 282) state:

> Sometimes, the risk of harm to the child is simply too great, pa-
> rental denial too entrenched or the likelihood of timely psycho-
> logical treatment too slim. For the children of these parents, it
> will be essential that protective action is taken at an early stage
> and a clear assessment of the reasons for this action is given. Not
> only does this afford maximum protection for the index child
> but it also ensures that appropriate consideration can be given to
> the welfare of siblings or future children born to the family.

In MBP cases, temporary or permanent custody with relatives
should be strongly resisted unless the relative evaluation discussed
earlier in this chapter results in a positive placement recommendation
and long-term agency monitoring is part of the court order. As long-
term planning is considered, keep in mind that even a relative who has

successfully completed the evaluation process may later die, become incapacitated, be successfully manipulated by the perpetrator, or otherwise be unable to continue as a caretaker. If this occurs, opportunity may arise for the perpetrator to access or resume custody of the victim or potential victims unless the child(ren) remain(s) in state custody.

When MBP maltreatment has occurred and reunification with the perpetrator is the goal, the case plan must contain elements specific to MBP. Even if an MMT has not been used previously, it is strongly recommended at this stage, since it is virtually impossible for one professional or agency to determine risk reduction independent of other involved professionals. Decisions about reunification, unsupervised visitation, and termination of parental rights are serious. The victim's life or health is potentially at risk. A team recommendation is much more powerful than that of one person or one agency. A team is able to consider more aspects of the case and provide more expertise. This is particularly true when difficult situations must be confronted.

Because significant changes are required before the perpetrator may be safe with the victim, the goal of reunification may not be attained. Kinscherff and Famularo (1991) believe that termination of parental rights is justified in the following four situations:

- Chronic and potentially lethal danger to the child, including cases of "extreme" MBP when the child is at "severe risk for death, disfigurement, invalidism, and massive impairment of psychological and social development." (p. 41)
- The perpetrator has psychological/behavioral problems for which no known effective treatments exist.
- Maltreatment continues even while the perpetrator is in therapy and the case is monitored.
- Neither the courts nor CPS can provide adequate long-term monitoring or services.

The recent emphasis on timely permanency planning suggests an additional criterion:

- Lack of progress with the case plan in a reasonable amount of time, or it is anticipated that reunification could occur safely only in the far distant future.

Some professionals associated with MBP cases believe that no MBP victim should ever be returned to the perpetrator (Seidl, 1995). Day (1998a,c) suggests that a true acknowledgment of the abuse on the part of the perpetrator often does not come until at least a year into therapy. Thus, there is a strong possibility that, in spite of everyone's best efforts, the MMT will ultimately have to recommend against reunification. They may not even be able to support placement with relatives or family friends. In coming to these conclusions, the team may have to resist a great deal of pressure from the perpetrator, relatives and friends, and even the court or child protective agency. An MMT, because of its composition, can speak persuasively. This can only occur, however, if a true MMT, familiar with MBP and the case, continues to be involved in the process of managing the case plan. The same results cannot be expected from a generic "review team" that is assembled just for decision making or for cases other than MBP.

Box 10.3 shows elements that must be completed before it is safe for the victim(s) to have unsupervised contact with the perpetrator and other significant adults, to return to the perpetrator's care or to return to the care of anyone who might be influenced by the perpetrator. Many of the elements in this reunification case plan are related to the risk assessment elements discussed in Chapter 9 and call for "sincerity" on the part of the perpetrator and other adults. Obviously, determining sincerity is a difficult task. The MMT can again be valuable as its members share information and look for inconsistencies.

Unless the perpetrator becomes the responsibility of the criminal justice system, she or he will generally be mandated to receive some form of psychotherapy. The child protective agency will be expected to monitor the course of this treatment, and to work toward a permanency plan for the victim(s) and possibly siblings. Many issues may be addressed in therapy, and MBP perpetrators may also have a variety of mental conditions (see Chapter 12). MBP perpetrator therapy includes three goals:

1. *The perpetrator must admit to the* pattern *of MBP and related behavior.* It is not enough for the perpetrator to concede that specific acts occurred on specific occasions. The perpetrator must be able to acknowledge the MBP behavior as a whole and the harm that it caused (Jones, Byrne, and Newbould, 2000). For example, the perpetrator might need to confront a pattern of attention seeking or using the child as an object that resulted in unnecessary medical care, place-

Box 10.3.
MBP Case Plan Recommendations to Be Completed Prior to Reunification

Part A: MBP Maltreatment Perpetrator

1. Perpetrator will sign necessary documents enabling agency responsible for the case to obtain written and verbal information regarding perpetrator and child(ren) from health care providers and others and to allow case team members, including mental health professionals, to share detailed case information with one another on an ongoing basis.
2. Perpetrator will undergo mental health therapy to address MBP behavior, any coexisting mental health problems, and other issues. This therapy will be provided by a therapist who has personally received MBP education and detailed case information, believes that the MBP maltreatment has taken place, is not challenging the MBP confirmation, and has been approved by the agency responsible for the case.
3. Perpetrator will undergo a comprehensive mental health evaluation to determine any coexisting mental health concerns.
4. Perpetrator will demonstrate basic understanding of MBP maltreatment.
5. Perpetrator will identify and sincerely admit to her or his pattern of MBP perpetration and related behavior.
6. Perpetrator will demonstrate a sincere understanding of how her or his victim(s) have been negatively impacted as a result of her or his MBP perpetration and related behavior.
7. Perpetrator will demonstrate a sincere understanding of how her or his MBP perpetration and related behavior could negatively impact victim(s) in the future.
8. Perpetrator will identify and sincerely demonstrate understanding of why her or his MBP perpetration and related behavior has happened, and the personal needs she or he has been trying to meet through use of the victim(s).
9. Perpetrator will sincerely identify past, present, and potential future MBP perpetration and related behavior "trigger situations."

(continued)

(Box 10.3, continued)

10. Perpetrator will sincerely identify, develop, and demonstrate use of alternative behaviors to substitute for MBP perpetration and related behavior.
11. Perpetrator will cooperate fully with and adhere to instructions given by the agency responsible for the case.

Part C: Nonperpetrating Spouse/Other Adults

This includes adults living in the home who are closely and consistently involved, or who seek unsupervised visitation with the victim(s)/potential victim(s).

1. Nonperpetrating spouse/other adults will sign necessary documents enabling the agency responsible for the case to obtain written and verbal information about themselves and their children from health care providers and others, and to allow case team members (including mental health professionals) to share detailed case information with one another on an ongoing basis.
2. Nonperpetrating spouse/other adults will demonstrate basic understanding of MBP maltreatment.
3. Nonperpetrating spouse/other adults will demonstrate a sincere belief in and understanding of the perpetrator's pattern of MBP perpetration and related behavior.
4. Nonperpetrating spouse/other adults will demonstrate a sincere understanding of the personal needs the perpetrator has been trying to meet through use of the victim(s).
5. Nonperpetrating spouse/other adults will demonstrate a sincere understanding of the perpetrator's past, present, and potential future MBP perpetration and related behavior "trigger situations."
6. Nonperpetrating spouse/other adults will demonstrate a sincere understanding of how the perpetrator's victim(s) has/have been negatively impacted as a result of his or her MBP perpetration and related behavior.
7. Nonperpetrating spouse/other adults will demonstrate a sincere understanding of how the perpetrator's MBP perpetration and related behavior could negatively impact victim(s) and/or potential victims in the future.
8. Nonperpetrating spouse/other adults will participate in meetings and/or mental health therapy as requested by the agency responsible for the case.

Part D: General Case Management

11. Prior to reunification or unsupervised visitation with anyone, the MMT, including the agency responsible for the case, will conduct a detailed case review to determine whether risk level is such that the proposed activity can take place, and under what conditions. Each plan component will be carefully evaluated to determine whether successful completion has occurred. The reasons for these decisions will be discussed and recorded. At least one professional who was a member of the MMT when MBP was confirmed will participate in this evaluation and in making recommendations. A credible MBP professional should be included. Evaluation and recommendations will be carefully documented, including any disagreements.

12. Throughout case activities, involved professionals will exercise great care in evaluating case information, in determining whether case plan components have been successfully completed and risk reduced, or whether apparent risk reduction actually reflects deception and/or manipulation by the perpetrator and/or others. The use of the word "sincere" in the case planning document, as well as the need for MMT members to share and carefully compare detailed case information on an ongoing basis, reflects this concern.

---

ment, etc. If the victim is to be safe, the perpetrator must develop sufficient insight that the general pattern leading to the behavior is understood. Otherwise, different forms of exaggeration, fabrication, or induction might be substituted.

2. *The perpetrator must understand how this pattern developed.* The perpetrator's behavior is not condoned, but—like all other forms of behavior—it developed for reasons. Little is known about why perpetrators choose MBP as their way of meeting needs. Some cases suggest an underlying lack of empathy or desire for attention combined with opportunity to produce MBP. Other cases suggest that perpetrators grew up in homes where attention or love came only with illness. Some evidence suggests that at least a few perpetrators were maltreated in this fashion. Unless the perpetrator truly understands the path that led to this situation, it is unlikely that she or he will be able to cope effectively with the needs that produced the behavior.

3. *The perpetrator must develop other ways to meet the needs that she or he was meeting or attempting to meet through MBP.* If reunification is to be possible, the perpetrator must be able not only to recognize the needs that led to MBP, but also to address those needs in a healthier way that does not include maltreatment of others. The perpetrator must be able to deal appropriately with the victim's realistic health care needs, evaluate the victim's symptoms, and allow the victim to grow and develop normally. This is asking a great deal of a perpetrator who may never have seen appropriate behavior modeled or who has little or no empathy for others.

Earlier in this chapter we discussed the need for regular evaluation of case progress, problems involved in assessing whether risk reduction has occurred, and the necessity for case information to be continually checked and not taken at face value. We discussed the need to assess whether the perpetrator is continuing attempts to deceive and manipulate others and to use the child(ren) and situations to meet his or her own needs. To determine these and related matters, professionals must share details of their ongoing case involvement, including detailed information derived from or about the perpetrator, with other professionals, hopefully in the context of an MMT. Although some may find the idea controversial due to confidentiality issues, this information exchange must include involved mental health professionals. They must be willing and able to participate fully in sharing, receiving, and comparing information. As a part of the case plan, the perpetrator must sign releases of information. Any hesitation should raise suspicion that the perpetrator has something to hide and does not sincerely wish to work toward accomplishing important elements of the case plan. A court order should also be obtained to ensure that all involved professionals have the legal obligation and authorization to participate in this way, even if someone (perpetrator or other) later decides not to share information. Professionals who are unwilling (for whatever reason) to participate in this manner may need to be excluded from the case management team.

Other Adults

Similar requirements must be met before reunification or unsupervised visitation for the nonperpetrating spouse, other adults in the home, relatives, or family friends. They, too, must understand the

MBP perpetration, believe in it, and have some insight into why it occurred. Like the perpetrator, these other adults must be willing to share information about themselves and their past and present health treatment. They must be willing to attend meetings and even seek mental health evaluation or therapy if the MMT considers it necessary. This may appear to be an invasion of their privacy, but it is vital to assess their suitability to care for the child(ren) affected by the MBP. If the child is to be returned to the home, as many people as possible in or near to the family must be able to aid in protection. This will not only extend the agency's ability to monitor, but will also build additional control for the perpetrator.

Therefore, relatives, friends, health care providers, teachers, etc., need to understand MBP, perpetrator-associated characteristics, and some details of the case. This education should be delivered in person so that the professional can also answer questions and assess whether it appears that the family and friends believe what is being said. As already discussed, those who do not believe or understand the seriousness of the situation will not assist effectively with protective activities.

Special attention must be paid to nonperpetrating parents or the perpetrator's "significant other." In the literature they are often described as trusting of the perpetrator and/or emotionally or physically distant. Each case is different. Sometimes it appears that MBP perpetration is initiated or escalates when the spouse or partner is out of the home (e.g., military assignment, divorce). This suggests that attention from the nonperpetrating parent is sometimes a motive or a contributor. The nonperpetrating parent or significant other will need solid education about MBP, and it is especially important that he or she believes that MBP has occurred. Some therapy may be necessary, directed to personal issues as well as to the relationship with the perpetrator. The nonperpetrator needs to understand, for example, why she or he did not suspect, remained silent, or denied the harm that was occurring to the child. Why did she or he not ask obvious questions? What qualities in the relationship may have led the perpetrator to be so desperate for attention? If the relationship is to continue, what will have to change in order for the nonperpetrator to spot the behavior and act effectively to prevent it? This is not to suggest that the spouse/partner be blamed for the maltreatment, although some responsibility may be present. Rather, this is intended to stress the seriousness and extent of change that must occur within the family as a whole if the victim is to be safe.

Selection of Therapists

> D3. Therapist selection for children or adults will be made after the potential therapist has personally received basic MBP education and detailed case information, has indicated belief in and is not challenging the MBP confirmation, and has (with appropriate legal authority) committed to participating as an MMT member and to sharing detailed case/client information.

Since so much of a successful case plan can depend on the perpetrator's progress in therapy, it is crucial to select an appropriate therapist for the perpetrator. This is equally true if therapy for the victim(s) or other adults is part of the case plan. In non-MBP child maltreatment cases, the perpetrator often selects her or his own therapist. Although the potential client may have input in MBP cases, the child welfare agency must make the final decision after discussion with the MMT. The recommended process and typical questions for the potential therapist are shown in Box 10.4 and discussed as follows. A therapist with credible MBP knowledge and experience is ideal, but few are available. Some therapists will say that they have extensive experience when they actually do not, so claims of experience should be checked carefully.

Therapists who will work with MBP cases need to be interested in learning about MBP, willing to take on a case of this difficulty and complexity, and willing to listen and work collaboratively with CPS and other MMT members. If no therapist with MBP experience is available, good candidates for the perpetrator's therapist might be those with experience in treating substance abusers, those with personality disorders, or sex offenders, and who also have a record of working well with other community professionals. Therapists who will be working with victims should have an understanding of and experience in other forms of child maltreatment or victimization.

Once possible therapists have been identified in the community, and have agreed to consider the case after a brief discussion, one or

Box 10.4.
Therapist Selection Process

1. Identification of possible therapists: Who is available in the community with appropriate qualifications and personal qualities?
2. Initial contacts to possible therapists: Do they have time available for a complex and challenging case that will require numerous contacts with other professionals? Can payment be arranged? Are they interested? Obtain curriculum vitae (résumés). Determine best candidates for follow-up.
3. Arrange interview between CPS and each potential therapist to determine interest and appropriateness and review MBP understanding.
   A. General: Education, training, experience, background. Types of cases the therapist usually works with and basic orientation/techniques.
   B. General case-related: Education, training, experience, background related to specific elements associated with the case at hand.
   C. Overall MBP knowledge and experience: Has the therapist had any training? When, where, and by whom? How extensive was it? Has the therapist read articles or books on MBP? Which ones? Has the therapist ever worked with an MBP case or known anyone who has? What was that experience like? Is the therapist willing to receive additional training if requested by CPS?
   D. Detailed information about the case and how it is being managed: Case outline, role of the MMT, expectations of the therapist (participation in the MMT, open communication with MMT and CPS, role in relation to case plan, e.g., risk reduction).
   E. Agreement about/legal releases of confidentiality, information about the case at hand, working with MBP perpetrators, and working with this perpetrator.
4. Final decision on the appropriateness of the therapist. The therapist is *not* appropriate if:
   A. Potential therapist presents self as an "expert" who is not open to learning and collaboration with the child welfare worker and others as a fellow professional.
   B. Potential therapist challenges the MBP confirmation/diagnosis or does not appear to believe that parents or this

(continued)

(Box 10.4 continued)

   perpetrator could have behaved in that fashion. This
   challenge can be overt or subtle.
C. Potential therapist is not willing to be part of/cooperate with
   the case plan and MMT.
D. Potential therapist requires absolute confidentiality with the
   perpetrator and is not willing to share information, even if a
   release is signed or court authority is in place.

---

more should be asked to meet (separately) with the assigned child welfare staff member to talk about potential involvement and to review their understanding of MBP. In this meeting, the potential therapist should be asked to discuss general background, the types of clients usually worked with, and basic therapeutic orientation/techniques. For MBP cases, therapists should be active in treatment and comfortable with confrontation. Do not use clinicians who will simply commiserate with the perpetrator. Therapists should clearly understand their role, which does not include case management activities. Apparent crises should be immediately reported to the assigned CPS worker or, if that worker is not available, to the on-call worker.

This discussion should be followed by a review of any education, training, experience, and background that may be related to or helpful with specific elements of the case. For example, has the therapist ever had any training in forensic interviewing that would help him or her with a client who is known to be deceptive? If the case includes sexual abuse, is the therapist competent in that area? If the case will involve issues related to health care, does the therapist have any medical background?

The therapist's MBP knowledge and experience must be assessed. Has the therapist had any training in MBP? When, where, and by whom? How extensive was it? Has he or she read articles or books on MBP? Which ones? (These questions may reveal specific theoretical orientations, as well as how current and correct their knowledge is.) Has the therapist ever worked with an MBP case or known another therapist who has? What was that experience like? (The therapist may anticipate a negative experience.) In his or her own words, what is known and understood about MBP? Is the therapist willing to receive additional training and consultation, comparable to that received by MMT members, if requested by CPS?

After this discussion, if the therapist still appears appropriate and interested, the CPS worker should discuss the agency's approach to the management of the case at hand. If the therapist already knows something about the case, this knowledge can be explored with particular attention to whether he or she seems to believe in the confirmation of MBP. With appropriate mutual agreement and legal protections for confidentiality, the CPS worker should provide detailed case information. In this discussion the role of the MMT in ongoing case management must be emphasized, along with expectations that the therapist involved with the perpetrator will participate as a member of the MMT. The need for open communication with the MMT and the CPS worker about the details of what is happening in therapy should be stressed. The potential therapist must understand that it is impossible for any one professional, in isolation from other involved case professionals, to make determinations about risk, "manage" the case, or offer a legitimate evaluation of the perpetrator's progress. That only comes from all involved professionals putting the pieces together. The MMT and MBP expert will also be available as a source of information and support to the therapist, and so will benefit the therapeutic process. The therapist must agree to be a part of the MMT and take part in regular meetings where details of what has been happening are exchanged. The therapist must also understand his or her role in relation to the child protective case; the therapist's job is not simply to provide therapy for the perpetrator, but to work toward risk reduction. This concept of risk reduction, and the risks specific to MBP and to the case, should also be explained, along with the goals of therapy related to MBP.

The realities of working with an MBP perpetrator should be discussed. The therapist should be prepared for the fact that the perpetrator may look, sound, and behave "normally." The perpetrator's psychological profile can be (or can appear to be) unremarkable. If the perpetrator admits to the behavior at all, there are likely to be rationalizations and explanations that sound so plausible that the therapist may doubt the MBP confirmation. The perpetrator is likely to be manipulative and perhaps seductive. The therapist should also take elementary safety precautions such as being careful about what personal information is revealed, since it is possible that the perpetrator could use this destructively (Day 1998c). All of these factors will make therapy more difficult.

Following this discussion, it should be clear whether the therapist being interviewed is a reasonable candidate for work on the specific case. A final decision can be reached by the child welfare agency in consultation with the MMT. Some elements will disqualify the therapist from consideration:

- The potential therapist presents himself or herself as an "expert" who is not open to learning and collaboration with the child welfare worker and others as an equal professional. Much of this will be revealed in the tone of the discussion between the potential therapist and the CPS worker. For example, the potential therapist may use a great deal of theoretical and technical language, may resist the idea that he or she must discuss case planning and management with the MMT, or may seem to feel that he or she should be the most important member of the MMT.
- The potential therapist makes incorrect statements about MBP and does not seem open to learning a "new approach."
- The potential therapist challenges the MBP confirmation or does not appear to believe that people in general or this perpetrator could have behaved in that fashion. This can be overt or subtle. For example, some therapists use a "postmodernist" approach that accepts a client's statements as reality. Whatever the objective truth might be, they focus on the client's "story" as what is true for him or her. This may be a useful approach in some circumstances, but can be problematic with a client who is a known deceiver. Also, when child protection is at issue, it is important to differentiate the client's subjective reality from objective reality.
- The potential therapist is not willing to be part of/cooperate with the case plan and especially with involvement in the MMT meetings.
- The potential therapist requires absolute confidentiality with the perpetrator and is not willing to share information, even if a release is signed or court authority is in place. (Note that signing such a release should be part of the case plan. If the perpetrator refuses to sign it, she or he is in violation of the case plan.)

In reality, the number of potential therapists may be limited and the therapist selected may be less than ideal. For example, the perpetrator may live in an area in which there are few therapists, or financial considerations may limit the choice. In such cases, the agency and MMT must do the best they can. One therapist should not, however, serve more than one party to the case. To do so raises the risk of conflict of interest. Nor is family therapy generally advisable as the initial method of treatment.

Initial and ongoing MBP education and periodic consultation for the selected therapist by a credible MBP professional should not be compromised. For example, the therapist may begin to lose objectivity about the case and become enmeshed with the perpetrator. The MBP expert consultant, who has been assisting throughout the case process, can help the therapist regain perspective. The expert consultant can also help the therapist when specialized questions arise.

Reunification

When (and if) CPS in consultation with the MMT believes that all elements of the case plan have been achieved, planning for reunification should begin. This may be done through the usual child welfare methods of gradually lifting restrictions on visitation, and allowing the child(ren) to spend progressively longer periods with the perpetrator. The foster parents should log the child(ren)'s physical and emotional state following each contact with the perpetrator, and—without being intrusive—should note what the child says about the visit. Anything of concern should be communicated to the CPS worker as quickly as possible. As this process continues, with regular review by the MMT, it may be possible to plan a date for a permanent return home. Even after that occurs, however, continued long-term monitoring of the case and close supervision by CPS must continue. The child's physical and mental health care should continue to be monitored by one person, as already described, and the MMT should continue to meet regularly to review the case status.

APPENDIX:
RECOMMENDED CASE PLAN ELEMENTS IN MBP

Part A: MBP Perpetrator

1. Perpetrator will sign necessary documents enabling agency responsible for the case to obtain written and verbal information regarding perpetrator and child(ren) from health care providers and others and to allow case team members, including mental health professionals, to share detailed case information with one another on an ongoing basis.

2. Perpetrator will undergo mental health therapy to address MBP behavior, any coexisting mental health problems, and other issues. This therapy will be provided by a therapist who has personally received MBP education and detailed case information, believes that the MBP maltreatment has taken place, is not challenging the MBP confirmation, and has been approved by the agency responsible for the case.

3. Perpetrator will undergo a comprehensive mental health evaluation to determine any coexisting mental health concerns.

4. Perpetrator will demonstrate basic understanding of MBP maltreatment.

5. Perpetrator will identify and sincerely admit to her or his pattern of MBP perpetration and related behavior.

6. Perpetrator will demonstrate a sincere understanding of how her or his victim(s) have been negatively impacted as a result of her or his MBP perpetration and related behavior.

7. Perpetrator will demonstrate a sincere understanding of how her or his MBP perpetration and related behavior could negatively impact victim(s) in the future.

8. Perpetrator will identify and sincerely demonstrate understanding of why her or his MBP perpetration and related behavior has happened, and the personal needs she or he has been trying to meet through use of the victim(s).

9. Perpetrator will sincerely identify past, present, and potential future MBP perpetration and related behavior "trigger situations."

10. Perpetrator will sincerely identify, develop, and demonstrate use of alternative behaviors to substitute for MBP perpetration and related behavior.

11. Perpetrator will cooperate fully with and adhere to instructions given by the agency responsible for the case.

Part B: Victims and Potential Victims

1. Victims and potential victims will undergo a mental health evaluation to determine if mental health intervention is presently needed.
2. Physical and mental health needs of victims and potential victims will be coordinated through one professional who has personally received MBP education and detailed case information, believes that the MBP maltreatment has taken place, is not challenging the MBP confirmation, and who has been approved by the agency responsible for the case.
3. MBP basic education and detailed case histories will be personally shared with all adults with whom victims or potential victims are placed.

Part C: Nonperpetrating Spouse/Other Adults

This includes adults living in the home or who are closely and consistently involved, or who seek unsupervised visitation with the victim(s)/potential victim(s).

1. Nonperpetrating spouse/other adults will sign necessary documents enabling the agency responsible for the case to obtain written and verbal information about themselves and their children from health care providers and others, and to allow case team members (including mental health professionals) to share detailed case information with one another on an ongoing basis.
2. Nonperpetrating spouse/other adults will demonstrate basic understanding of MBP maltreatment.
3. Nonperpetrating spouse/other adults will demonstrate a sincere belief in and understanding of the perpetrator's pattern of MBP perpetration and related behavior.
4. Nonperpetrating spouse/other adults will demonstrate a sincere understanding of the personal needs the perpetrator has been trying to meet through use of the victim(s).
5. Nonperpetrating spouse/other adults will demonstrate a sincere understanding of the perpetrator's past, present, and potential future MBP perpetration and related behavior "trigger situations."
6. Nonperpetrating spouse/other adults will demonstrate a sincere understanding of how the perpetrator's victim(s) have been negatively impacted as a result of his or her MBP perpetration and related behavior.
7. Nonperpetrating spouse/other adults will demonstrate a sincere understanding of how the perpetrator's MBP perpetration and related

behavior could negatively impact victim(s) and/or potential victims in the future.

8. Nonperpetrating spouse/other adults will participate in meetings and/or mental health therapy as requested by the agency responsible for the case.

Part D: General Case Management

1. A multiagency-multidisciplinary team (MMT) comprised of case-involved professionals and others as appropriate, who have personally received basic MBP education and detailed case information, will meet regularly (at least every four to six weeks) to share and compare detailed case information, evaluate progress toward attainment of case goals and risk reduction, discuss concerns, and make recommendations. If composition of the MMT changes, new members will be personally provided with basic MBP education and detailed case information prior to their official involvement as a team member.

2. If possible, a credible MBP expert will frequently consult with the MMT and/or agency responsible for the case.

3. Therapist selection for children or adults will be made after the potential therapist has personally received basic MBP education and detailed case information, has indicated belief in and is not challenging the MBP confirmation, and has (with appropriate legal authority) committed to participating as an MMT member and to sharing detailed case/client information.

4. Unsupervised contact with anyone will not take place unless the case plan elements in parts A and C have been satisfied. Unsupervised contact will also not take place until it has been approved by the MMT, including the agency responsible for the case.

5. Supervised visitation, if necessary to meet the needs of the child, will take place under the following conditions:
   A. Visitation will take place in a controlled setting (e.g., not in the home).
   B. Visitation will be supervised by a staff member of the agency responsible for the case. This person will have personally received basic MBP education and detailed case information as well as specific instructions for monitoring and logging.
   C. The visitation supervisor will remain in the room where the visitation is occurring at all times, with attention directed only toward supervision.
   D. No activities may occur during the visitation that the supervisor cannot hear or see.

E. Anything brought to the visit must either be left outside the visitation area or be searched.

F. No food, drink, medications, gum, candy, or anything else that can be ingested will be allowed during visitation unless absolutely necessary. If these must be provided, they must be prepared by an agency staff member using material supplied by the agency responsible for the case, and given to the child by the visitation supervisor at least several feet away from the visitor(s).

G. No discussion of the case, health care issues, or related subjects will be allowed during the visitation.

H. Prior to each visit, visitors will sign an agreement indicating their understanding of these rules.

6. Telephone contact will be allowed only under the following conditions:

A. Telephone contact will be monitored from both ends of the conversation by a staff member of the agency responsible for the case who has personally received basic MBP education and detailed case information as well as specific instructions for monitoring and logging.

B. No discussion of the case, health care issues, or related subjects will be allowed during the telephone contact.

C. Individuals approved for telephone contact will sign an agreement indicating their understanding of these rules.

7. Contact by mail will be allowed only under the following conditions:

A. Mail will be directed to the child(ren) in care of the agency responsible for the case.

B. Letters and packages will be opened and inspected by an agency staff member who has personally received basic MBP education and detailed case information.

C. Letters and packages will be sent to the child(ren) only if they are believed to be beneficial.

D. No discussion of the case, health care issues, or related subjects will be allowed in letters.

E. No gifts of food, drink, medications, gum, candy, or anything else that can be ingested will be allowed.

F. Individuals approved for mail contact will sign an agreement indicating their understanding of these rules.

8. Placement with relatives or friends of the family is potentially dangerous in MBP cases and will be allowed only after a specialized process (over and above what is normally done in approving relatives) and recommendation from the MMT, including the agency responsible for the case.

9. Foster parents will be considered part of the MMT.
10. Foster parents will have no contact with the perpetrator, nonperpetrating spouse, other adults in the home, or other friends and relatives of the family. If such contact occurs, it will be limited to necessary formal discussion. The location of the foster home will not be divulged. Transportation to/from any visits will be performed by the agency responsible for the case.
11. Prior to reunification or unsupervised contact with anyone, the MMT, including the agency responsible for the case, will conduct a detailed case review to determine whether the risk level is such that the proposed activity can take place, and under what conditions. Each plan component will be carefully evaluated to determine whether successful completion has occurred. The reasons for these decisions will be discussed and recorded. At least one professional who was a member of the MMT when MBP was confirmed will participate in this evaluation and in making recommendations. A credible MBP professional should be included. Evaluation and recommendations will be carefully documented, including any disagreements.
12. Throughout case activities, involved professionals will exercise great care in evaluating case information, in determining whether case plan components have been successfully completed and risk reduced, or whether apparent risk reduction actually reflects deception and/or manipulation by the perpetrator and/or others. The use of the word "sincere" in the case planning document, as well as the need for MMT members to share and carefully compare detailed case information on an ongoing basis, reflects this concern.

Part E: Other Case Plan Elements

Specific elements should be added to meet the needs of the case.

Chapter 11

MBP Maltreatment Legal Activities and Considerations

As discussed in Chapter 1, "The desired outcome with MBP cases, as in any form of child maltreatment, is the identification and protection of victims and the avoidance of false accusations. It is very important that MBP neither be missed nor falsely confirmed." Effective legal involvement is necessary if victims of genuine MBP are to be protected and if erroneous MBP suspicions or allegations are to be identified and refuted. From earliest suspicion, those involved in an MBP case should consider the legal activities and issues that may arise. This kind of planning plays an important part in a thorough and appropriate confirmation-disconfirmation process and legal activities.

This chapter is not intended to be a discussion about "the law," nor is it intended to take the place of the involved attorney or of a careful reading of this book as a whole. The purpose of this chapter is to identify and discuss major legal activities and issues that are common to MBP cases.

ATTORNEY SELECTION

As discussed in Chapters 4 and 8, one of the essential elements in a suspected or confirmed MBP case is a competent, correctly MBP-educated attorney. This attorney provides legal advice, takes legal action as necessary to assist the investigation, and prepares thoroughly for court and related activities. Throughout the case, the attorney and the MBP expert should work together as a team. When CPS becomes involved in a suspected or confirmed MBP case, a CPS attorney must become involved very quickly. Persons suspected or accused of MBP maltreatment should also seek legal counsel as soon as they learn of the suspicions or accusation.

Another essential element is the attorney's acceptance of the participation of an MBP expert. Credible MBP experts should work personally with involved attorneys to provide initial and ongoing education as well as other expert activities. Attorneys or other professionals should not try to learn about MBP on their own in the course of a case. It is simply too much for them to master the information, separate correct information about MBP from incorrect information, and still attend to the work that needs to be done. Furthermore, the attorney should receive MBP education from the same source and ideally at the same time as other case-involved professionals. This will help to ensure that all are on the "same page."

The attorney's job is to combine correct MBP information with legal knowledge and skills to provide high-quality legal representation. If this does not happen, the whole case process can be undermined. This requires teamwork between the attorney and the MBP expert. For example:

1. A court order is often necessary to obtain information needed in the confirmation/disconfirmation process. Either side may need this information. If the attorney does not have an adequate understanding of MBP including the investigative process, it is less likely that motions to procure such court orders will be obtained. The attorney and MBP expert should work together in framing or responding to motions.

2. During the case, numerous statements may be made, even by supposed experts, about what criteria and methods must be used for a finding of MBP. If the attorney does not have a clear, correct understanding of MBP identification, intervention, and case management, false information may go unchallenged. This can easily result in mistakes, either finding MBP maltreatment when it is not present, or failing to confirm it when it is present. If the attorney and MBP expert are working closely together, it is much more likely that false information will be uncovered in time for appropriate response.

3. During the investigation and court process, a great deal of information will be presented from seemingly authoritative sources. If the attorney has not been correctly educated about MBP, and is not working closely with the MBP expert, he or she may as-

sume that information contained in health care and other records is true, objective, and unassailable.

4. During an MBP case, a great deal of information will come from a variety of sources. Some information derived from records will seem true, but will need to be verified. Some professionals will present themselves as knowledgeable and experienced in MBP even though they are not. If the attorney has a solid, basic MBP education, and receives and reviews the same information as the MBP expert, the attorney will be less likely to accept and even pass along incorrect information.

In the "real world" it is not always possible to choose one's attorney. Attorneys are usually assigned ahead of time to represent child protective agencies. Persons accused of MBP who do not have funds to pay for private counsel may be assigned a public defender. If the agency or individual has the opportunity to choose an attorney, openness to learning and working closely with an MBP expert throughout the case should be one of the criteria for selection. If legal counsel is assigned, every attempt must be made to convince the attorney that MBP is different from other forms of maltreatment and that specialized basic and continuing education, expert assistance, and teamwork will be needed throughout the case. If it becomes obvious that an attorney is not willing to work in this way, and if attempts to talk over the situation do not improve it, then that person is not appropriate for the case. If the attorney was hired privately, he or she will need to be replaced. If the attorney was assigned, the problem must be brought to the attention of those who have the power to deal with it. Those taking such action should be prepared to include basic MBP education, and seek the advice of the MBP expert in preparing for the discussion.

THE MBP EXPERT

Two of the essential elements in working with suspected or confirmed MBP cases, as discussed in Chapter 4, are an MBP expert and expert witness. In MBP cases, the same person usually fills both roles, mainly because there are few credible MBP experts, and also because of associated costs. Although the MBP expert may become involved at any stage of the case, it is important to do this as quickly as possible after initial MBP suspicion. This will reduce the chances of mistakes early in the investigation and confirmation/disconfirmation process.

If the MBP expert becomes involved after MBP has been confirmed or disconfirmed, for example to provide a second opinion or to make case recommendations, the expert must review all case information. The expert should determine whether or not she or he agrees or disagrees with the opinion, criteria and methods used, recommendations, present case management, etc. This new, independent review should be completed, regardless of what has been accomplished previously in the case, and regardless of the assumed competence of the people who have confirmed or disconfirmed MBP.

The importance of this review is illustrated by the following case in which CPS staff believed that MBP had been correctly confirmed, but the expert witness's independent review led to a different conclusion.

Case 11.1 MBP Erroneously Confirmed by a Pediatrician

A well-regarded pediatrician telephoned CPS. He reported that a nurse had walked into a hospital room and discovered a grandfather forcing a pillow into his ten-year-old granddaughter's face. The pediatrician reported this as confirmed MBP maltreatment, stating that it accounted for some breathing irregularities that the child had experienced in the hospital. CPS accepted the pediatrician's MBP confirmation and did no further investigation or confirmation/disconfirmation process activities.

The grandfather admitted to attempting to kill the child. With tears in his eyes he described the girl's repeated and anguished pleas that he "stop" her terrible pain. However, the pediatrician continued to insist that the grandfather had perpetrated MBP maltreatment. Based on the pediatrician's affidavit, the court granted CPS an emergency order granting temporary legal custody to CPS and ordering that there be no contact between the grandfather and the child. CPS also began proceedings to gain legal custody of the child including a permanency plan of terminating the grandfather's custody of the child.

At this point, the grandfather's attorney retained an MBP expert who completed a thorough and objective MBP investigation and confirmation/disconfirmation process. The expert concluded that the grandfather had engaged in "MBP-like behavior" (attempting to smother his granddaughter), but there was no reason to conclude that MBP maltreatment was involved. No evidence had been found that the grandfather had a deceptive pattern of behavior, either in relation to his granddaughter or otherwise. Problem induction appeared to be limited to the one event, to which the grandfather had admitted. Interviews with hospital staff, including the pediatrician, revealed that the grandfather had been distraught over his grandchild's condition. Staff had heard the child repeatedly ask the grandfather to "help." The breathing problems had, in fact, worsened since the grandfather was denied contact with the girl.

At the next hearing, the MBP expert provided MBP education, related the education to the case, and explained why evidence did not support a confirmation of MBP. Although acknowledging the seriousness of the grandfather's actions, the expert stated why, in her opinion, it was in the best interest of the now dying child that supervised contact between the child and grandfather be allowed. The court agreed with the expert, and the grandfather was able to be with the girl until her death.

In this case a report of maltreatment and even criminal charges would have been appropriate. In disconfirming MBP, the expert was not excusing the grandfather's conduct. However, even if one wrong has been committed, it is not correct to find a person guilty of a different wrong, particularly one that carries the implications and case plan elements of MBP.

SELECTING THE MBP EXPERT

No universally accepted criteria or certifications for MBP experts exist. The hiring professional must assess the candidate's qualifications and decide whether these meet the requirements of the case. The court will determine whether a person will be allowed to testify as an expert witness. Prior to the judge's decision, it is likely that each attorney will challenge the qualifications of the other side's expert. Thus it is essential that a person with the highest possible MBP qualifications be chosen, and that the qualifications be fully and accurately presented to the court.

There are three important criteria for an MBP expert:

1. credible, skills-based knowledge and experience specific to MBP maltreatment;
2. sound, basic, general investigative skills; and
3. working knowledge of the various forms of child maltreatment.

Those seeking an expert must realize that expertise in MBP maltreatment is not gained solely by virtue of being a health, mental health, or other kind of professional. Some professionals may have been introduced to the subject of MBP in the course of their training, or may have attended workshops or read articles about MBP, but this does not make them experts. This was one key problem in Case 11.1; the pediatrician erroneously believed he was sufficiently knowledgeable about MBP. The second key problem in Case 11.1 occurred when CPS accepted the pediatrician's finding uncritically. Even though an individual may have read extensively about MBP and have been involved in a few cases, the lack of significant actual experience in working with a variety of suspected and confirmed MBP cases would be concerning.

Questions to Determine an Expert's Qualifications

Box 11.1 provides important questions to determine an individual's MBP qualifications. These questions may be used as a part of selecting an MBP expert, for attempting to qualify the professional as

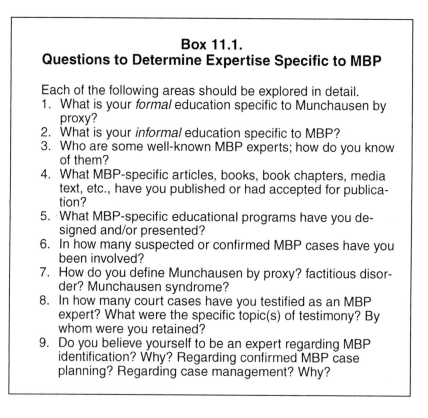

Box 11.1.
Questions to Determine Expertise Specific to MBP

Each of the following areas should be explored in detail.
1. What is your *formal* education specific to Munchausen by proxy?
2. What is your *informal* education specific to MBP?
3. Who are some well-known MBP experts; how do you know of them?
4. What MBP-specific articles, books, book chapters, media text, etc., have you published or had accepted for publication?
5. What MBP-specific educational programs have you designed and/or presented?
6. In how many suspected or confirmed MBP cases have you been involved?
7. How do you define Munchausen by proxy? factitious disorder? Munchausen syndrome?
8. In how many court cases have you testified as an MBP expert? What were the specific topic(s) of testimony? By whom were you retained?
9. Do you believe yourself to be an expert regarding MBP identification? Why? Regarding confirmed MBP case planning? Regarding case management? Why?

an expert in court, or for use in assessing and potentially challenging the MBP expert qualifications of others. Answers to these questions will lead to further questions. In addition, sources of information such as the Internet, reference books, and publication abstracts should be investigated for what they may reveal about the candidate.

1. *What is your formal education specific to Munchausen by proxy? (Classes, workshops, seminars, etc.) Who presented the educational programs? Who sponsored the programs? What topics were included? How long were the programs?*

Explanation: There is no specific training program or academic degree in MBP. Professionals may not have been exposed to the topic in their training. However, a person with true expertise in MBP will have a combination of formal and informal education and experience that adds up to extensive engagement with the subject. Information about the programs attended may reveal not only thoroughness and accuracy, but also specific interests or even biases of the individual under consideration.

2. *What is your informal education specific to MBP?* (Specific books and articles read, authors, etc.)

Explanation: (same as for Question 1).

3. *Who are some well-known MBP experts? How do you know of them?*

Explanation: The potential expert should have knowledge of major MBP professionals. As with the first two questions, this may also reveal specific areas of interest or bias. The potential expert should not be expected to know everyone who has written or spoken about MBP, and all details of their work.

4. *What MBP-specific articles, books, book chapters, media text, etc., have you published or had accepted for publication? What topics were included? Where were they published (etc.)?*

Explanation: A record of publication probably indicates a scholarly and substantial interest in MBP and worthwhile contributions to knowledge about it. However, the mere fact of having written about MBP is not significant if these writings were never published, or if there is not a definite commitment from a publisher. The quality of publication should also be taken into account. Publications in peer-reviewed journals and mainstream book publishers, for example, are more credible than publications only in the popular press or self-published books.

5. *What MBP-specific educational programs have you designed and/or presented? Where were they presented (including national/ international professional meetings)? What topics were included?*

Explanation: If the potential expert has designed and presented credible educational programs to a variety of respected organizations, this attests to the respect with which the expert is regarded.

6. *In how many suspected or confirmed MBP cases have you been involved? What was your specific role? At what point did you become involved? At what point did your involvement cease? In how many cases did you confirm MBP? In how many cases did you disconfirm/not find it? What criteria do you use to confirm/disconfirm MBP? What methods are appropriate to the MBP investigation and confirmation-disconfirmation process? (Review of records? What kinds of records? Records regarding whom? Interviews? Of whom? Mental health testing or evalution? Of whom? Why? Anything else?)*

Explanation: As already discussed, the potential expert should have considerable experience in a variety of cases. Be concerned if involvement in most cases was only brief, if the potential expert always or never confirms MBP in cases, and if the potential expert cannot articulate clear criteria and methods for deciding if MBP is present. It is also concerning if the person appears to confirm or disconfirm MBP without having completed a confirmation/disconfirmation process using multiple sources of information, or by basing the opinion on an inappropriate methodology. For example, it would clearly be *unacceptable* if the candidate depends heavily on a mental health evaluation that includes testing and interviews of the suspected perpetrator to determine whether the person "has" MBP.

7. *How do you define Munchausen by proxy? factitious disorder? Munchausen syndrome?*

Explanation: The potential expert should be able to distinguish among these terms easily.

8. *In how many court cases have you testified as an MBP expert? What were the specific topic(s) of testimony? Who retained you?*

Explanation: Find out in how many cases the potential expert was qualified as an expert by the judge and whether this person generally speaks to only one aspect of a case or to one point of view, and if so, why.

9. *Do you believe yourself to be an expert regarding MBP identification? Why? Regarding confirmed MBP case planning? Regarding case management? Why?*

Explanation: The potential expert's areas of strengths should match the needs of the case.

As part of the selection process, it must be agreed that two basic activities will occur as quickly as possible. First, the MBP expert should personally provide at least basic MBP education to the attorney and other case-involved professionals. This is necessary if they are to begin working as a team, and so that the attorney and others can incorporate vital information into case activities from the beginning. Additional education should be provided as needed. Second, the MBP expert should review all available case information and provide initial impressions and recommendations verbally or in writing. This should be accomplished quickly, since it is likely that initial recommendations will include the need for further information. Because written documents are potentially available to the other side through the process of "discovery," there must be a clear understanding between the expert and the attorney about what information the attorney does and does not want in writing. Even e-mail may be "discoverable," depending on the particular area and court, and it cannot be regarded as secure.

COMMON MBP MALTREATMENT LEGAL STRATEGIES

Following are a number of common strategies used specifically in MBP court cases. Because these are so common, persons preparing for an MBP court hearing should be ready to respond to them.

Common MBP maltreatment legal strategies include:

- attempts to disqualify the other side's MBP expert;
- use of "hired gun" experts;
- assertion that Munchausen by proxy does not exist or is just a theory that has not been "proven";
- assertions based on deliberate or unknowing misuse of DSM-IV;
- assertion that MBP is or is not involved because the alleged perpetrator does or does not fit a "profile";

- assertion that the alleged perpetrator is merely overanxious or overprotective;
- other assertions that the alleged MBP behavior has been misinterpreted and is not really deliberate exaggeration and/or fabrication and/or induction;
- assertion that the perpetrator merely followed doctor's orders or recommendations;
- assertion that others saw the "problem";
- assertion or appearance that this is a good, loving caregiver who would never deliberately harm or cause harm;
- assertion that MBP perpetration is not involved because a mental health evaluation of the alleged perpetrator is "normal";
- attempts to limit time allocated for the court hearing;
- attempts to keep the MBP label from being used;
- misuse of terminology;
- assertion that MBP is so rare that it is very unlikely to be involved in this case;
- assertion that, because a professional made a physical or mental health diagnosis, the diagnosis must be true;
- assertion that because there is a divorce/custody dispute or domestic violence, the MBP suspicions or allegations have been "trumped up";
- assertion that the MBP opinion was not based on a thorough and appropriate investigation and confirmation-disconfirmation process;
- assertion that the child has not been in the hospital very often, or has never been in the hospital, so MBP cannot be involved;
- assertion that the accused caretaker and child love each other; therefore, the caretaker could not have maltreated the child; and
- assertion that a professional has alleged MBP because he or she can't find out what is the matter.

1. *Attempts to disqualify the other side's MBP expert.* Questions in Box 11.1 can be used to determine the depth and breadth of a person's MBP-specific knowledge and experience. Often a person who is reputed to be an MBP expert turns out to have only limited actual knowledge and experience. Potential testimony by such a supposed "expert" should be vigorously challenged.

Unfortunately, in some MBP cases, serious personal attacks may be made against the MBP expert. These may include false allegations—sometimes scathing and prolonged ones—that the expert's opinion was bought, that the expert is biased, that the expert has personal problems that render the expert's testimony suspect, or even that the expert enjoys breaking up families and the attention of court testimony. Persons who will be testifying in MBP cases should not underestimate the possibility that this may occur.

2. *Use of "hired gun" experts.* Unfortunately, there are people in the field of MBP, as elsewhere, who deliberately attempt to twist facts, misinterpret information, disregard information, etc., to provide an opinion that is sympathetic to the side that is paying them. Some people may be retained because their testimony is highly predictable—for example, because they are known to assert that MBP does not exist or has not been "scientifically proven." Again, knowledge about the witness prior to the court hearing will help the side to anticipate and counter testimony.

3. *Assertion that Munchausen by proxy/factitious disorder by proxy does not exist or is just a theory that has not been "proven."* This defense strategy is used frequently, and some "hired guns" are well-known for this argument. A discussion of this issue appears in Chapter 1.

Those who advance this argument often build a plausible-sounding case based on technical interpretations of words such as "theory," "science," and "proven." For example, they exploit the popular belief that "theory" means something that has no evidence to support it. Because, strictly speaking, "proof" only occurs when there has been a formal experiment, they may say that the existence of MBP has never been "proven." Of course, this argument ignores the many ways that a pattern of behavior can be demonstrated to have occurred. If this line of reasoning were followed to its absurd conclusion, no disease (for example, cancer) could be "proven" to exist since no disease has been validated by formal experimental findings.

If a side anticipates that this argument will be used, they should attack the argument directly rather than trying to advance "proof" that the witness will never accept. They should consider an expert witness (probably not an MBP expert) with specific training in scientific standards of proof. A university professor who teaches research or the philosophy of science (courses available at most universities) would be one example of such an expert.

4. *Assertions based on deliberate or unknowing misuse of DSM-IV.* As discussed in Chapter 1, professionals frequently misunderstand the DSM-IV, and may use it in court to "prove" either that MBP is involved or that it is not involved. The attorney and MBP expert should be alert for assertions based on the "invoking" of the DSM-IV. These assertions can be countered by correct understanding and testimony regarding this area including reference to the definition of "research criteria" contained in the DSM-IV itself, or by the published views of experts in the field about problems with the criteria for MBP as it appears in the DSM-IV (see, for example, Meadow, 1995b; Schreier, 2002).

Two commonly heard assertions related to the DSM-IV are that MBP is a mental illness that a perpetrator "has," and that the alleged perpetrator has engaged in this behavior because of mental health problems; therefore this is not MBP maltreatment. These ideas have been discussed in detail in Chapter 1. It requires careful listening to "catch" each instance in which a witness or discussant refers to a person (perpetrator or victim) who "has" MBP. Misuse of language must not be allowed. The argument can be countered on two levels. First, as discussed repeatedly throughout this book, MBP is not "in" the DSM-IV as a recognized form of mental illness, but as a category for further study. Second, even if a mental illness is listed in the DSM-IV it does not necessarily render a person incapable of knowing right from wrong or incapable of controlling his or her behavior. For example, stuttering, nicotine withdrawal, depression, anxiety, lack of sexual desire, and insomnia are all "mental disorders" included in the body of the DSM-IV. The safest strategy is to insist, throughout proceedings, that MBP is not a mental health diagnosis.

5. *Assertion that MBP is or is not involved because the alleged perpetrator does or does not fit a "profile."* This assertion is sometimes based on incorrect information or selective reading of the literature. For example, the stereotype of MBP perpetrators is that they are female and that they "doctor shop." As discussed in Chapter 2, no set of traits can infallibly distinguish perpetrators from nonperpetrators. Certain indicators may add to suspicion, but do not constitute proof. The important issue is whether the case, as a whole, constitutes or does not constitute a provable pattern of behavior that fits the defini-

tion of MBP. Details in the literature or elsewhere, particularly if they are outdated or incorrect, should not be allowed to distract from that issue.

6. *Assertion that the alleged perpetrator is merely overanxious or overprotective.* This strategy is so common that it should be anticipated, and ample evidence should be prepared to show a pattern of truth telling or deception. As discussed in Chapter 2, overanxious/ overprotective caretakers stick close to the truth about their child's problems or perceived problems, and they are sincerely concerned that something is or might be wrong with the child. One does not find the pattern of deception with regard to the child's health care (and often in other aspects or their lives) that is found with an MBP perpetrator. If a thorough and appropriate investigation and confirmation-disconfirmation process is completed, either a *pattern* of deliberate deception appears or it does not.

7. *Other assertions that the alleged MBP behavior has been misinterpreted and is not really deliberate exaggeration and/or fabrication and/or induction.* MBP perpetrators usually can provide seemingly plausible reasons for their questionable behaviors. Although explanations of individual situations can be persuasive, the pattern (if present and identified) should speak for itself.

8. *Assertion that the perpetrator merely followed doctor's orders or recommendations.* This is an attempt to shift the responsibility for the maltreatment from the perpetrator to the health care (or other) provider. It should be clear from the confirmation-disconfirmation process whether the professional relied on accurate information, or was manipulated through inaccurate information. If inaccurate information was provided or manipulation occurred, the professional was only the instrument of the perpetrator.

9. *Assertion that others saw the "problem."* As discussed in Chapter 6, such "eyewitnesses" cannot be taken at face value, and specialized interviews must occur. Even if someone saw a genuine problem at some point (for example, a demonstrably real illness), that does not invalidate other instances of demonstrated or likely exaggeration and/or fabrication and/or induction.

10. *Assertion or appearance that this is a good, loving caregiver who would never deliberately harm or cause harm.* MBP perpetrators are often excellent actors and usually look like normal, even exemplary people and caregivers. Friends, neighbors, relatives, and profes-

sionals will likely come to court to testify on their behalf. However, "character witnesses" in MBP cases are no more reliable than in sexual offense cases, where they also are frequently used to suggest that the perpetrator is incapable of doing what is alleged. The truth is that anyone can have a hidden side.

This is equally true even if the child victim or other children of the perpetrator testify in court that the alleged perpetrator has done no wrong. As discussed in Chapters 2 and 13, children's statements may represent a lack of knowledge, having been misled by the perpetrator, or having been manipulated to lie.

11. *Assertion that MBP perpetration is not involved because a mental health evaluation of the alleged perpetrator is "normal."* As discussed in Chapter 6, there is no mental health test or evaluation that establishes to a level of certainty the presence or absence of MBP.

12. *Attempts to limit time allocated for the court hearing.* Ample time must be allowed to thoroughly present the case (frequently much more time than other kinds of hearings). Without sufficient time, the court may not be provided with the education and evidence necessary for a fair decision.

13. *Attempts to keep the MBP label from being used.* The accused's side may ask for "deals" or "stipulated agreements" in which the alleged perpetrator will admit to non-MBP maltreatment. Sometimes the agreement is to something more general such as "the child is deprived" or "is a child in need of care." The label MBP must be included in the finding of facts in court so that the appropriate case plan, along with appropriate case management, can be justified. Also, the MBP maltreatment should always be linked to the type of abuse/ neglect defined in the state's statutes. For example: "In this case, Munchausaen by proxy maltreatment has manifested as physical abuse, emotional abuse, and health care neglect."

14. *Misuse of terminology.* Cases can be substantially weakened, lost, or even dismissed if terminology is not used correctly. This may be due to an incorrect understanding of the terminology, or it may be deliberate. For example, cases have been dismissed because the term "Munchausen syndrome" or "factitious disorder" was used on legal documents rather than "Munchausen by proxy" or "factitious disorder by proxy." Another example is confusion between the terms "rule out" and "ruled out." The former means that a problem is under consideration, while the latter means that it is not. If the two are con-

fused, the conclusion, resulting report, and court testimony may contain information that the problem has been resolved.

15. *Assertion that MBP is so rare that it is very unlikely to be involved in this case.* This issue was discussed in Chapter 1. MBP is often more common than some of the rare diagnoses the victim is alleged to "have."

16. *Assertion that, because a professional made a physical or mental health diagnosis, the diagnosis must be true.* As previously discussed, even expert professionals can be duped through word or deed. Diagnoses in suspected or confirmed MBP cases must be scrutinized with reference to the possible MBP. The conclusion must not be drawn that, because one diagnosis in a case situation is valid, others are also.

17. *Assertion that because there is a divorce/custody dispute or domestic violence, the MBP suspicions or allegations have been "trumped up."* Child maltreatment often does occur in the context of these kinds of situations, and MBP maltreatment may occur and/or be identified during or as a result of these situations. Several large-scale studies have shown that other types of allegations of maltreatment (e.g., sexual abuse), are equally likely to be validated in custody and noncustody contexts (see, for instance, Thoennes and Tjaden, 1990). Each piece of a situation must be evaluated on its own merits.

18. *Assertion that the MBP opinion was not based on a thorough and appropriate investigation and confirmation-disconfirmation process.* This may be true, and if so, the opinion is suspect. However, inappropriate objections or other delaying tactics related to the opinion may also be raised. For example, the other side may try to discredit the opinion by pointing out that a specific mental health evaluation was not done (when it would not show whether MBP has occurred) or by impugning the credentials of the person who performed an evaluation. The integrity of the confirmation/disconfirmation process as a whole should be kept in focus.

19. *Assertion that the child has not been in the hospital very often, or has never been in the hospital, so MBP cannot be involved.* Children do not have to be hospitalized to be MBP victims. Many MBP cases involve outpatient, rather than inpatient settings.

20. *Assertion that the accused caretaker and child love each other; therefore, the caretaker could not have maltreated the child.* Examples demonstrating this assertion may be courtroom behavior, pic-

tures, videos, witness testimony, etc. At issue is what has occurred, not emotions.

21. *Assertion that a professional alleges MBP because he or she can't find out what is the matter.* It may be claimed that MBP is only a self-protective label used by professionals to cover up their own failure to diagnose the genuine problem. A thorough confirmation/disconfirmation process should reveal the truth: that the professionals have found out what is the matter, and it is MBP.

MOTIONS

Various kinds of legal motions are likely to be made throughout the case and by both sides. When writing or arguing for or against a particular motion in an MBP case, correct education and strong rationale must be provided. Otherwise, the argument may be lost, and the case with it. Typical motions include the following:

1. Motions requesting court orders to obtain various kinds of records necessary to the MBP confirmation/disconfirmation process. Often, necessary records are not obtainable without a court order. One example would be the perpetrator's health care records, which she or he has refused to release.
2. Motions for a court order requiring the suspected/alleged perpetrator and/or others to be interviewed by the MBP expert, and under what conditions. Again, these people may not consent to interviews. An example of a condition that might be court ordered is the interview with the suspected perpetrator alone, without the presence of attorneys.
3. Motions for a court order enabling other professionals to communicate freely, personally or in writing, with the MBP expert about the case and family. Without such an order, professionals or their agencies may refuse to communicate with the MBP expert because of laws or ethics about confidentiality. For example, although records may have been released, a court order may be required for the MBP expert to talk with professionals to clarify details of the records or secure additional information.
4. Motions for the suspected or alleged perpetrator and/or others to have mental health evaluations. Such evaluations do not determine whether the person has perpetrated MBP, but may be use-

ful for obtaining additional information, or for case planning and management. The perpetrator or others may not agree to these evaluations without the court order.

5. Motions to exclude the MBP label. As already discussed, this is a common legal strategy in MBP cases. If MBP is present, such a motion should be vigorously opposed.

6. Motions for a court order that case-involved professionals personally receive MBP education. As important as this education is, some professionals may resist it and not attend unless they are forced to. Case 11.1 is an example of the damage that can be done when professionals do not have complete and correct information about MBP.

7. Motions for a court order that case-involved professionals form a multiagency-multidisciplinary team (MMT), or for certain professionals to be involved in the MMT. Sometimes professionals will resist forming an MMT because of confidentiality or other concerns. Some of those who need to be involved in the MMT may also resist unless their participation is mandated. Case 4.1 in Chapter 4 shows the impact of one professional's refusal to participate. A motion requiring the psychologist's involvement would have been helpful.

8. Motions regarding out-of-home placement, visitation, or other contact. The MBP-specific details of such placement and contact are vital to the protection of the victim(s) (see Chapter 10). This is particularly important in jurisdictions where child protective agencies do not have the authority to specify such details, or where the court must approve any changes in the placement. For example, a motion may be necessary to specify if and when contact is to occur and under what circumstances.

EDUCATING THE COURT ABOUT MBP MALTREATMENT

Regardless of the kind of hearing, the court must receive education regarding MBP maltreatment in order to make fair and appropriate decisions. As stated by Stern (1997), "The quality of the decisions made by judges and jurors is largely dependent upon the quality of education they receive from expert witnesses" (p. 1). This educational process is important in anticipating and diffusing strategies of the other side. The questions in the following list can be asked of the expert witness to educate the court about MBP basics and to attempt to neutralize anticipated strategies of the other side.

1. Are you familiar with the term factitious disorder?
2. What is factitious disorder?
3. Is factitious disorder the same thing as Munchausen syndrome?
4. Is there a difference between hypochondria and factitious disorder including Munchausen syndrome? Please explain.
5. Are you familiar with the term Munchausen by proxy or MBP?
6. Are there other terms that mean the same thing as Munchausen by proxy or MBP?
7. What is the definition of Munchausen by proxy?
8. What does "exaggerate" mean in the context of MBP?
9. What does "fabricate" mean in the context of MBP?
10. What does "induce" mean in the context of MBP?
11. Are physical abuse, emotional abuse, sexual abuse, and neglect related to MBP? Please explain.
12. Please explain how each of those kinds of maltreatment can manifest through MBP maltreatment.
13. What is the *Diagnostic and Statistical Manual of Mental Disorders,* commonly known as the DSM-IV?
14. Is factitious disorder (Munchausen syndrome, or any term that means the same) mentioned in the DSM-IV? Is it a formal DSM-IV mental health diagnosis?
15. Are there any problems with using information about MBP contained in DSM-IV? Please explain.
16. Should MBP be considered something someone "has" or "suffers from"? In other words, should MBP be considered a person's diagnosis? Please explain.
17. Is Munchausen by proxy a recognized kind of maltreatment—meaning abuse/neglect?
18. Is there any mental health evaluation or test that can determine whether MBP is or is not present?
19. Is there any profile or combination of personal characteristics or traits that can determine whether someone is or is not an MBP perpetrator?

20. What criteria must be met in order to confirm MBP maltreatment?
21. What methods should be used in determining whether the case situation meets the criteria?
22. Does working with suspected or confirmed MBP cases require specialized knowledge and experience? Please explain.
23. Is there a difference between an overanxious/overprotective caretaker and an MBP perpetrator? Please explain.
24. Are there any situations that should cause at least suspicion that MBP maltreatment might be occurring? Please describe some of the major MBP suspicion indicators.
25. Should cases involving suspicion or confirmation of exaggeration and/or fabrication be considered less dangerous than cases in which suspicion or confirmation of inducing problems is involved? Please explain.
26. Is MBP a dangerous kind of maltreatment? Please explain.
27. Does a person with expertise regarding factitious disorder, including Munchausen syndrome, necessarily have expertise with regard to Munchausen by proxy? Please explain.
28. How does deception relate to MBP? Please explain.
29. If professionals and others observe the suspected or alleged perpetrator as a good, loving caretaker, and the dynamics between the suspected or alleged perpetrator and the alleged victim appear appropriate, should suspicion or confirmation of MBP maltreatment be ruled out? Please explain.
30. If friends, neighbors, and relatives state or even testify that the suspected or alleged MBP perpetrator is a good, loving caretaker who has never mistreated the child, should suspicion or confirmation of MBP be ruled out? Please explain.
31. Do methods of MBP perpetration necessarily remain the same throughout a particular case? Please explain.
32. Is there any change to victim risk when a suspected or alleged perpetrator learns of the suspicion? Please explain.
33. Should it be expected that catching and confronting an MBP perpetrator will cause victim or potential victim risk to cease? Please explain.
34. Does an MBP perpetrator usually admit to the MBP perpetration?

35. If an MBP perpetrator admits to perpetrating MBP, should it be expected that the perpetrator will admit to the entire pattern of MBP and related behavior? Please explain.
36. Is determining victim risk in MBP maltreatment cases different from other kinds of maltreatment cases? Please explain.
37. Is it safe for MBP victims or potential victims to remain under the care, custody, control, or influence of the suspected perpetrator or anyone who might be influenced by the perpetrator? Please explain.
38. Are there any special considerations regarding placing MBP victims or potential victims with relatives?
39. Are there any other special considerations regarding out-of-home placement of MBP victims or potential victims?

Some questions will be more appropriate to various phases of the case, for example, the evidentiary stage where one side is attempting to prove or disprove MBP, or the dispositional phase where case planning and case management are argued. These questions can be asked of any others who are testifying in any way regarding factitious disorder, including Munchausen syndrome, as well as MBP. Attorneys must be careful not to underestimate the importance of taking the time for educational testimony. Evidence brought forth without the court's understanding of this kind of maltreatment may be of little influence.

Exhibits

An especially effective method of educating the court about the particular case is through use of visual and audiovisual aids ("exhibits"). These are often very effective in clarifying aspects of these complicated cases, as well as conveying specific information. A variety of exhibits may be appropriate to MBP cases as adjuncts to testimony by the expert witness and other professionals. Following are some possible exhibits.

1. A listing of every unnecessary health care visit, procedure, medicine, etc., that the victim has experienced. These can be placed on one large chart, perhaps separated by type. Such a chart can be very effective in conveying to the court the massive number

of unnecessary procedures and interventions the victim has endured.
2. A listing of the pain, suffering, and harm experienced by the victim. This should include past, present, and projections for the future. Detailed descriptions should be provided in testimony.
3. A listing of each type of child maltreatment recognized by the state (e.g., physical, emotional, sexual, neglect) and how these relate to the MBP maltreatment in the case.
4. If important patterns have been identified (for example, victim having problems only when the father is on military duty, or only when in the custody of the perpetrator), time lines or graphs can be very useful. Figure 11.1 shows information about the frequency of episodes for a child while at home with the perpetrator and while in placement. Use of such visual aids can bring data to life and show relationships clearly, in this case, the relationship between exposure to the perpetrator and the occurrence of events.
5. Video and/or audiotapes of actual perpetration or other MBP behavior are, of course, vital evidence.
6. Videotapes or photos that counter the perpetrator's assertions about the victim's condition can also be very powerful. For example, in one case the grandparents stated that the victim was very frail. A videotape was presented in court that showed the child running and playing.

Such exhibits must be testified to and visible in court. Efforts to simply place them into evidence or stipulate to them should be resisted. Even if there are handouts of the exhibits, they should be enlarged and placed on an easel or played on a large screen during testimony.

When exhibits are going to be used that could be subject to tampering, such as tapes, "chain-of-evidence" procedures must be followed. The attorney should be consulted for assistance with this.

THE PROBABLE CAUSE HEARING

After a child is taken into protective custody, a probable cause hearing is almost always held within a certain length of time, typi-

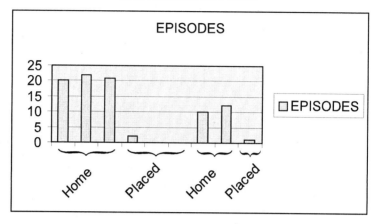

FIGURE 11.1. Episodes When at Home and in Placement

cally twenty-four to seventy-two hours. In this hearing the court decides whether it was appropriate to take the child into custody and whether reasonable efforts were made to keep the child with the family (or if it was in the best interest of the child not to make such efforts). The court will also decide whether the child should remain in out-of-home placement and, if so, it will decide issues such as visitation or other contact. Non-MBP probable cause hearings do not usually include expert testimony. However, since MBP is unique and often misunderstood, it may be wise for the MBP expert to provide basic MBP education and testify to the case process so far. The questions in the following list can be useful for this process, and will supplement any written report. Even if an expert witness is not available, these issues should be addressed in the probable cause hearing.

1. Are you suspicious, or have you provisionally confirmed, that Munchausen by proxy has been perpetrated in this case? (If the expert is not testifying: Is there suspicion or has there been a provisional confirmation that MBP has been perpetrated in this case?)
2. Who is the suspected/confirmed/provisionally confirmed perpetrator?
3. What is the basis for your suspicion/provisional confirmation? (If the expert is not testifying: What individual(s) have been in-

volved in formulating MBP suspicion or provisional confirmation?)

4. What activities must still be accomplished for a definitive opinion to be provided regarding the presence or absence of MBP in this case?
5. Are there any current or anticipated problems relating to completion of these activities?
6. What would be the risk to the child(ren) if returned to the home today? When MBP has been confirmed or provisionally confirmed, an MBP risk assessment work sheet for each child should be submitted as an exhibit. If MBP maltreatment is in the suspicion stage, a careful statement should be made or submitted about present risk. If concerns exist regarding the health or safety of the child (or children) under the present circumstances, those concerns should be clearly stated and, if appropriate, motions should be made to address the concerns.
7. What are your present recommendations?

A FINAL OBSERVATION ON THE IMPORTANCE OF THE COURT PROCESS

For many professionals, going to court is seen as time-consuming and stressful. Professionals often do not understand the proceedings or the specialized vocabulary that accompanies court hearings. These feelings are natural, but must be overcome if the victim is to be protected. As stated at the beginning of the chapter, effective legal involvement is necessary if victims of genuine MBP are to be protected and if erroneous MBP suspicions or allegations are to be identified and refuted. Although the attorney and MBP expert should take the lead in legal involvement, each professional involved in the case bears a responsibility to help as needed and, if called to testify, to prepare and present testimony to the best of his or her ability. This is the only way that both victims and those accused of victimization can be protected.

Chapter 12

Therapeutic Considerations with Perpetrators

The authors of this book had reservations about addressing the topic of therapy with perpetrators. The medical and social science literature do not present a comprehensive theoretical or practical approach to this topic, nor do the authors know of any clinician who has published or presented extensive and specific methodologically oriented work related to MBP. Many of the journal articles and book chapters cited in this chapter are based on work with a small number of cases. However, a synthesis of the literature and some approaches to this topic may be useful both to clinicians who are seeing their first MBP perpetrator, and to the field in suggesting lines for future investigation.

Two basic approaches will be discussed in this chapter. First, the literature on therapy with MBP perpetrators will be reviewed. Therapeutic approaches found in the literature and the claims made for them are presented.* The form of therapy used in any case depends on careful consideration of the specific issues and personalities involved. In MBP cases, the need for victim protection must not be compromised. The training, experience, and competence of the therapist will also influence the choice of method.

In the second part of the chapter, the mental health diagnoses often associated with MBP and the therapeutic approaches often associated with these diagnoses are reviewed. A cautionary note is necessary. There is an old joke, "How many therapists does it take to change a lightbulb?" The answer is, "Only one, but the lightbulb must want to change." This joke points out a truism: therapists, no matter how con-

---

*The authors of this book do not endorse any specific approach and do not have independent knowledge about the efficacy of any of these methods.

scientious or talented, do not change people. Their skills may help to engage the client in the change effort. They may work hard to understand the client's psychosocial dynamics, and point these out in ways that the client can accept. But they cannot "make" people do the internal and interpersonal work necessary for true change to occur. Only the individual can do that. If the person is not willing or able to be honest and open, if he or she is not motivated to change or does not have the capacity to change, change will not occur. Polledri (1996, p. 554) states, in relation to MBP:

> Success in therapy will ultimately depend on the individual dynamics of the patient, her willingness to acknowledge the fabricating behavior and its destructiveness and, equally importantly, on the therapist's ability to work supportively with the patient without being deceived by her cheerful surface presentation. In most cases this presents a highly challenging task for even the most experienced of health professionals.

Rand (1990, pp. 88-89) believes that psychotherapy is so prone to difficulties that case management is more appropriate:

> Traditional individual psychotherapy has, by and large, been found to be ineffective in the treatment of MSP. . . . In theory, at least, enlightened therapy of less severe cases may be helpful if the mother is motivated, if she exhibits minimal antisocial tendencies, and the therapy is part of a holistic, *well-supervised* case plan monitored by the court or child protective services. . . . When all is said and done, however, these families remain, as Meadow so simply and eloquently states, "exceedingly difficult and stressful to manage." [Emphasis in original]

Schreier and Libow (1993, p.162) caution that therapists working with MBP perpetrators must be prepared for a challenging experience. "MBPS patients," they state, "are masterful at evoking the sympathy, doubt, and narcissism of their caretakers." As a result, therapists may be influenced to doubt the accusations made against the perpetrators, even when adequate proof is offered. These "countertransference" reactions (in the wider sense of feelings evoked in the therapist by the perpetrator) may result from the perpetrator's ability to deceive, or even from the malleability of the perpetrator to "become" whatever is called for in the situation. To prevent this, the therapist must be extremely self-aware, firmly grounded in the practice of psychotherapy, and knowledgeable about MBP (Szajnberg et al., 1996). Schreier and Libow (1993) recommend that all professionals active in the case communicate with one another, and receive consultation or supervision. This supports the participation of therapists in the MMT.

In the absence of extensive literature specific to treatment of MBP perpetrators, clinicians and theorists may find some models in work with other groups, particularly those in which there is often a mixture of personal mental illness and the exploitation of others. For example, similarities exist among sexual predators, criminal psychopaths, and MBP perpetrators. Sexual offenders, for example, are predominantly from one gender (male) and gratify their own needs at the expense of others. Like MBP perpetrators, they often have histories that appear to include abuse or sad life circumstances. Their sexual desires, like an MBP perpetrator's involvement with the victim's problem(s), often consume and structure their lives. Hare and Hart (1993, p. 104) describe psychopaths, who are also predominantly male, as characterized by: "a glib and superficial charm; egocentricity; selfishness; lack of empathy, guilt, or remorse; deceitfulness and manipulativeness; lack of enduring attachments to people, principles, or goals; impulsive and irresponsible behavior; and a tendency to violate explicit social norms." This description has many elements similar to MBP perpetrators. Perhaps there is a common core, still unknown, in the development of these disorders. Unfortunately, although mental health has a long and varied history of attempting to treat sexual predators and criminal psychopaths, little success has been reported. In fact, some practitioners believe that the only effective "treatment" is lifelong monitoring.

THERAPY IN THE MBP LITERATURE

A review of the limited literature on MBP reveals the following treatment approaches.

Feminist Therapy

According to Robins and Sesan (1991, p. 288), the principles of feminist therapy include:

> (a) recognizing the harmful effects of sexism in society; (b) exploring costs, consequences, and contradictions in prescribed sex roles for women; (c) valuing and supporting women's inner resources and their capacity for nurturance and healing; (d) maintaining a nonsexist frame of reference; (e) demystifying the power relationship in therapy; (f) encouraging women to look elsewhere for help, for example, [to] support groups; and (g) using social change as a source of empowerment for women.

Robins and Sesan believe that MBP perpetration by women is one result of social roles that give women: power in the home but little elsewhere; excessive responsibility for child care while leaving men underinvolved; and little opportunity to care for themselves while mandating that their needs should be met through addressing the needs of others.

In this conceptualization, MBP is a behavior of women (predominantly) who have accepted society's view that they should be little more than nurturing wives and mothers. They cannot ask for care for themselves, so they present a proxy—a child—for care. Through overinvolvement with the child's purported problems and treatment, they act out the role of the good, caring, and self-sacrificing mother. Leeder (1990, p. 80) suggests that a mother's special knowledge and role in management of the problem(s) provide her with "credibility and attention" that she might otherwise not be able to achieve. Her role both within the family and with health care professionals is enhanced.

If the female perpetrator herself was maltreated, especially at the hands of men, she may have internalized anger. She may also be angry at social values that seem to give a child's needs more legitimacy than a mother's. Traditionally, however, society has not permitted women to express anger. Covert abuse of the child may be a means of expressing this anger while still apparently conforming.

Nicol and Eccles (1985, p. 347), although not writing from the perspective of feminist therapy, describe the childhood of one perpetrator:

There can be no doubt that the [abuse of the child] was totally conscious; however, it was based on motivations that arose from a deeper disturbance. The patient realized that her family of origin had been built on a pattern of dominance and submission. Dominant family members [especially the father] raged and bullied, singled out favorites and rejects, and took total control of all family decisions. . . . [The perpetrator's] mother was characterized as a timid placating soul, chronically overconcerned with her own and her children's health.

To the feminist therapist, therefore, major issues to be addressed in therapy with the female MBP perpetrator are her rage at objectively unfair conditions (including her own abuse and victimization, if present), and learning better ways to get her own needs met. Through therapy, it is hoped, the MBP perpetrator can understand her unmet needs from childhood, learn to nurture herself, and claim more power than is offered by the traditional female role. She can express her rage and learn to direct it more appropriately. Participation in a women's group can also be a vital means of helping the perpetrator see that she is not alone in facing gender-role issues, and in providing a supportive, nurturing, and empowering environment. At an appropriate time, couples therapy can be useful, especially if it is directed toward rebalancing issues of power within the family so that the father can be more nurturing and the mother's needs can be addressed directly. Leeder states (1990, pp. 83-84),

Eventually, [the father] will have to take some responsibility for the problems, perhaps because of his absence on a physical or emotional level as a partner and certainly because of his absence in the role of parenting. He is not to blame for her actions; they are hers. . . . Nonetheless, real communication and understanding of each other's needs is essential to a healthy relationship.

Without an improvement in the couple relationship, Leeder (1990) states that the chances for therapeutic success in MBP cases are poor. If the perpetrator does not have a partner, it will also be more difficult for her to find resources to meet her emotional needs, and this will affect the outcome.

Once the therapeutic relationship is established, Leeder (1990) also finds it useful to help perpetrators understand the extent to which communication and concern in their present family, and probably in their family of origin, center around medical issues. This approach again helps the perpetrator to put behavior in context.

The feminist perspective makes sense of the MBP behavior without labeling it as a sickness. It appears to provide a hopeful direction for therapy with female MBP perpetrators, although much more experience will be necessary before firm conclusions can be drawn. However, at least in MBP, it is not a "quick fix." Leeder (1990) believes that at least a loose long-term relationship with a therapist may be necessary so that a resource may be available if symptoms recur.

Intergenerational Approaches

Rappaport and Hochstadt (1993) share some of the feminist perspective in that they conceptualize MBP as a means used by perpetrators to get their own needs met. Perpetrators displace ("project") these needs, which often stem from "profound emotional deprivation and abuse," onto their victims. Although the children are harmed, or at least exposed to the possibility of harm, when they are in the hospital the perpetrator is in a "safe and nurturing environment," one that also allows the perpetrator to be distracted from her or his own needs. The perpetrator's role is then clear—to nurture the sick child. He or she receives approval for this nurturing even if it is deceptive. This approval tends to perpetuate the behavior.

Similarly, Grand (2000) discusses the "catastrophic loneliness" of the trauma victim, and theorizes that traumatized perpetrators may induce trauma in others, particularly those they love, in order to force the others to join them emotionally. The original emotional reaction is thus "recognized" and can be better owned.

Dowling (1998, pp. 325-326) presents another intergenerational formulation in her discussion of a family in which the mother poisoned a six-year-old girl. The father failed to protect the child. Dowling states:

> It seems that the parents' hatred and despair with each other were projected on the child and the child's body, which was attacked by the mother to eliminate these unbearable feelings. This became more understandable when we learned that both

parents had been abused as children, and in attacking Loretta [the victim] the mother was also trying to eradicate feelings of vulnerability and dependency. . . . Work with the parents to enable them to separate and own their own feelings eventually made it possible for Loretta to have a sense of herself as an individual. . . . What became clear in our work with the family was that the poisonous feelings belonged to the parents' relationship. If they could be helped to face their fury with each other that each could not meet the other's great feelings of deprivation, then Loretta could be released from carrying these feelings.

In therapy, Rappaport and Hochstadt suggest (pp. 285, 288): "These families present many challenges because they are highly resistant and deny [MBP]. Issues of dependency, lack of personal competence, denial, avoidance, and resistance often need to be addressed as part of the psychotherapeutic process." Thus, treatment should focus on "issues of what [MBP perpetrator] parents received as children from their parents . . . and how this affects their own child-rearing methods. Their understanding of this, and their willingness to change their behavior, is vital to treatment."

Lyons-Ruth et al. (1991, p. 317) suggest another implicitly intergenerational approach. They believe that an infant mental health service is an appropriate vehicle for offering help to MBP perpetrators because "infant mental health services tend to be characterized by greater outreach capability, an orientation toward treating the mother-child relationship rather than a single individual, and a preventive focus." Furthermore, they believe that:

Treating the relationship rather than the mother and child separately is uniquely suited to the treatment of mothers with Munchausen by Proxy behavior because the mother's psychopathology is vividly expressed in her relationship with her child. The simultaneous somatizing and projecting onto the child of the mother's emotional needs is dramatic testament to the mother's difficulties in recognizing and verbalizing her emotional experiences within a traditional psychotherapy format. . . . [T]he preventive rationale . . . often leads to an initial approach to families based on identifying and supporting strengths. . . . Because serious psychopathology is usually accompanied by an extremely damaged and unstable sense of self-esteem, the first task is to demonstrate that the client's precarious defenses and damaged self-esteem will not be devastated further.

Lyons-Ruth et al. (1991) caution that the task of uncovering and working through defenses, or even achieving a full admission of what happened and why, may be a long one.

Sanders (1996) presents another family approach in which a team provides therapy to all family members, using multiple modalities. An important focus is on uncovering the family's "story" of the illness and MBP behavior, then replacing this with a more correct family narrative based on health. For example, the family's initial story may be that the child has multiple allergies and that the perpetrator has saved his or her life. The family's story could also be that the family is a happy and loving one, when relationships are actually cold and distant. This story is, of course, built on falsehoods and deception. It may take on a compulsive quality. It must be worked through if the MBP behavior is to resolve.

According to Sanders (1996), this approach can be done within family therapy, which allows the family to consider both positive and negative outcomes of their preoccupation with illness. This treatment approach works toward not just a new view of the MBP behavior, but of the whole family's identity and function.

Inpatient Whole Family Therapy

Two specialized treatment programs are described in the literature in which the whole family is the focus of treatment. Intensive therapy as well as child protection is provided by admitting the whole family to an inpatient psychiatric unit. Dowling (1998) describes the case of a child who had been poisoned by her mother. The goal of this inpatient treatment (which had a psychoanalytic focus [Flynn, 1998]) was to decide if it would be safe for the child to return home or whether an adoptive placement would be necessary. Individual, couples, and community milieu therapy were provided to the victim and her parents. After twenty months in therapy, it was deemed safe for the child victim to go home with her parents. On follow-up three years later she was reportedly safe and doing well. The family as a whole, including the child victim, tended to keep family secrets and to become ill under stress.

Berg and Jones (1999) describe outcomes with sixteen families treated in an inpatient psychiatric program. They believe that a trial of psychotherapy in selected MBP cases is indicated because it offers the hope that victims can return safely to their own homes. This not only avoids the risks of foster placement but may also protect siblings, including those born later. The inpatient program is described as multidisciplinary, with individual "focal" and cognitive therapy as well as family systems therapy. All cases manifested serious abuse, but were also selected as potentially responsive to treatment. Therapeutic procedures were described as (pp. 466-467):

> Psychological interventions targeted at: the parent-child relationship, the quality of the child's attachment to each parent, the abuser's own childhood experiences, and the current social network and family dynamics, together with work with the parental couple. In addition, intensive liaison work was undertaken with key professionals from the family's local area.

In thirteen families treated (versus just assessed) by this program, two mothers were continuing to somatize at follow-up, and in one family the mother continued to take the child for unnecessary doctor visits. In none of these cases were parents continuing to induce or falsify symptoms, as they had previously. In all but one of the treatment cases, the perpetrators eventually acknowledged that they had, indeed, harmed their children. Concerns remained about many of the children and their families, but the situation appeared improved in the treatment group at follow-up. Berg and Jones (1999) state (p. 470):

> We cautiously conclude that psychiatric treatment has had the desired effect on the factitious illness by proxy process, but for a minority of parents the effect has been to shift their tendency to somatise along the continuum . . . from factitious production of symptoms toward more normal health-seeking behavior, while not fully achieving that goal.

Berg and Jones (1999) also believe that the following factors contributed to good outcomes. Some of them are similar to the tasks to be accomplished prior to unsupervised visitation or reunification, as discussed in Chapter 10.

1. The perpetrator is willing to acknowledge that the MBP abuse occurred and the factors that contributed to it.
2. The family as a whole becomes more open in its communications (a point also made by Dowling, 1998).
3. The parents become more aware of the child as an individual with needs.
4. The perpetrator recognizes that he or she must take steps to prevent recurrence of MBP in the future.

Jones, Byrne, and Newbould (2000) believe that the multidisciplinary and comprehensive nature of the inpatient program is an important part of its success, and that no single element can be isolated as more important than the others. They conclude (p. 293):

> While awaiting the outcome from long-term follow-up of successfully treated cases, it may still be concluded that the goal of family reunification is feasible for a selected minority of cases, provided a long-term approach to risk management can be mustered by the professionals and the family itself.

Individual Insight-Oriented Therapy

Individual therapy with the perpetrator, with a goal of uncovering the roots of underlying behavior, is implied or included in all these forms of treatment. Because of the realities of working with MBP perpetrators, the therapeutic stages of engagement (relationship formation), assessment/diagnosis, and evaluation (checking to see how well the treatment is working) are crucial. These are especially true because MBP perpetrators are likely to come to therapy involuntarily (e.g., because of court order), and because they are already known to be deceptive.

Therapy with MBP perpetrators is outlined by Nicol and Eccles (1985, p. 348). They believe that it is appropriate in patients:

> [W]hose behavior seems motivated by severe neurotic conflicts but who seem otherwise well socialized . . . and where the patient is reasonably well motivated in trying to confront his or her difficulties, is of average intelligence, and not beset with family and social problems.

Feldman and Ford state (2000, p. 1543):

> Ideally, the therapy [with the perpetrator] will focus on teaching the parent adaptive ways to get her needs met, including expressing painful affects in words rather than with abusive actions. However, no author has yet described a consistently effective or specific treatment program for the factitious disorder by proxy maltreater, especially if an acknowledgment of culpability is not forthcoming.

Probably the most complete description of therapy with MBP perpetrators has been provided by Day (1998a,b,c). She identifies issues for the beginning, middle, and late stages of therapy. In the first stage, the main challenge is for the therapist to build a trusting relationship with the perpetrator. Setting boundaries is also an important task, as MBP perpetrators can be demanding and are highly focused on themselves and their own needs. Day believes that in order to understand and help an MBP perpetrator, it is necessary to understand the perpetrator's family of origin—which has often been dysfunctional and which may have included MBP. Ultimately, after trust has been formed, exploring the meaning of these early experiences and "family secrets" will form the core of treatment.

Day sees manipulation as a "survival strategy" (1998a, p. 176) that many perpetrators adopt to deal with the numerous stresses in their lives. Day also believes that, without losing touch with reality, many MBP perpetrators distort reality in ways that provide them comfort. When they begin to understand, in concrete terms, the realities of their lives and what they have done to their children, they can be flooded with guilt and even become suicidal. Often, as the problem with the child victim resolves, other issues such as eating disorders may emerge and require specialized treatment (Day, 1998c).

An important part of the therapist's task, Day feels, is to help the perpetrator reconnect emotionally with the child victim. Empathy can be built by helping the perpetrator understand the child's experience. Only when this is done, and the perpetrator is no longer afraid of reabusing, can the perpetrator safely have unsupervised visits with the child.

Success, Day feels, comes when the perpetrator is able to acknowledge the abuse and recognize that it was potentially life threatening. This acknowledgement should include appropriate feelings of guilt, horror, and empathy for what the child victim endured. The perpetrator should have grieved the sadnesses in her or his own life and feel ready to move forward with appropriate life plans and supports. If a caretaker, the perpetrator should feel ready to meet the child's needs even before her or his own. From the standpoint of child protection, success is also the achievement of the case management goals discussed in Chapter 10. Regardless of theoretical orientation, these should also be included in the goals of therapy.

DIAGNOSIS AND PROGNOSIS IN MBP

A different approach to treatment of MBP perpetrators is to consider implications of mental health diagnoses that have been assigned to them. Diagnosis should occur only after a thorough assessment that takes into account the whole situation of MBP perpetration and the perpetrator's life experiences. This is *not* the same as saying that MBP is a "disease" that a perpetrator "has." Nor is it attributing MBP maltreatment solely to mental illness. But it does recognize that the factors that led up to the MBP maltreatment may include psychological problems. If a competent and thorough evaluation reveals that to be the case, then the implications of the diagnosis ought to be taken into consideration when therapy and future planning are designed.

Many MBP perpetrators may not receive a mental health diagnosis, even though they may have significant mental illness. A brief diagnostic process, consisting of one or two interviews and perhaps psychological testing, may not be enough to reveal underlying cognitive and emotional disorders. This is especially true if the mental health professional is not well informed about MBP, the MBP case, and the purpose for the diagnostic assessment. MBP perpetrators have the deceptive skills to convincingly deny the extent of their problems, and to answer psychological test items in a socially approved way (Baute, 2000). A review of records pertaining to the case and especially to the perpetrator is necessary as part of the mental health evaluation. If the investigation has been done thoroughly, these should be easily available.

Mental health diagnosis serves many purposes, but the most basic is its role in guiding therapy. If a person is known to have a particular form of mental disorder, the therapist should understand, based on that diagnosis, some things (not all) about the person's behavior, the types of interventions that are likely to be useful in therapy, the likelihood that the person will improve, and the length of time that such improvement might take. Individual issues and responses will still need to be considered and clinicians must always recognize the limits of knowledge, but this accumulated professional wisdom means that each case does not have to be approached in a vacuum.

In her review of the MBP literature, Sheridan (2003) found that several mental health disorders had been reported for MBP perpetrators. However, relatively few journal articles about MBP include information about any mental health diagnoses. Some form of personality disorder was by far the most frequently reported, with approximately sixty-four cases (about half of which were not identified by subtype). This finding is not surprising, as Feldman and Lasher (1999, p. 26) state, "Psychopathology—particularly personality disorders such as borderline, histrionic, narcissistic, and antisocial—often coexists with and contributes to the MBP behavior." Twenty-three other perpetrators were reported to be depressed. Seven had been formally diagnosed with factitious disorder or somatization disorder, although the review of the literature suggests that the actual number with at least some features of factitious disorder is considerably higher. Each of these diagnoses will be discussed, and its implications for treatment of MBP perpetrators will be considered. All discussions will reflect the categorization and definitions of the *Diagnostic and Statistical Manual of Mental Disorders,* Fourth Edition (American Psychiatric Association, 1994), which is considered the standard for mental health diagnosis in the United States.

Personality Disorders

Feldman states (1994, p. 126), "Personality disorders seem generally to underlie the MSBP behavior." If a full diagnostic process were undertaken, the majority of MBP perpetrators would probably be found to have a personality disorder. This category of psychiatric diagnosis does not encompass acute mental illnesses in which a person suffers from temporary and intrusive symptoms. Rather, personality disorders are long-term and pervasive behavioral and emotional characteristics that keep a person from functioning normally or optimally. These disorders may affect thinking, feeling, behavior, and relationships with others. People with personality disorders often are described as having "been that way" since childhood, and in a wide variety of situations. People with this disorder do not necessarily experience—or experience fully—that their behavior gets them into trouble. They often secretly think that they are smarter than others. For these reasons, they are reluctant to change. Even if they become motivated, change is difficult because the patterns are so much a part of who they are.

One way to think of personality disorders is as "smoldering" forms of mental illness. They are not as florid as full-blown insanity, but they often lead to a person being regarded as "different" or "eccentric." As an example, normal people occasionally think they hear their name called on the street. They turn, see no one they know, conclude that they were mistaken, and think no more about it. Persons with a paranoid personality disorder will, throughout their lives, be unjustifiably suspicious. If they hear their name on the street, they will be convinced that people are talking about them, and cannot be dissuaded from this belief. They will be difficult to get along with because they suspect spouses of being unfaithful, bosses of evaluating them unfairly, and neighbors of deliberately causing them trouble. These patterns will persist across multiple marriages, jobs, and neighborhoods.

The DSM-IV identifies ten personality disorders (APA, 1994). (An additional category, "Personality Disorder Not Otherwise Specified," also exists for individuals who have characteristics of a personality disorder but do not fit the specific categories.) In Sheridan's (2003) review, MBP perpetrators were found in the following categories:

1. *Borderline personality disorder,* which is characterized by a poor sense of personal identity, brief and intense relationships with others, a fear of losing those relationships, impulsive and self-destructive behavior, and intense emotions such as anger. People with borderline personality disorder often feel "empty" inside, and may use intense sensations to fill the emptiness. The disorder often improves as persons with it enter their forties. In Sheridan's review, nine perpetrators were found to have been diagnosed with borderline personality disorder.

2. *Paranoid personality disorder,* which is characterized by a generalized suspiciousness and inability to trust others. People with paranoid personality disorder are often excessively sensitive,

quick to have feelings hurt, and persistent in carrying a grudge. In Sheridan's review, eight perpetrators were found to have been diagnosed as paranoid or with paranoid features, although these diagnoses may or may not be paranoid personality disorder.

3. *Histrionic personality disorder,* which is characterized by frequent attention-seeking behavior. People with histrionic personality disorder are likely to be happier, sadder, or more excited than the situation calls for, but these emotions are often shallow. In Sheridan's review, four perpetrators were found to have been diagnosed with histrionic personality disorder.

4. *Narcissistic personality disorder,* which is characterized by an unwarranted belief in one's own importance, good qualities, and entitlement to service from others. At the same time, people with narcissistic personality disorder are unable to recognize others' needs and feelings. Such people cannot empathize with a child because they cannot put themselves in the child's emotional position. Narcissistic personality disorder is not just good self-esteem. People with this disorder have perceptions that are unrealistically high, and they are willing to exploit others. In Sheridan's review, three perpetrators were found to have been diagnosed with narcissistic personality disorder.

5. *Dependent personality disorder,* which is characterized by an excessive desire to be cared for, and a willingness to do a great deal to ensure that care is forthcoming. People with dependent personality disorder have difficulty making decisions on their own or disagreeing with others. For this diagnosis to be fair, the person must seek or accept dependence because of personal needs, not because circumstances such as an abusive spouse or social roles (e.g., for women) demand it. In Sheridan's review, two perpetrators were found to have been diagnosed with dependent personality disorder.

6. *Obsessive-compulsive personality disorder,* which is characterized by an excessive and involuntary desire for things to be in good order, neat, and "right." People with obsessive-compulsive personality disorder are worriers (obsessional) and/or perfectionists who need to follow rules (compulsive). In Sheridan's review, two perpetrators were found to be "obsessional," although it is not clear whether this is meant as obsessive-compulsive personality disorder. It may have referred to obsessions in another

diagnostic sense, that of being excessively preoccupied with one subject—in the case of the MBP perpetrator, that subject being the child's problem(s).

7. *Antisocial personality disorder,* which is characterized by behavior that does not take others into consideration, and is often unlawful. People with antisocial personality disorder are often reckless, do not think through the consequences of behavior, and are not genuinely sorry afterward even when others have been harmed. In Sheridan's review, one perpetrator was found to have been diagnosed with antisocial personality disorder.

Many characteristics of these personality disorders are reminiscent of some MBP perpetrator-consistent characteristics discussed in Chapter 2.

1. "MBP perpetrators often present initially and on the surface as 'normal,' 'good' caretakers." Those with personality disorders often appear to be no different from anyone else. Persons with a paranoid personality disorder may appear "odd" in their thinking, but may also be so convincing in their (false) reasoning or explanations that these are taken at face value. For example, a perpetrator's statements about being falsely accused "because the doctors are frustrated and need someone to blame," uttered with sincerity, may sound reasonable to others. Persons with antisocial personality disorder are known to be superficially friendly, charming, and easy to get along with. "Glibness/superficial charm" is one of the items in the Hare Psychopathy Checklist (Hare and Hart, 1993) (psychopathy is a concept similar to antisocial personality disorder). Persons with borderline personality disorder characteristically form intense personal relationships in which they idealize others. Until the relationship breaks down they may appear to be the best of friends. Others may question their judgment, but usually do not consider them to be abnormal or mentally ill. This unwillingness to consider people mentally disordered may also extend to persons with histrionic, narcissistic, dependent, and obsessive-compulsive personality disorders. They may be considered theatrical, self-absorbed, submissive, or "one-track," respectively, but these are not completely negative traits. The entertaining friend, the parent who has reason (such as a critically ill child) for self-

preoccupation, and the "perfect wife" may be admired from a distance for qualities that would be seen as pathological if the truth were known. This can explain another MBP perpetrator-consistent characteristic: "MBP perpetrators may appear to be overanxious, overprotective, mistaken, or deluded. On closer observation, however, their concern is of a different quality."

2. "MBP perpetrators are accomplished liars, deceivers, and manipulators." This is particularly consistent with antisocial personality disorder. "Pathological lying," and "conning/manipulative" are items on the Hare Psychopathy Checklist. Persons with borderline personality disorder are frequently manipulative when they fear that a relationship may end; it is not uncommon for them to harm themselves or threaten to harm themselves under these circumstances. Persons with dependent personality disorder are also often experienced as manipulative because of their constant efforts to obtain and keep the care and attention of others. Similarly, those with histrionic or narcissistic personality disorder may exaggerate (at least) in order to keep the spotlight on them.

3. "MBP perpetrators may seek attention from a variety of people." As already indicated, this need for attention in one form or another is characteristic of several personality disorders. Those with borderline or dependent personality disorder have a strong need for relationships. The core of histrionic personality disorder is the need for attention from others. People with paranoid personality disorder may seek attention to confirm beliefs or even make "converts." People with antisocial personality disorder may seek attention as part of a "con."

4. "MBP perpetrators may deny all or part of what they have done, even when there is overwhelming evidence." This, again, is characteristic of persons with antisocial personality disorder. One of the Hare Psychopathy Checklist items is, "failure to accept responsibility for actions." Persons with other forms of manipulative personality disorders may also lie and/or deny because of the consequences of telling the truth. For example, an MBP perpetrator who has borderline or dependent personality disorder may fear the loss of a spouse if the abuse is revealed or if the victim's problems no longer summon the partner.

5. "MBP perpetrators do not necessarily stop their behavior when they are suspected or caught." Hervey Cleckley summarizes a description of psychopaths (cited in Schwartz, 2000, pp. 426, 428):

> When confronted with evidence of their misbehavior, psychopaths first try to blame others. When this fails, they may admit their misdeeds and feign regret, but their remorse and concern for their victims is not genuine, and their misbehavior is often repeated. Punishment does not deter them. In fact, psychopathic people engage in antisocial behavior even when they are almost certain to be caught and punished. It is as if they cannot see the future. When they are apprehended, psychopaths remain self-centered. Some have even been known to ask employers for references after being caught for stealing.

The Hare Psychopathy Checklist (Hare and Hart, 1993) also includes items such as "need for stimulation/proneness to boredom, lack of remorse or guilt, poor behavioral controls, and impulsivity." Together, these characteristics suggest that the MBP perpetrator with some personality disorders is likely to go for the "rush" without evaluating the consequences. If the MBP perpetration has obsessive-compulsive components, the perpetrator may not feel capable of controlling the impulses to harm the victim. If the perpetration includes manipulative components, the perpetrator may continue MBP maltreatment to achieve goals such as maintaining a relationship with a physician or spouse.

Those working with MBP perpetrators must be prepared for the possibility that the individuals will be diagnosed as having personality disorders. If that occurs, specific implications for therapeutic methods and outcome are indicated based on the diagnosis. However, because personality disorders are "the way the person is" rather than recent and intrusive symptoms, they are considered resistant to treatment. Evidence suggests genetic factors, personality characteristics, dysfunctional family life, a history of child abuse, and learned behavior as contributors to the development of personality disorders. A single definitive cause or combination of causes has not been established. Some of these factors, such as genetics, are not presently curable. Other factors, such as the damage done by early abuse, may be overcome—but with difficulty, and probably only partially. Learned behaviors can be unlearned, but the difficulty of this is proportionate to how entrenched and satisfying they are.

For those who are receiving attention because of a personality disorder, it may be difficult to trade the gratification for a quieter and more "normal" life. For example, an MBP perpetrator who is receiving a great deal of attention from professionals, family, and even the media will lose this if the child "recovers." Even when the MBP perpetration appears to bring negative consequences, the perpetrator can often use the situation to gain even more attention. For example, the "unjustly accused" MBP perpetrator may rally supporters among the media or in cyberspace.

Treatment for Personality Disorders

Barlow and Durand (1995, p. 544) comment that therapy with these clients

> [U]sually involves a focus on their problematic interpersonal relationships. They often manipulate others through emotional crises, using charm, sex, and seductiveness, or complaining . . . . [They] often need to be shown how the short-term gains derived from this interactional style result in long-term costs, and they need to be taught more appropriate ways of negotiating their wants and needs.

Sperry (1995) is no more than "cautiously optimistic" about the effectiveness of treatment with patients who have antisocial personality disorder. He divides these patients into two categories: those with poor prognosis and those with somewhat better prognosis. Particularly pertinent to MBP, he believes that patients have a poor prognosis if they have committed sadistic and violent acts toward others and do not sincerely regret this behavior. The prognosis is also poor if they have difficulty forming genuine relationships with others.

Perry, Bannon, and Ianni (1999) are somewhat more optimistic about the use of therapy with people who have personality disorders. As a result of their literature review, they estimated that 25.8 percent of personality disorder patients recover per year of therapy, in contrast to the 3.7 percent of untreated patients estimated to recover per year. In cases of child maltreatment, however, the federal mandate of permanency planning for children means that there is a limited time for therapeutic results before the decision must be made as to whether the child can return to the home. Many of the therapeutic modalities used with personality-disordered patients envision treatment extending across years.

Persons with borderline personality disorder may be more likely to enter therapy. But they may not persist because of the disease's pattern of relationships that are first idealized, then devalued. In other words, the therapy may start well, but when the real work of therapy begins, the person with borderline personality disorder may find fault with the therapist and no longer be open to intervention.

Treatment: Borderline Personality Disorder

Sperry (1995) believes that individual therapy is most appropriate for patients with borderline personality disorder, However, he is no more optimistic about the outcome than with antisocial personality disorder. Even if the patient accepts treatment, it is likely to take a long time. In borderline personality disorder, the therapist must be active, enforcing structure and limits in therapy, and oriented toward helping the patient make connections between actions and feelings in the present time. Because people with borderline personality disorder frequently use self-destructive behavior or threats to manipulate, the therapist must structure therapy so that this strategy does not "pay off." The therapist must also be particularly in touch with his or her personal feelings and issues (countertransference) during treatment. Cognitive strategies and a focus on strength building may be effective in addressing behavioral issues, especially at the beginning of therapy, because persons with borderline personality disorder have difficulty building trust. Later, the more core beliefs about personal worthiness and the fear of abandonment can be addressed. Group therapy has been demonstrated to be successful when used as an adjunct to individual therapy with persons who have borderline personality disorder. Family therapy may be useful in helping to keep borderline patients in therapy, improving relationships among family members, and helping family members set relationship limits. When medication is used, it should be targeted toward specific symptoms. Combined therapies probably offer a higher chance of success than individual therapy.

Treatment: Paranoid and Antisocial Personality Disorders

According to Schwartz (2000), few people with paranoid or anti-social personality disorder seek treatment. By nature, they are suspicious. If ordered into therapy by a court or other agency, the nature of the personality disorder will work against their forming a relationship with a therapist. Barlow and Durand (1995) state that goals in therapy with persons who have a paranoid personality disorder are to form a trusting relationship and to challenge (often using cognitive therapies) the patient's distorted view of the world. But, they add (p. 524), "to date there are no clear-cut demonstrations that *any* form of treatment can significantly improve the lives of people with paranoid personality disorder." They are no more optimistic about work with those who have antisocial personality disorder.

Sperry (1995) recommends that the therapist not take a neutral stance about the harmful behavior of patients with antisocial personality disorder, because this would seem to endorse what they are doing. Rather, the therapist must confront any efforts to minimize or deny the behavior, and must be alert to the client's manipulation. The content of therapy, according to Sperry, should be the present rather than the distant past, and the acquisition of specific coping skills. Group therapy or activities may be useful in helping people with antisocial personality disorder to bond with others. Family therapy may also be useful, especially to help family members (in the case of MBP, other adults in the home) learn to set limits and improve communication patterns. If medication is used, it should not be the only modality of treatment.

Treatment: Histrionic Personality Disorder

Persons with histrionic personality disorder are more likely than those with other personality disorders to seek treatment, but they are difficult to engage in true therapy because of their need to "perform." The therapist's office may simply be another "stage." Barlow and Durand (1995) state that there has been a good deal of theorizing about ways to work with histrionic patients, but little testing of these theories.

For histrionic personality disorder, Sperry (1995, p. 105) suggests that "general treatment goals include helping the individual to integrate gentleness with strength, moderating emotional expression, and encouraging warmth, genuineness, and empathy." Counseling goals include helping them focus on important issues rather than trivia, and become more empathic toward others (a goal appropriate for any MBP perpetrator). Because persons with histrionic personality disorder use threats of self harm to manipulate (as do those with borderline personality disorder), therapists must set clear limits from the beginning of therapy. Long-term psychoanalytic psychotherapy is, according to Sperry, considered the best modality for those with histrionic personality disorder, but shorter-term therapies may also be used. Patients with histrionic personality disorder usually form relationships quickly with therapists, and these relationships may be deep. The therapist's goal, however, is not to assuage the histrionic patient's neediness by gratifying it, but to help the patient learn to challenge her or his core beliefs about inadequacy and dependence on others. Some indications suggest that both group and family therapy may be useful with persons who have histrionic personality disorder. Medications may be useful for specific symptoms, or if other forms of mental illness are present. As with the other forms of personality disorder, combined modalities may be more effective than single interventions.

Treatment: Narcissistic Personality Disorder

Barlow and Durand (1995) believe that both research and reports of therapeutic success are lacking in narcissistic personality disorder. They state that therapy often focuses on helping patients to correct distorted notions about themselves and become more satisfied with the reality of their lives. Specific coping techniques may also help persons modify their expectation that others accept them uncritically. The developing of empathy for others is also important in work with persons who have narcissistic personality disorder.

Treatment: Dependent Personality Disorder

Because of the nature of their disease, patients with dependent personality disorder tend to form at least superficially good relationships. However, they may be reluctant to improve, and thus risk losing the relationship with the therapist. Barlow and Durand (1995) state that overdependence is always a danger with such patients, whose tendency to be submissive works against the therapeutic goal of their taking responsibility for meeting their own needs. Barlow and Durand also conclude that most of the literature on treatment of depressive personality disorder is descriptive, so little is known about how well therapy really works.

Depression

The second most frequent mental health diagnostic category among perpetrators of MBP, according to Sheridan's (2003) review of the literature, is mood disorder. The DSM-IV identifies several forms of depression. The exact diagnosis depends on the severity of the depression, the length of time that it has been present, and the symptoms associated with it. For example, when it alternates with an unnaturally euphoric mood, it is part of bipolar (manic-depressive) disorder. The term depression is also often used in a generic sense.

Depression is at the far end of the spectrum that begins with normal "blues" and reactions to the happenings of everyday life, including the tragic ones. It is a relatively common disorder. Up to 20 percent of the population is estimated to experience a major depressive episode at some time in their lives (Schwartz, 2000). Theories about the cause of depression include genetics and biology, social opportunities and roles, learning and thinking processes, and access and openness to social support. Depression is diagnosed twice as often in women as in men (Schwartz, 2000), but this may reflect women's greater frequency of coming for help. Modestin, Hug, and Ammann (1997) theorize that men's ways of coping with depression (substance abuse, criminal behavior) are more likely to result in their being diagnosed with antisocial personality disorder, while women's coping behaviors (crying, talking about their sad feelings) are more likely to result in their being diagnosed with depression. The idea that there might be a common core of depression under both diagnoses is intriguing. It goes counter to some of our present understandings of personality disorder, and is worthy of further study especially in relation to its implications for diagnosis and treatment of MBP perpetrators who have been diagnosed with personality disorder.

People with depression endure deep sadness, lack of energy, and a sense that they are personally worthless or unworthy. Life may seem hopeless, even when an observer would say that it is going well.

Eating and sleeping patterns are often disrupted. Considerable anxiety may accompany the depressed mood, and those with depression may feel that disaster is impending. In its severe forms, depression is disabling and potentially fatal.

Fortunately, with the development of modern antidepressants, many patients with depression can recover from or at least live with the disease. Depression also responds to "talk" therapy. Combinations of therapies, for example, drugs plus counseling, may have higher rates of success than single methods alone (Schwartz, 2000). Episodes of depression also tend to get better on their own, with the main goals of therapy being to shorten the suffering, disability, and risk of suicide associated with the disease, and to prevent or delay future episodes. Because of this positive outlook, if an MBP perpetrator has been correctly diagnosed with depression, the chances are good that it will respond to treatment.

It must be repeated, however, that one hallmark of MBP perpetrators is their ability to deceive. They are often highly perceptive, and even flexible, appearing to be what they think others want. By the time an MBP perpetrator or suspected perpetrator is referred to a mental health professional for assessment or therapy, evidence shows that this person has the potential to be deceptive. Mental health diagnosis depends on what the patient reports and on observation of behaviors. A person with knowledge of mental health diagnosis, which is easy enough to obtain, could probably report convincingly whatever symptoms he or she chooses. Mental health professionals must be alert to this possibility.

Factitious Disorder/Munchausen Syndrome

Frequently, MBP perpetrators have behavior that suggests they have at least some features of factitious disorder/Munchausen syndrome. One of the MBP perpetrator-consistent characteristics in Chapter 2 is, "MBP perpetrators may have a personal history of symptom/illness exaggeration, fabrication, or induction." A similar preoccupation with illness may be seen in the parents of MBP perpetrators, suggesting that this disorder may be multigenerational and thus learned in a family context. Some child victims of MBP continue the feigning of problems into their adult lives as factitious disorder/Munchausen syndrome patients.

The distinction between factitious disorder/Munchausen syndrome and Munchausen syndrome by proxy must be repeated. Factitious disorder or Munchausen syndrome is the term given to people who create problems or the appearance of problems in themselves. Munchausen by proxy or factitious disorder by proxy is the term given to people who create illness or the appearance of illness in others. The two sets of terms must *not* be confused. The terms "factitious disorder" and "Munchausen syndrome" should not be used instead of "Munchausen syndrome by proxy" or "factitious disorder by proxy."

Many similarities exist between persons with factitious disorder and MBP perpetrators. For example, persons with factitious disorder often present their problems knowledgeably and with dramatic detail. They are often skilled deceivers, and often seek multiple sources of care. In the literature, men are considered to have factitious disorder/Munchausen syndrome more commonly than women. Feldman and Ford (2000, p. 1536) divide Munchausen patients into two categories:

> middle-aged men who are unmarried, unemployed, and estranged from their families [and] women aged 20-40 years. A number of reports suggest that those in the second group are commonly employed in or intimately familiar with health care occupations such as nursing and physical therapy.

Factitious disorder/Munchausen syndrome is often believed to be rare, although its true incidence is unknown because it has the same research and epidemiological difficulties as MBP. Schwartz states (2000, p. 309):

> [Factitious disorder] seems to begin in early adulthood and is typically difficult to treat. Although it is the subject of much speculation . . . , there are no generally accepted etiological theories or treatment programs for factitious disorder. Many professionals are reluctant to expend their energies on people who are faking their symptoms, so the factitious disorders have received little clinical attention. However, some treatment success has been reported using a combination of behavioral, cognitive, and insight-based approaches.

When a client comes to a mental health professional for assessment and/or therapy, and some features of factitious disorder/Munchausen syndrome are present, the clinician must consider other possibilities. These include true physical or psychological problems (especially in their early stages). Other forms of mental illness that mimic physical illness must also be considered, including somatoform disorder, in which the patient unconsciously produces symptoms, and malingering, in which there are monetary or other concrete motives for reporting problems. Feldman and Ford (2000) also state that clients who have factitious disorder/Munchausen syndrome frequently meet the criteria for antisocial, borderline, histrionic, and other personality disorders. They often abuse substances and are at risk for suicide. As with MBP, the clinician must gather or review records and talk with family and friends to determine the truth of the perpetrator's condition and its severity. Feldman and Ford (2000) state that persons with more severe forms of factitious disorder/Munchausen syndrome rarely seek treatment on their own, and rarely remain in or benefit from it. Patients with this condition, like child victims of MBP, are at risk for injury or death from the mechanisms they use to produce their problems (Feldman and Ford, 2000).

Feldman and Ford (2000) recommend that when factitious disorder/Munchausen syndrome is suspected by health care providers, a multidisciplinary approach should be used to coordinate the efforts of involved health care professionals. If the disorder is confirmed, the patient should be confronted supportively, and the problem presented as a psychological rather than a physical one. A psychological evaluation should then follow if the patient is willing, with treatment of any mental illness (e.g., depression). Feldman and Ford comment (2000, p. 1542), "The psychotherapist who treats these patients must have modest expectations, anticipating relapse and accepting periods of symptomatic relief rather than 'cure.' It is the relationship itself that at least transiently serves to provide the nurturance that these patients crave." General therapeutic techniques, according to Feldman and Ford, are the same as with the personality disorders. Family therapy may help relatives learn to meet the patient's needs in ways other than responding to his or her physical symptoms.

If factitious disorder or Munchausen syndrome is diagnosed in an MBP perpetrator, this would suggest that using problems to get needs met is an entrenched means of coping. Although every effort to engage the patient in productive therapy should be made, the mental health professional should bear in mind that the outlook is guarded at best. Again, the capacity of the MBP perpetrator to make gains in therapy must be considered in light of child protective agencies' mandate to make permanent plans for children within specific time periods.

CONCLUSION

Many of the ideas discussed in this chapter are speculative or based on very limited clinical experience. Thus these conclusions must also be speculative. However, it appears that the following are useful approaches when therapy is attempted with MBP perpetrators:

1. Therapists must recognize that work with MBP perpetrators is difficult and that the outcome is uncertain. There are no "recipes" for success. It may not be possible to completely resolve the problem, so therapists should celebrate small improvements. Therapists must remain objective even while forming a therapeutic alliance with the perpetrator. Neither they nor the MMT can accept what the client says in therapy at face value. Statements must be evaluated and compared with what has been verified from other sources. The therapist should not attempt to perform investigative activities, but should bring this material to the MMT.

2. Because of the difficulty of the therapeutic task, consultation with other professionals who have credible MBP training and experience is highly advised. Even experienced therapists may lose their objectivity. Some therapists think of their role as advocating for the perpetrator. They must be helped to make the distinction between advocating for the perpetrator's mental health and joining her or his "cause."

3. Without excusing the harm caused by the behavior, the therapist should strive to place it in a context that makes sense to the perpetrator. The context and approach may be framed in terms of women's roles in society, family dynamics (couples, parent/child), or personal concerns. Hopefully, this will help the perpe-

trator recognize that the MBP perpetration was purposeful, and that there are better ways to get needs met.

4. A thorough and fair assessment process should be conducted to reveal whether the perpetrator warrants a DSM-IV diagnosis. (Remember that MBP/FDP is *not* an appropriate diagnosis). If so, knowledge about treatment techniques for the diagnosis can be used to guide therapy. The presence of such a diagnosis can be used to explain part of the *context* in which the MBP perpetration took place, but should not be considered as the *cause* of the MBP behavior. A mental health diagnosis also affects case planning and management.

5. Multiple modalities—group, family, or couples therapy—may usefully be considered as adjuncts to individual therapy. However, all personnel interacting with the family must have basic MBP education and detailed case information, and serve as members of the ongoing MMT. Family therapy should *not* include the perpetrator before he or she has honestly and remorsefully admitted what she or he has done. The focus on family dynamics and communication problems may appear to (or may be manipulated by the perpetrator to) move the focus away from the perpetrator's taking personal responsibility for the behavior and the harm that has occurred. Family therapy prior to an honest admission also provides the perpetrator with a continuing opportunity to manipulate the other members of the family in relation to past, present, or potentially future problems. For example, the victim(s) may be cued to continue reporting problems. The same therapist should not provide services to both perpetrator and victim(s), as this is likely to raise either the appearance or reality of conflicts of interest.

6. Successful work with MBP perpetrators is likely to require long-term therapy if the patient is willing to persist, and long-term involvement of the therapist in the deliberations of the MMT. This may work against the requirement that CPS make timely permanency plans for the child victim. (The authors of this book know of no research about how loss of a child might impact therapy with an MBP perpetrator.) In other forms of child protection, the prospect of reunification often motivates parents to make positive changes in their lives. However, some MBP perpetrators whose parental rights have been terminated

continue to obtain significant attention from their situation. At the very least, the loss of the child would have to be considered along with other issues in therapy.

This chapter has raised difficult issues about mental illness and personality disorders. Theory suggests that some of these psychological conditions may be, at least in part, the result of complex biological processes as well as abuse. At the same time, persons with these disorders have a responsibility to control their behavior. Mental health theory cannot yet account for why some people respond to family and societal conditions dysfunctionally, while others are normally or highly functional. Nor can it be explained why a few persons with these diagnoses perpetrate MBP, while the vast majority do not. Balancing fairness and compassion toward the perpetrator with justice, compassion, and protection for the victim is not easy.

Chapter 13

Implications for Intervention
with Victims

Less information is in the professional literature about work with victims of MBP than about work with perpetrators of MBP. As a whole, the literature has focused primarily on medical manifestations of MBP, and then on perpetrators. Even when the literature discusses the relationship between perpetrator and victim, the focus is generally on the perpetrator. Sometimes the role of mental health clinicians on behalf of victims is described primarily as the education, consultation, and advocacy that advance child protection. Effective methods of intervening with victims represents an area for future growth for the field. Such intervention does not only mean psychotherapy. Not all victims will need therapy. Rather, the term "intervention" as used in this chapter includes all the actions taken to ensure and improve the welfare of the victim. These include foster placements with support to foster parents, appropriate case plans and case management, medical rehabilitation, and other such activities, as well as short- or long-term counseling.

A review of the consequences of child maltreatment as a whole is beyond the scope of this book. Nor is it possible to review all that is known about medical rehabilitation of victims who have suffered a wide variety of problems from the maltreatment and its consequences. This must be decided based on the victim's situation after an adequate period of evaluation. The areas of screening, preparing, and supporting foster parents have been dealt with elsewhere in this book, as has the development of case plans and case management. This chapter will review what is known and hypothesized about assessing the need for and delivering of psychotherapy to MBP victims. It will also make an analogy with child sexual abuse that may be useful in therapy with victims and in suggesting future directions. But this information must be seen as limited and preliminary.

Hobbs, Hanks, and Wynne (1993, p. 259) state that "children who have experienced abuse or maltreatment need help." This is true of victims of MBP maltreatment. However, the form of help that is needed depends on the individual and situation. Chaffin (2000, p. 409) states, "It is not correct to assume . . . that abused children always need therapy any more than it would be to assume that all children who have suffered automobile accidents need stitches." The fact that a child has been the victim of MBP does not, of itself, mean that the child requires psychotherapy or requires it immediately. Many elements of the case plan may be therapeutic for the victim. Fisher (1995, p. 388) states, "A long-term, secure, consistent, nurturing, and warm environment is treatment in itself for infants and very young children." Throughout the life of the case, the child's needs (physical, social, psychological, etc.) should be assessed. A variety of interventions (medical, environmental, recreational, therapeutic, etc.) should be considered as warranted by those needs. This should be one of the regular tasks of the MMT. The application will be specific to the MBP case, but the concept is the same as in other forms of maltreatment.

ASSESSING THE VICTIM'S NEED
FOR PSYCHOSOCIAL TREATMENT

The immediate need for medical stabilization and protection may preclude addressing psychological needs in-depth early in the case, and rightly so. The provision of needed health care and safety are the forms of intervention appropriate at the time. The victim also may or may not immediately exhibit psychological/behavioral problems or emotional distress that suggest a need for counseling. The unique experience of the maltreatment; the relationship with the perpetrator; and the victim's age and personality characteristics may also affect the need for treatment, timing of treatment, or the type of treatment that is needed.

The victim's need for counseling or other therapeutic services depends, in part, on his or her developmental stage. Most typically, MBP begins when victims are under five years of age. Often, they are infants when the maltreatment starts, but they may come for help at any age, even into adulthood. The victim's subjective experience of maltreatment is determined, in part, by his or her psychological and cognitive development at: the time of the maltreatment, the time the victim becomes aware of the maltreatment, and the time the victim comes for help. The ability to understand or interpret the maltreatment is very different at the age of five months from what it will be at the age of five years. Likewise, the victim's personal coping abilities and receptivity to intervention are determined, in part, by age. Some problems may only become apparent as the individual reaches specific developmental stages. For example, help may be needed as the victimized teenager begins to form loving relationships or the adult begins to parent (Hobbs, Hanks, and Wynne, 1993). So, again, the determination of whether intervention is needed, and what form it might take is complex and must be reevaluated throughout the life of the case.

Bonner (2000) gives some practical suggestions on when a maltreated child (not specifically a victim of MBP maltreatment) should be referred for evaluation and treatment. Referral is indicated when major problems occur, or when problems do not improve with behavioral strategies, they get worse, or they last longer than six to eight weeks. Referral should also be made before problems have become so serious that the child's stability and important role functioning (e.g., as student, sibling, foster child, church member, etc.) are threatened. For example, problems should be addressed before they become so serious or frustrating to foster parents that the child may need new placement. These guidelines and this preventive strategy appear appropriate for victims of MBP.

Day and Ojeda-Castro (1998) believe that MBP victims should have a complete psychosocial evaluation at least initially and before reunification (if reunification is to occur.) The focus on "psychosocial" implies that multiple areas of functioning are assessed, with the potential for multiple means of intervention if necessary. This should include a review of all available records from the child's eye view (Jones, 1997), supplemented as appropriate by psychological testing of the victim, psychiatric evaluation of victim and/or perpetrator, and possibly behavioral inventories completed by foster parents or others who know the child well. (Day and Ojeda-Castro [1998] suggest that parents can fill out such inventories, but this only invites further exaggeration and/or fabrication.) Psychological testing should assess "the cognitive, academic, and personality development of the child" (p. 210) as appropriate to the child's age. Day and Ojeda-Castro (1998) go on to describe this testing in more detail (p. 210):

> The elements evaluated include social development, fine and gross motor skills, expressive and receptive language skills, and developmental achievement. The intellectual portion of the evaluation includes the use of standardized test instruments appropriate to the child's age . . . multiple objective and projective test instruments.

Dey and Ojeda-Castro acknowledge, however, that the user of such instruments must understand that their validity and specificity may decrease with the age of the child.

Fisher (1995) adds several components to this evaluation. Observational data contributed by those who have interacted with the child can be very useful. This may include hospital staff if the child has been an inpatient, school or preschool staff, and foster parents. An observation of child/parent interaction by the child psychiatrist that may include feeding as well as playing is often part of a non-MBP child psychiatric (or other mental health) evaluation. However, in MBP cases it is risky to allow a perpetrator this kind of contact with a victim. The perpetrator will almost certainly try to look like a loving parent, and may attempt to create problems during the session. This could be done in ways that an observer might not recognize. For example, a perpetrator could try to poison the infant during feeding, using a bottle brought from home or prepared out of the observer's line of sight. The usefulness of watching this imposture is questionable, and the safety of the victim might be compromised. It may be better to defer this part of the evaluation until the child has formed a relationship with a foster parent or is in a permanent living situation.

For MBP victims from about age two on, Fisher (1995) states, the child should be interviewed directly, using art and play materials as appropriate. A childhood mental status examination can be administered. The child can be asked to draw a picture of himself or herself. The clinician should be alert for themes related to the MBP abuse (e.g., playing out themes of illness), but should also probe for other forms of abuse that may have occurred. This may also lead to suggestions for other forms of evaluation that may be helpful, such as specific testing or consultation with other specialists. The evaluator should be alert to the possibility that the victim has difficulty socializing, and to features of post-traumatic stress disorder, which is known to occur in children who have been through extended experiences of maltreatment.

Hobbs, Hanks, and Wynne (1993, pp. 260-261) also list questions that may be useful in understanding the effect of maltreatment on any child victim who is verbal. Some of these questions, derived from work with abused and sexually abused children, appear particularly appropriate for use (in language appropriate for the child's age and development) with victims of MBP. However, it should be remembered that victims of MBP may not know that they have been maltreated. For example, they may be too young to understand what has happened, or may believe the perpetrator's story of their problems. It is simplistic to believe that victims will be fully aware of their victimization and grateful to be rescued from it. From the child's point of view, the most serious part of the situation may be placement outside of the home. For this reason, these questions have been rewritten in a more neutral and less "leading" fashion.

- How does the victim perceive and understand what has happened? What changes have occurred to the victim's situation? How does the victim explain it to himself herself?
- Does the victim feel that what has happened is his or her fault?
- Is the victim experiencing unpleasant feelings such as anxiety, sadness, fear, etc.? How troublesome are these? Are there problems at home, in school, or at other places?
- How does the victim feel about himself herself?
- Is the victim is aware of the maltreatment? To what extent did the victim "cooperate" with or remain passive during the maltreatment? To what extent was the victim manipulated or forced? What threats were used? How does the victim feel about this? (Note that the issue of cooperation raises both practical and philosophical questions. Realistically, the victim may not have had a free choice about cooperating. However, even if coercion occurred, it is useful to understand the victim's perceptions about this cooperation and choice.)
- If the victim is aware of the maltreatment: Did the victim attempt to disclose the maltreatment at any point? If so, what happened? How does the victim feel about this?

The relationship between the perpetrator and the victim should also be assessed. Often, the relationship is one of close psychological allegiance. Two explanations for this are raised in the literature: symbiosis and Stockholm syndrome.

Crouse (1992) states that MBP victims who are maltreated by their mothers have a symbiotic relationship with them. This means that the two are almost as close as though they were, psychologically, one person. Symbiosis should be understood in developmental context. Infants normally have a symbiotic relationship with their mothers, and the normal task of childhood is to gradually separate and become an individual. Given what is known of the psychodynamics of MBP maltreatment, the symbiosis may be abnormally strong and/or prolonged—a failure in development. This should be seen as bidirectional. From the perpetrating mother's perspective (assuming the mother is the perpetrator), there may be little desire for a child who is a person in his or her own right. The child is an object for her gratification. From the child's side, the symbiotic relationship may be a consequence of this unvoiced expectation or a consequence of the maltreatment. According to family theory, all children try to meet their parents' needs and expectations in order to get their own needs met. Thus, if symbiosis is present, it is likely that the child victim is highly invested in maintaining it. The child will probably be reluctant to give it up.

In contrast to the theory of symbiosis, other authors (see, for example, Goddard and Stanley, 1994) view the relationship between perpetrator and victim as one of "captor and hostage." They apply the Stockholm syndrome theory which suggests that, as a survival method, victims take on the perspective of their captors and form a strong, even consuming relationship with them. An example of this is the Patty Hearst case in which the heiress was kidnapped by a radical group and allegedly then became a member of the group. Many elements of the MBP situation predispose to such an "identification with the aggressor," including the child victim's dependence on the adult, the frequent isolation of the victim, the length of time that maltreatment often occurs, and the almost ideological quality of the perpetrator's "story."

Such a strong relationship between perpetrator and victim, either because of Stockholm syndrome or symbiosis, will be important when intervention is considered. It may explain a victim's seeming cooperation or collusion in the MBP. It is one reason why evaluators and therapists should not simply take what a victim says at face value, uncritically, as has been done in cases of child sexual abuse. Rather, while the victim's statements must be taken seriously, they must also be seen in context.

At the end of the evaluation, the assessing professional should identify areas of strength and concern. These should be communicated to the MMT, and can be integrated with other past and present information about the victim's situation and functioning. From this whole picture, decisions should be made about how best to meet the victim's needs.

CONSEQUENCES OF MBP TO VICTIMS

What issues and feelings might victims of MBP bring to therapy? Again, the literature is limited. Bools, Neale, and Meadow (1993) report on fifty-four children followed up one to fourteen years after their MBP abuse. Only five of thirty children who remained with their mother (the perpetrator) and six of twenty-four children in placement were judged to have "no disorder." For the remainder, behavioral difficulties and physical consequences of the abuse were found. For example, a number of the children had attendance, concentration, or achievement difficulties in school. A few had problems with lying, stealing, or other conduct disorders. There was some indication that, when children received good parenting from their fathers or other relatives, when the perpetrator's life situation stabilized, or when the children were placed in stable foster or adoptive homes, this mitigated some of the damage. But, again, this is probably individualized. Some child victims understand and welcome placement, while others grieve the loss of the family (Fisher, 1995) or experience guilt. Some are old enough to understand what is happening when they are placed, and some understand only the loss of the familiar.

Byrk and Siegel (1997) report on the experiences of one victim (now an adult) who suffered serious and disfiguring abuse over many years. After individual and group therapy, she has "built a new life based on truth and love" (p. 5). During the maltreatment, in addition to years of physical suffering, the victim reported fear of her mother, low self-esteem, a lifelong desire for loving parental relationships, and guilt when her brother became the target of abuse and she was too frightened to protect him. This brother is described as for "many years a lost soul, wandering from job to job, starting and never completing college classes" (p. 4) and abusing substances. Her sister, who was never physically maltreated but who must have suffered greatly in this family, is described as chronically angry; the victim also felt guilty over this.

In her summary of ten adults who identified themselves as victims of MBP during childhood, Libow (1995) found self-reports of depression or its elements—"feelings of helplessness, poor self-esteem, and self-destructive ideation" (p. 1136) as well as fear and anxiety which often continued into adulthood. As adults they also experienced symptoms of post-traumatic stress disorder and:

> [A] struggle to avoid playing the victim role, difficulty maintaining relationships, insecurity, . . . a fruitless search for mother's love, and difficulty separating fantasy from reality. . . . This intensity of confusion, "paranoia," and self-doubt about their bodies, feelings, and relationships is hardly surprising given their almost impossible childhood dilemma of reconciling an experience of illness and betrayal with seemingly devoted caregiving by an admired parent. (p. 1137)

Other victims acknowledged rage toward their families. It came as a relief to these adults, whose abuse often had occurred before widespread knowledge about MBP, that there was a name for what they had experienced and that they were not unique (see also Richardson, 1999). However, the victims known to Libow (1995) do not represent a cross section of all adult MBP victims. At least some may have been referred to her specifically because they were having problems.

In their review of the literature, Day and Ojeda-Castro (1998) link behavioral problems such as hyperactivity, withdrawal, and oppositional behavior (problems found by Bools, Neale, and Meadow [1993] among MBP victims) to a failure of individuation. This is the other side of the symbiosis already discussed. One can also speculate that the "hothouse" and isolated atmosphere in which many MBP victims live is simultaneously "special" (Briere [1996] refers to this as "negative specialness") and objectified (see Warner and Hathaway, 1984) and may also harm their ability to socialize with others and, perhaps, to interact in a group. Victims of MBP may have learning difficulties, perhaps as a result of brain damage in the process of abuse, missed school, or for other reasons.

It is believed that children who have been victimized are at greater risk of developing factitious disorder/Munchausen syndrome as children or adults, or may themselves become MBP perpetrators. This is not unexpected, as it is well-known that some (certainly not all) victims of abuse grow up to become abusers. In their follow-up study, Bools, Neale, and Meadow (1993) found that some victims of MBP were, themselves, "somatizing" (expressing emotions through physical symptoms). Sigal, Gelkopf, and Meadow (1989) state that some children abuse themselves because they fear loss of the perpetrator's love and attention if they are not sick. Conway and Pond (1995) describe a victim's progression from ignorance of the abuse through complicity, and finally, as a young adult, to persistently presenting herself as having a diagnosis that had repeatedly been refuted. Therapeutic work is thus seen as having a preventive aspect. Rappaport and Hochstadt (1993), for example, conceptualize MBP using an "intergenerational perspective." That is, they recognize that this generation's perpetrators may have been the last generation's victims, and today's victims may be tomorrow's perpetrators. Therefore, without being specific, they advocate "treatment" for these victims as a "preventive measure" (p. 288).

THERAPEUTIC APPROACHES DESCRIBED
IN THE LITERATURE

Methods of intervention with victims should flow from the problems that have been discovered in assessment (Jones, 1997). For the victim who needs treatment, Fisher (1995) states that all forms of therapeutic intervention should be considered, both direct (i.e., with the victim) and indirect (i.e., with others such as foster parents on behalf of the victim). These indirect methods are often especially appropriate for infants and toddlers.

Individual Inpatient Therapy

Dowling (1998) describes a twenty-month process of psychotherapy (apparently involving both talk and play) with a girl who had been poisoned by her mother at the age of four. This therapy occurred within the context of a specialized, comprehensive inpatient family mental health unit in England; settings of this type probably do not exist, or are extremely rare, in the United States. Dowling describes therapeutic themes of difficulty trusting/relating to others, poor self-esteem related to her mother's hostility, and a difficulty in separating/individuating that may have mirrored the perpetrator's use of the victim as an object of convenience. Progress for the child also depended on the parents' making progress in their own treatment and thus being able to tolerate her anger, regression, and individuation. The perpetrator had to face her own feelings, and presumably her culpability in the child's abuse. For the child, thinking about her maltreatment and experiencing the associated feelings was frightening. Again, the ability of the parents to tolerate these things and to separate themselves from her was key in helping the child acknowledge and feel the sequelae of maltreatment, and give up her own perceived role as the "sick one."

This case is an example from the literature, and both the case and the treatment setting may be unique. This kind of family-based treatment should be undertaken only if it appears warranted by an MBP-specialized case plan. It should be based on the achievement of case plan elements that allow extended contact between the perpetrator and the victim leading to reunification.

Individual Outpatient Therapy

Sanders (1996) suggests that the need of MBP victims for therapy should be evaluated, and that they will generally need some assistance to deal with the trauma they have experienced. She sees relationship as one focus of therapy: rebuilding the child/parent relationship if the child will be returning home; or, building a new relationship with foster or adoptive parents if the child will not be returning home. She recommends play or talk therapies as appropriate for the age of the child. As to therapeutic goals, she recommends that they be:

> [S]imilar to those found in other therapies of abused children . . . which include engaging with an adult who models a healthy caretaking relationship . . . and encourages mastery of conflictual relationship and medical traumas. . . . Therapy would help [MBP victims] understand the role of illness in their lives and

begin to explore alternative stories that would include reclaiming their lives from illness and engaging in more social, recreational, and developmentally appropriate activities. (p. 324)

Play Therapy

In play therapy, children are allowed to express their feelings and concerns not only through verbalization but through selected toys and art materials. Day and Ojeda-Castro (1998) describe their experience with six young victims of MBP maltreatment. They found that the children's ability to bond appeared intact, although these children had been betrayed by (in these cases) their mothers. With their mothers, they appeared insecurely attached, clinging, and anxious. The children exhibited problems in trusting, both in the generalized sense and specifically in trusting health care professionals, including therapists. They sometimes dealt with the paradox of a loving yet maltreating mother by imagining that they had two mothers, one good and one bad.

In play therapy, the children often acted out regressive themes, as though they needed to reexperience infancy, this time without maltreatment. The children also needed to work through images of themselves as having the problem(s) on which the perpetrator focused. Since the problems were a significant source of attention, the victims had to learn new ways to obtain attention when they needed it. A major therapeutic goal was for victims to move from acting out their maltreatment through play to being able to talk about it. Finally, if victims were to return home, they had to have "the cognitive skills, verbal capacity, and emotional strength to report any induction of illness or to resist any pressure within the mother-child relationship to resume the sick role" (Day and Ojeda-Castro, 1998, p. 209).

Family Therapy

Inpatient or outpatient family approaches to MBP are described by several authors (Berg and Jones, 1999; Coombe, 1995; Dowling, 1998; Sanders, 1996). In general, family therapy looks not only at the problems of each family member, but also uses systems theory to understand and intervene in the relationships among family members. Some settings have been structured to provide intensive treatment of families or mothers with children on an inpatient basis, as already described. Small studies of single or carefully selected small series of patients have described successful outcomes, but this has also depended on the ability of the perpetrators to admit what they had done (Berg and Jones, 1999). Most professionals dealing with cases of MBP will not have access to such intensive therapeutic settings or funding to pay for extended whole-family inpatient treatment. Unless the proposed setting can demonstrate successful experience both with family selection and family treatment in MBP cases, inpatient family treatment is not recommended. Outpatient family treatment is also not recommended until, possibly, very late in an MBP case process when most goals for reunification have already been met. From the standpoint of the victim, there are many ways in which a persisting perpetrator can manipulate the family treatment to the detriment of the therapeutic process. Also, the prognosis for maltreating families in therapy differs by the type of maltreatment that has occurred (Hobbs, Hanks, and Wynne, 1993). At present, little is known about the prognosis for family treatment in MBP. Therefore, clinicians using family treatment should be particularly cautious. They should consider consultation with a colleague experienced in family therapy and child maltreatment, and participate regularly and nondefensively with the MMT. The following case may be an extreme example, but demonstrates some of the problems that can be associated with family therapy if used before the perpetrator has progressed to the point that she or he has admitted to the MBP behavior and its consequences.

Case 13.1

A family therapist undertook work with a mother and her two children. MBP had recently been confirmed. The family therapist held sessions with all three members present. Her focus was on understanding and affirming each family member's perception of reality, and on improving the relationships among the family members. She soon became convinced that the mother's stories about the children's illnesses were "her truth," and defined her role as advocating for the mother. This even extended to her calling the foster family and giving instructions without the knowledge or approval of CPS. Family therapy sessions became an opportunity for the mother to seek attention from the therapist, while reminding the children that they "had" various illnesses and problems—which they promptly began to display in foster care. When the children agreed with the mother that they "had" these problems, the therapist defined that as "their reality" and did not work toward establishing the objective truth. Family therapy sessions became, in effect, unsupervised visitation in which the children were subjected to subtle, con-

tinuing MBP perpetration, including emotional abuse and behavioral induction tactics. The therapist refused to take part in the MMT. Major problems
were posed by the family therapist's uncritical acceptance of reunification as
a goal, her lack of demand for meaningful change in the perpetrator prior to
contact with the children, and her insistence that this family's problems were
due to "family system factors." Because the family therapist was well respected in the community and presented herself as an expert, the child protection agency refused to make changes. They persisted in this stance even
after a nationally recognized MBP expert reviewed the case and identified
lack of progress during therapy due to inappropriate therapeutic goals and
incorrect knowledge about MBP.

MBP AND CHILD SEXUAL ABUSE: AN ANALOGY

Similarities exist between MBP maltreatment and the sexual abuse
of children (Griffith, 1988; Lasher and Feldman, 2001; McGuire and
Feldman, 1989). Like MBP, sexual abuse involves a particular violation of trust between perpetrator and victim. Sexual abusers, like
MBP perpetrators, have done something that is contrary to world-
wide notions of adult moral conduct. MBP, like sexual abuse, involves the invasion or potential invasion of the victim's body and the
objectification of the victim as a source of illicit gratification. Sexual
abuse, like MBP, also frequently involves deception, as sexual abusers create a secret life with the victim, and other family members remain ignorant of the truth. Given what is known today, there is a poor
outlook for perpetrators of sexual abuse and for perpetrators of MBP.
Thus, reunification of children with perpetrators in either form of
maltreatment must be undertaken with extreme caution. This analogy
to MBP is imperfect, however, since men are more commonly sexual
predators and women are more commonly MBP perpetrators.

The field of MBP today is also similar to the field of sexual abuse
twenty to thirty years ago. That is, MBP has only recently begun to be
widely recognized. People still have limited and, often, incorrect information about it. It is as difficult for people to recognize the reality
of MBP today as it was for them to recognize the reality of sexual
abuse a quarter century ago. There is a strong need for correct knowledge about MBP, and for appropriate child protective policies to respond to it. If this analogy holds, the extensive literature on sexual
victimization and treating victims of sexual abuse, as well as the history of policy development in the field of sexual abuse, may offer in-

formation and suggestions for those who are working with victims of MBP.

Information from the field of sexual abuse supports findings about the damage to victims of MBP.

Gilmartin (1994, pp. 120-152) has summarized the reported effects of incest and child sexual abuse upon victims. These effects are similar to those reported for victims of MBP. Although the data are imperfect, Gilmartin concludes that children who were sexually abused show immediate problems in the following areas:

- Psychological/emotional, including feelings about the self (e.g., low self-esteem)
- Physical, especially in relation to the injured parts of the body
- Behavioral; for example, regression, aggression, or withdrawal and clinging
- Interpersonal relationships; for example in trusting others
- Cognitive, including difficulty in understanding what is real, and distorted bodily image
- Sexual, with problems such as inappropriate sexualization and confusion. (This may be analogous to the MBP victim's problems with medicalization and confusion over health.)
- Spiritual, with victims often believing that they are to blame for their maltreatment or that they are "bad" in some way

To this list many would add symptoms associated with post-traumatic stress disorder. Gibson and Hartshorne (1996) also found that women who had been sexually abused as children were more likely to be lonely in adulthood. This may also be related to the isolating effect of such abuse, which is also characteristic of MBP.

Information from the field of sexual abuse suggests that damage to victims is long-lasting and may be multigenerational.

Gilmartin (1994) summarizes the long-term effects of sexual abuse on victims, particularly women.

Time does not cure the effects of incest. Although the memories go underground, the consequences of the abuse flourish. Sometimes they are buried under other problems. . . . But they lie waiting, waiting for the clarity that sobriety brings; waiting for release from thought confusion and phobias, the lifting of depression, the opening that comes through therapy or intimacy. They also may erupt on their own. . . . And, in the saddest paradox of all, the aftereffects . . . usually spell continuing victimization for the survivor herself, for her lovers, even her children. (Blume, p. 15, as cited in Gilmartin, 1994)

Again, although it has not been demonstrated that the long-term consequences (including substance abuse) are the same for MBP, this forms a reasonable hypothesis.

Experience with sexual abuse suggests that victims of MBP may be especially stigmatized by the type of maltreatment they have experienced, and may blame themselves.

In her discussion of treatment for sexually abused children, Kempe (1997) points out that the horror with which society regards incest, and society's denial that it occurs at all, result in

> an atmosphere of shock and disapproval which increases the social isolation of the victim and his or her family. . . . Disclosure threatens the security of the entire family. . . . The child faces loss or disruption of the family, often with the additional burden of being told it is his (or her) fault. (p. 559)

Society also regards MBP with shock and horror. Communities find it hard to believe that apparently exemplary caretakers can behave in this way. Often a result is a pulling away from the family, and that may include the victim and siblings. They may face some of the same stigma as anyone whose family situation is seen as deviant. The victim very frequently faces the loss or disruption of the family, often being removed from it permanently. In addition, victims of sex abuse may blame themselves for the destruction of the family. This could be expected if the victims of MBP believe that their problems are genuine. Probing for such feelings should be part of both the assessment and interventive processes in MBP.

Special circumstances of the abuse may heighten damage to the victim.

1. Deliberateness and malevolence: In relation to incestuous families, Gelinas (1993) asserts that emotional reactions are heightened if a victim experiences deliberate behavior, and especially malevolent behavior, in the context of a relationship. Deliberateness is a defining characteristic of MBP. Malevolence is present in some (but not all) cases of MBP (Bools, Neale, and Meadow, 1994).

2. Characteristics of the maltreatment may lead to confusion over what is real. Gelinas (1993) states that it can be very frightening for sexual abuse victims when the familiar parent becomes, intermittently, the abuser. This may lead the child victim, who cannot see things as an adult would, to question his or her own perceptions of reality. How is it possible that the "good" parent (and the victim needs to see the parent as good) is sometimes behaving in a "bad" way? During the times when maltreatment is not occurring, or if the perpetrator denies the maltreatment, the victim may question his or her own experience and wonder if it really occurred. The victim may see the situation as unbelievable, and may doubt that anyone else would believe it either. (If the victim discloses and is not believed, this sense of unbelievability is reinforced.) The victim may have only the perpetrator to turn to for help or confirmation of reality, and so receive additional distorted messages. Thus the maltreatment may seem at once very real, and also very unreal. This confusion over reality is an additional source of suffering for the victim.

For these reasons, Gelinas (1993) states, adult incest survivors repeatedly deal in therapy with the question of whether their memories are real, and can even sometimes be persuaded that their memories are false. Gelinas summarizes (p. 9):

> Usually the child's feelings of security and safety oscillate hopefully for a time with feelings of fear and disbelief. But with repeated turnings and trauma, security and safety become the hypervigilant scanning of the parent and the environment. Trust is seriously compromised, and this distrust generalizes to all relationships. . . . Dependency becomes a baffled depression, and joy seems to wither and become foreign. More importantly, the child finds that she is being abused *within* what had been her safe base, and so she no longer has a safe base in the world.

Although it is speculative, these dynamics seem to apply to MBP as well. In MBP, the positive attention so frequently given to the perpetrator could also contribute to this sense of unreality.

3. Prolonged and multiple forms of abuse have serious consequences and may lead to adoption of the maltreating behavior. Bagley, Wood, and Young (1994) found that young adults who reported experiencing multiple events of sexual abuse were more likely to be depressed, anxious, or suicidal. When emotional abuse accompanied the sexual abuse, damage was even more likely. Eight of 117 identified victims of sexual abuse were identified as pedophiles. Harrison, Fulkerson, and Beebe (1997) found that students in grades six, nine, and twelve were more likely to use drugs if they had been sexually abused, and far more likely to use drugs if they had been both physically and sexually abused. Similarly, Jasinski, Williams, and Siegel (2000) found that African-American women who had been sexually abused as children were more likely to abuse alcohol. In this study, multiple episodes of abuse were more highly correlated with alcohol abuse than the severity of individual episodes.

For MBP, this leads to the speculation that multiple forms of maltreatment and multiple incidents of maltreatment are more likely to be damaging. The Bagley, Wood, and Young (1994) study suggests that the concern about victims becoming MBP maltreaters may be justified. However, as in other forms of maltreatment, it also suggests that experience is not destiny, since the majority of victims, although multiply abused, did *not* go on to abuse others (see also Knutson, 1995). As the number of identified victims of MBP increases, and as they move through middle and high school, it would be of research interest to see if they also use drugs or alcohol as a means of escape. Unfortunately, there appears to be little interest in conducting such research (M. Feldman, personal communication). Until more is known, those working with MBP victims should be alert to the possibility.

Some techniques useful with victims of sexual abuse may also be useful with victims of MBP.

1. Crisis intervention: Gilmartin (1994) summarizes treatment soon after victimization as incorporating the following general approaches, largely derived from crisis intervention (p. 267, ordering altered):

- Helping the victim express her or his feelings about the experience
- Letting the victim know that her or his responses are normal
- Cognitive restructuring (looking at things in a different way), especially to help the victim recognize that she or he is not to blame for the abuse
- Helping the victim link current symptoms to the experience of abuse
- Helping the victim to cope with symptoms related to the abuse
- Helping the victim to incorporate the experience into her or his overall view of life and self, and perhaps to take specific action related to this experience

These approaches would appear useful with victims of recent MBP if their age and abilities make talk therapy (or brief therapeutic conversations) appropriate.

2. Coming to terms with reality: Gilmartin (1994) believes that treatment of the many problems that follow sexual victimization, especially for the adult abused as a child, must focus on the core issue: accepting the fact that the maltreatment occurred. Once this occurs, attention can be turned to relegating the experience to the past, and to "develop[ing] a new world view which includes awareness of [everyone's] vulnerability to victimization and a realistic view of the randomness of negative life events" (p.169). This should help develop a sense that one is in reasonable control of one's life (internal locus of control), positive self-esteem, and nurturing relationships.

3. Becoming a "survivor" and not a "victim": Ultimately, the goal of treatment in cases of sexual abuse is for the victim to be a survivor who has found her or his sense of self and "voice." The field of sexual abuse has developed and advocated for the language of survival rather than victimization. This is an area almost untouched in the field of MBP. It is an important concept for future exploration.

Briere (1996, p. 81) states that the experience of therapy for sexual abuse should not repeat the "powerlessness, intrusion, and authoritarianism" of the original assault. This is an important part of rejecting victimhood. Although challenged to do the difficult self-examination of the therapeutic process, the victim of maltreatment should feel safe and supported in therapy by a caring professional. Thus the therapist should not present the image of an "all-knowing expert" who blames the victim or forces interpretations. Rights and boundaries should hold an important place in sessions. Therapist and client should work collaboratively and from a strengths perspective. Briere also suggests an educational component, in which the client is encouraged to learn the social/cultural aspects of maltreatment and victimization.

All of these approaches would seem appropriate for victims of MBP. Without denying the abuse that has occurred, therapists can empower victims within the therapeutic setting. Although more is known about the social/cultural aspects of sexual abuse and of abuse and oppression in general than is known about MBP, the information that is available can be shared.

   4. Group therapy: Therapeutic and/or support groups have proven useful in a variety of situations that elicit specific responses. Among these is sexual abuse. Kempe (1997), for example, states that group therapy is the treatment of choice for child victims of sexual abuse. In a group of peers, victims learn that their responses to trauma are not unique, and can be understood and shared by others. Group members can be honest about feelings and experiences that might not be understood by outsiders. They gain support and encouragement from one another in their efforts to understand their problems. Group therapy is appropriate for both adults and children. It has been found appropriate for sexually abused children as young as three years old, using play therapeutic techniques (Gallo-Lopez, 2000).

There has never been a sufficient number of MBP victims identified in one area to make group support feasible. This remains an interesting and useful idea for the future. The Internet appears to offer an opportunity, if access is limited to persons who have been screened for appropriateness (including verification of their status as victims) and leadership is provided by credible professionals knowledgeable about MBP.

   5. Confrontation of the perpetrator: According to Gelinas (1993), confrontation of the abuser helps the victim reclaim a sense of power, reality, and self-worth. The old denial is broken, and people—or at least the therapist helping with this process—believe the victim. According to Gelinas, it is the action of the victim rather than the response of the abuser that is effective. The confrontation itself requires lengthy and thorough preparation on the part of the victim. (The authors of this book are not aware of confrontation being done by adult survivors of MBP.) Some activities such as writing (unmailed) letters

to the perpetrator and placing the perpetrator in the "empty chair" (a therapeutic technique in which the client pretends that the perpetrator is present in the session) may be worthy of trial. Given the denial that is so pervasive with perpetrators, and the difficulties in confrontation even for professionals, an in-person confrontation may not be desirable.

Caution about reunification and parental involvement in therapy is justified.

Hobbs, Hanks, and Wynne (1993) are cautious about reunification and parental involvement in therapy when sexual abuse has occurred. They state (p. 277, ordering altered):

> Not all adults are capable of giv[ing] up those behaviors that contribute to, or are a consequence of, the abuse. . . . When both parents have been involved in their child's sexual maltreatment it will not be appropriate to involve them in therapy with the child. Also, when the nonabusing parent is denying the abuse the child may need space and the experience of an adult who can be more accepting of the child's experience and help the child to express this. Because of the almost addictive quality of behavior in the adults when they have sexually abused the child, it will simply not be safe for the child to be in the abusive parent's presence until major changes have occurred in the abusing adult's life.

It is difficult for MBP perpetrators to give up their abuse or their assertions about health problems in the victim or in themselves. As has been previously stated in this book, the perpetrator's denial and the denial of the nonperpetrating friends and relatives also places the victim at risk. MBP victims often need to be placed with an adult who is more able to meet their needs until major change occurs—if it does—in the perpetrator and family.

Gelinas (1993) also reports on the rigidity of the incestuous family, the difficulty of involving them in family therapy, and the poor likelihood that the family will be able to translate insight into change. Similarly, as has already been stated, families in which MBP is occurring are resistant to involvement in therapy, insight, and change.

Work with victims takes its toll on professionals.

The stress on those investigating MBP and pursuing cases through court has been discussed elsewhere in this book. As more professionals become involved in work directly with victims, they will likely experience similar problems. Those working with childhood trauma (not specifically sexual abuse) are affected by victims' stories. As they identify with the victims, especially in the first six months of work, therapists may come to experience some of the same posttraumatic symptoms that victims experience. This is discussed extensively as "countertransference" by Dalenberg (2000). Support from other staff, consultation, and considerable self-awareness are necessary for therapists to succeed and persist in this field. Therapists should be aware of this possibility and take steps to build their own supports.

The use of this model derived from sexual abuse is admittedly speculative. It may not be the model that the field will be using twenty years from now (M. Feldman, personal communication). However, it does provide a starting place, and a set of observations to test as work with victims begins.

References

Allison, D. B. and Roberts, M. S. (1998). *Disordered mother or disordered diagnosis?* Hillsdale, NJ: Analytic Press.

American Counseling Association (1995). *The code of ethics and standards of practice.* Alexandria, VA: ACA.

American Medical Association (1996). *Principles of medical ethics.* Chicago: AMA.

American Medical Association (1998). *E-principles of medical ethics.* Retrieved May 15, 2002 from <http://www.ama-assn.org/appf>.

American Nursing Association (1985). *Code for nurses with interpretive statements.* Washington, DC: ANA.

American Psychiatric Association (1994). *Diagnostic and statistical manual of mental disorders,* Fourth edition. Washington, DC: APA.

American Psychological Association (1995). *Ethical principles of psychologists and code of conduct.* Washington, DC: APA.

American Public Human Services Association (1999). *Guidelines for a model system of protective services for abused and neglected children and their families.* Washington, DC: APHSA.

Ayoub, C. C. and Alexander, R. A. (1998). Definitional issues in Munchausen syndrome by proxy. *The APSAC Advisor, 11,* 7-10.

Bagley, C., Wood, M., and Young, L. (1994). Victim to abuser: Mental health and behavioral sequels of child sexual abuse in a community survey of young adult males. *Child Abuse and Neglect, 18,* 683-697.

Barlow, D. H. and Durand, V. M. (1995). *Abnormal psychology: An integrative approach.* Pacific Grove, CA: Brooks/Cole.

Baute, P. (2000). Expert witnessing and Daubert: Is your expert witness prepared for a Daubert/Kumho challenge? *Forensic Examiner, 9*(3/4), 15-20.

Berg, B. and Jones, D. P. H. (1999). Outcome of psychiatric intervention in factitious illness by proxy (Munchausen syndrome by proxy). *Archives of Disease in Childhood, 81,* 465-472

Blix, S. and Brack, G. (1988). The effects of a suspected case of Munchausen's syndrome by proxy on a pediatric nursing staff. *General Hospital Psychiatry, 10,* 402-409.

Bonner, B. (2000). What are effective strategies to address common behavior problems? In H. Dubowitz and D. DePanfilis (Eds.), *Handbook for child protection practice* (pp. 414-419). Thousand Oaks, CA: Sage.

Bools, C. N., Neale, B. A., and Meadow, S. R. (1993). Follow-up of victims of fabricated illness (Munchausen syndrome by proxy*). Archives of Disease in Childhood, 69,* 625-630.

Bools, C. N., Neale, B. A., and Meadow, R. S. (1994). Munchausen syndrome by proxy: A study of psychopathology. *Child Abuse & Neglect, 18,* 773-788.

Briere, J. (1996). *Therapy for adults molested as children: Beyond survival.* New York: Springer.

Brown, M. L. (1997). Dilemmas facing nurses who care for Munchausen syndrome by proxy patients. *Pediatric Nursing, 23,* 416-418.

Byard, R.W. and Burnell, R. H. (1994). Covert video surveillance in Munchausen syndrome by proxy: Ethical compromise or essential technique? *Medical Journal of Australia, 160,* 352-356.

Byrk, M. and Siegel, P. T. (1997). My mother caused my illness: The story of a survivor of Munchausen by proxy syndrome. *Pediatrics, 100,* 1-7.

Chaffin, M. (2000). What types of mental health treatment should be considered for maltreated children? In H. Dubowitz and D. DePanfilis (Eds.), *Handbook for child protection practice* (pp. 409-413). Thousand Oaks, CA: Sage.

Child Abuse Prevention and Treatment Act, As Amended. NCCAN: US DHHS, 1996, Sec. 111.2.

Conway, S. P. and Pond, M. N. (1995). Munchausen syndrome by proxy abuse: A foundation for adult Munchausen syndrome. *Australian and New Zealand Journal of Psychiatry, 29,* 504-507.

Coombe, P. (1995). The inpatient psychotherapy of a mother and child at the Cassel Hospital: A case of Munchausen's syndrome by proxy. *British Journal of Psychotherapy, 12,* 195-207.

Corey G., Corey, M. S., and Callanan, P. (1998). *Issues and ethics in the helping professions.* Pacific Grove, CA: Brooks/Cole.

Crouse, K. A. (1992). Munchausen syndrome by proxy: Recognizing the victim. *Pediatric Nursing, 18,* 249-252.

Dalenberg, C. J. (2000). *Countertransference and the treatment of trauma.* Washington, DC: American Psychological Association.

Davies, N. (1993). *Murder on ward 4.* London: Chatto and Windus.

Davis, P., McClure, R. J., Rolfe, K., Chessman, N., Pearson, S., Sibert, J. R., and Meadow, R. (1998). Procedures, placement, and risks of further abuse after Munchausen syndrome by proxy, non-accidental poisoning, and non-accidental suffocation. *Archives of Disease of Childhood, 78,* 217-221.

Day, D. O. (1998a). The initial therapeutic stage: Trust. In T. F. Parnell and D. O. Day (Eds.), *Munchausen by proxy syndrome: Misunderstood child abuse* (pp. 167-182). Thousand Oaks, CA: Sage.

Day, D. O. (1998b). Later therapeutic stage: Identity formation. In T. F. Parnell and D. O. Day (Eds.), *Munchausen by proxy syndrome: Misunderstood child abuse* (pp. 193-201). Thousand Oaks, CA: Sage.

Day, D. O. (1998c). The middle therapeutic stage: The secrets. In T. F. Parnell and D. O. Day (Eds.), *Munchausen by proxy syndrome: Misunderstood child abuse* (pp. 183-192). Thousand Oaks, CA: Sage.

Day, D. O. and Ojeda-Castro, M. D. (1998). Therapy with family members. In T. F. Parnell and D. O. Day (Eds.), *Munchausen by proxy syndrome: Misunderstood child abuse* (pp. 202-215). Thousand Oaks, CA: Sage.

Dowling, D. (1998). Poison glue: The child's experience of Munchhausen syndrome by proxy. *Journal of Child Psychotherapy, 24,* 307-326.

Eminson, M. (2000). Background. In M. Eminson and R. J. Postlethwaite (Eds.), *Munchausen syndrome by proxy abuse: A practical approach* (pp. 17-70). Oxford: Butterworth Heinemann.

Facey, S. (1993). Munchausen syndrome by proxy. *Nursing Times, 89*(4), 54-56.

Feldman, M. D. (1994). Denial in Munchausen syndrome by proxy: The consulting psychiatrist's dilemma. *International Journal of Psychiatry in Medicine, 24,* 121-128.

Feldman, M. D. (1997). Canine variant of factitious disorder by proxy. *American Journal of Psychiatry, 134,* 1316-1317.

Feldman, M. D. (2000). Munchausen by Internet: Detecting factitious illness and crisis on the Internet. *Southern Medical Journal, 93,* 669-672.

Feldman, M. D., Bibby, M., and Crites, S. D. (1998). 'Virtual' factitious disorders and Munchausen by proxy. *Western Journal of Medicine, 168,* 537-539.

Feldman, M.D. and Brown, R. (2002). Munchausen by proxy in an international context. *Child Abuse and Neglect, 26,* 509-525.

Feldman, M. D. and Ford, C. V. (1994). *Patient or pretender: Inside the strange world of factitious disorders.* New York: Wiley.

Feldman, M. D. and Ford, C. V. (2000). Factitious disorders. In Sadock, B. J., Sadock, V. A. (Eds.), *Kaplan and Sadock's comprehensive textbook of psychiatry,* Volume 1 (pp. 1533-1543). Philadelphia: Lippincott Williams and Wilkins.

Feldman, M. D. and Hamilton, J. C. (2001). "Chest pain" in patients with Munchausen syndrome. In J. W. Hurst and D. C. Morris, (Eds.), *Chest pain* (pp. 457-467). Armonk, NY: Futura.

Feldman, M. D. and Lasher, L. J. (1999). Munchausen by proxy: A misunderstood form of maltreatment. *The Forensic Examiner,* September/October, 25-29.

Firstman, R. and Talan, J. (1997). *The death of innocents: A true story of murder, medicine, and high-stakes science.* New York: Bantam.

Fisher, G. C. (1995). The role of psychiatry. In A. V. Levin and M. S. Sheridan (Eds.), *Munchausen syndrome by proxy: Issues in diagnosis and treatment* (pp. 369-398). New York: Lexington.

Fisher, G. C. and Mitchell, I. (1995). Is Munchausen syndrome by proxy really a syndrome? *Archives of Disease in Childhood, 72,* 530-534.

Flynn, D. (1998). Psychoanalytic aspects of inpatient treatment. *Journal of Child Psychotherapy, 24,* 283-306.

Ford, C. V. (1996). Ethical and legal issues in factitious disorders: An overview. In M. D. Feldman and S. J. Eisendrath (Eds.), *The spectrum of factitious disorders* (pp. 51-64). Washington, DC: American Psychiatric Press.

Gallo-Lopez, L. (2000). A creative play therapy approach to the group treatment of young sexually abused children. In H. G. Kaduson and C. E. Schaefer (Eds.), *Short-term play therapy for children* (pp. 269-295). New York: Guilford.

Gelinas, D. J. (1993). Relational patterns in incestuous families, malevolent variations, and specific interventions with the adult survivor. In P. L. Paddison (Ed.), *Treatment of adult survivors of incest* (pp. 1-34). Washington, DC: American Psychiatric Press.

Gibson, R. L. and Hartshorne, T. S. (1996). Childhood sexual abuse and adult loneliness and network orientation. *Child Abuse and Neglect, 20,* 1087-1093.

Gilmartin, P. (1994). *Rape, incest, and child sexual abuse: Consequences and recovery.* New York: Garland.

Goddard, C. R. and Stanley, J. R. (1994). Viewing the abusive parent and the abused child as captor and hostage: The application of hostage theory to the effects of child abuse. *Journal of Interpersonal Violence, 9,* 258-269.

Grand, S. (2000). *Reproduction of evil.* Hillsdale, NJ: Analytic Press.

Griffith, J. L. (1988). The family systems of Munchausen syndrome by proxy. *Family Process, 27,* 423-437.

Guerisik, U. E. (1997). Challenges to the ambulatory treatment process and how to survive them: A case study. In H. J. C. van Marle (Ed.), *Challenges in forensic psychotherapy* (pp. 43-52). London: Jessica Kingsley.

Guyer, B., Hoyert, D. L., Martin, J. A., Ventura, S. J., MacDorman, M. B., and Strobino, D. M. (1999). Annual summary of vital statistics 1998. *Pediatrics, 104,* 229-1246.

Hare, R. D. and Hart, S. D. (1993). Psychopathy, mental disorder, and crime. In S. Hodgins (Ed.), *Mental disorder and crime* (pp. 104-115). Thousand Oaks, CA: Sage.

Harrison, P. A., Fulkerson, J. A., and Beebe, T. J. (1997). Multiple substance abuse among adolescent physical and sexual abuse victims. *Child Abuse and Neglect, 21,* 529-539.

Hobbs, C. J., Hanks, H. G. I., and Wynne, J. M. (1993). *Child abuse and neglect: A clinician's handbook.* Edinburgh: Churchill Livingstone.

Hochhauser, K. G. and Richardson, R. A. (1994). Munchausen syndrome by proxy: An exploratory study of pediatric nurses' knowledge and involvement. *Journal of Pediatric Nursing, 9,* 313-320.

Jasinski, J. L., Williams, L. M., and Siegel, J. (2000). Childhood physical and sexual abuse as risk factors for heavy drinking among African-American women: A prospective study. *Child Abuse and Neglect, 24,* 1061-1071.

Jones, D. P. H. (1997). Treatment of the child and family where child abuse or neglect has occurred. In M. E. Helfer, R. S. Kempe, and R. D. Krugman (Eds.), *The battered child* (pp. 521-542). Chicago: University of Chicago Press.

Jones, D. P .H., Byrne, G., and Newbould, C. (2000). Management, treatment, and outcomes. In M. Eminson and R. J. Postlethwaite (Eds.), *Munchausen syndrome by proxy abuse: A practical approach* (pp. 276-294). Oxford: Butterworth Heinemann.

Jones, J. G., Butler, H. L., Hamilton, B., Perdue, J. D., Stern, P., and Woody, R. C. (1986). Munchausen syndrome by proxy. *Child Abuse and Neglect, 10,* 33-40.

Jones, V. F., Badgett, T. J., Minella, J. L., and Schuschke, L. A. (1993). The role of the male caretaker in Munchausen syndrome by proxy. *Clinical Pediatrics, 32,* 245-247.

Kaufman, K. L., Coury, D., Pickrel, E., and McCleery, J. (1989). Munchausen syndrome by proxy: A survey of professionals' knowledge. *Child Abuse and Neglect, 13,* 141-147.

Kempe, R. S. (1997). A developmental approach to the treatment of abused children. In M. E. Helfer, R. S. Kempe, and R. D. Krugman (Eds.), *The battered child* (pp. 543-565). Chicago: University of Chicago Press.

Kinscherff, R. and Famularo, R. (1991). Extreme Munchausen syndrome by proxy: The case for termination of parental rights. *Juvenile and Family Court Journal, 40,* 41-53.

Knutson, J. F. (1995). Psychological characteristics of maltreated children: Putative risk factors and consequences. *Annual Review of Psychology, 46,* 401-431.

Lasher, L. J. and Feldman, M. D. (2001). Munchausen by proxy (MBP) maltreatment manifesting as child sexual abuse. In *Child sexual abuse investigations: Multidisciplinary collaboration.* Retrieved April 15, 2002 from <http://childabuse.gactr.uga.edu>.

Leeder, E. (1990). Supermom or child abuser? Treatment of the Munchausen mother. *Women and Therapy, 9*(4), 69-88.

Levin, A. V. and Sheridan, M. S. (1995). *Munchausen syndrome by proxy: Issues in diagnosis and treatment.* New York: Lexington Press.

Libow, J. A. (1995). Munchausen syndrome by proxy victims in adulthood: A first look. *Child Abuse and Neglect, 19,* 1131-1142.

Libow, J. A. and Schreier, H. A. (1986). Three forms of factitious illness in children: When is it Munchausen syndrome by proxy? *American Journal of Orthopsychiatry, 56,* 602-611.

Light, M. J. and Sheridan, M. S. (1990). Munchausen syndrome by proxy and apnea (MBPA). *Clinical Pediatrics, 29,* 162-168.

Lloyd, H. and MacDonald, A. (2000). Picking up the pieces. In M. Eminson and R. J. Postlethwaite (Eds.), *Munchausen syndrome by proxy abuse: A practical approach* (pp. 295-314). Oxford: Butterworth Heinemann.

Lyons-Ruth, K., Kaufman, M., Masters, N., and Wu, J. (1991). Issues in the identification and long-term management of Munchausen by proxy syndrome within a clinical infant service. *Infant Mental Health Journal, 12,* 309-320.

Masterson, J. (1988). Extreme illness exaggeration in pediatric patients: A variant of Munchausen's by proxy? *American Journal of Orthopsychiatry, 58,* 188-195.

McClure, R. J., Davis, P. M., Meadow S. R., and Sibert, J. R. (1996). Epidemiology of Munchausen syndrome by proxy, non-accidental poisoning, and non-accidental suffocation. *Archives of Disease in Childhood, 75,* 57-61.

McGuire, T. L. and Feldman, K. W. (1989). Psychological morbidity of children subjected to Munchausen syndrome by proxy. *Pediatrics, 83,* 289-292.

Meadow, R. (1977). Munchausen syndrome by proxy: The hinterland of child abuse. *Lancet, 2,* 343-345.

Meadow, R. (1985). Management of Munchausen syndrome by proxy. *Archives of Disease in Childhood, 60,* 385-393.

Meadow, R. (1990). Suffocation, recurrent apnea, and sudden infant death. *Journal of Pediatrics, 117,* 351-357.

Meadow, R. (1995a). The history of Munchausen syndrome by proxy. In A. V. Levin and M. S. Sheridan (Eds.), *Munchausen syndrome by proxy: Issues in diagnosis and treatment* (pp. 3-12). New York: Lexington Press.

Meadow, R. (1995b). What is and what is not "Munchausen syndrome by proxy." *Archives of Disease in Childhood, 72,* 534-538.

Mercer, S. O. and Perdue, J. D. (1993). Munchausen syndrome by proxy: Social work's role. *Social Work, 38,* 74-81.

Mian, M. (1995). A multidisciplinary approach. In A. V. Levin and M. S. Sheridan (Eds.), *Munchausen syndrome by proxy: Issues in diagnosis and treatment* (pp. 271-286). New York: Lexington Press.

Mitchell, I., Brummitt, J., DeForest, J., and Fisher, G. (1993). Apnea and factitious illness (Munchausen syndrome) by proxy. *Pediatrics, 92,* 810-814.

Modestin, J., Hug A., and Ammann, R. (1997). Criminal behavior in males with affective disorder. *Journal of Affective Disorders, 42,* 29-38.

Morley, C. J. (1995). Practical concerns about the diagnosis of Munchausen syndrome by proxy. *Archives of Disease in Childhood, 72,* 528-538.

Mother of the year tried on child abuse charges. (1996). *San Diego Daily Transcript,* May 9. Retrieved May 20, 1997 from <http://www.sddt.com/files/librarywire/96wireheadlines/05_96>.

My sister-in-law was starving her baby (1991). *Good Housekeeping, 213*(4), 26-29.

National Association of Social Workers (1996). *Code of ethics.* Washington, DC: NASW.

National Center for Hearing Assessment and Management (2000). A brief history of UNHS legislation. Retrieved June 26, 2000 from <http://www.infanthearing.org/legislative/index.html>.

Nicol, A. R. and Eccles, M. (1985). Psychotherapy for Munchausen syndrome by proxy. *Archives of Disease in Childhood, 60,* 344-348.

Orenstein, D. M. and Wasserman, A. L. (1986). Munchausen syndrome by proxy simulating cystic fibrosis. *Pediatrics, 78,* 621-624.

Ostfeld, B. A. and Feldman, M. D. (1996a). Factitious disorder by proxy: Clinical features, detection, and management. In M. D. Feldman and S. J. Eisendrath (Eds.), *The spectrum of factitious disorders* (pp. 83-108). Washington, DC: American Psychiatric Press.

Ostfeld, B. A. and Feldman, M. D. (1996b). Factitious disorder by proxy: Medical awareness among mental health practitioners. *General Hospital Psychiatry, 18,* 113-116.

Parnell, T. E. (1998). Defining Munchausen by proxy syndrome. In T. F. Parnell and D. O. Day (Eds.), *Munchausen by proxy syndrome: Misunderstood child abuse* (pp. 9-46). Thousand Oaks, CA: Sage.

Pasqualone, G. A. and Fitzgerald, S. M. (1999). Munchausen by proxy syndrome: The forensic challenge of recognition, diagnosis, and reporting. *Critical Care Nursing Quarterly, 22,* 52-64.

Perry, J. C., Bannon, E., and Ianni, F. (1999). Effectiveness of psychotherapy for personality disorders. *American Journal of Psychiatry, 156,* 1312-1321.

Polledri, P. (1996). Munchausen syndrome by proxy and perversion of the maternal instinct. *Journal of Forensic Psychiatry, 7,* 551-562.

Rand, D. C. (1990). Munchausen syndrome by proxy: Integration of classic and contemporary types. *Issues in Child Abuse Accusations, 2,* 83-89.

Rand, D. C. and Feldman, M. D. (1999) Misdisgnosis in Munchausen by proxy: Literature review and four new cases. *Harvard Review of Psychiatry, 7*(2), 94-101.

Rappaport, S. R. and Hochstadt, N. J. (1993). Munchausen syndrome by proxy (MSBP): An intergenerational perspective. *Journal of Mental Health Counseling, 15,* 278-289.

Richardson, J. (1999). My mother was making me sick. *Mademoiselle, 105*(2), 125-127, 146.

Robins, P. M. and Sesan, R. (1991). Munchausen syndrome by proxy: Another women's disorder? *Professional Psychology: Research and Practice, 22,* 285-290.

Rosen, C. L., Frost, J. D, and Glaze, D. G. (1986). Child abuse and recurrent infant apnea. *Journal of Pediatrics, 109,* 1065-1067.

Rosenberg, D. A. (1987). Web of deceit: A literature review of Munchausen syndrome by proxy. *Child Abuse and Neglect, 11,* 547-563.

Rosenberg, D. A. (1995). From lying to homicide: The spectrum of Munchausen syndrome by proxy. In A. V. Levin and M. S. Sheridan (Eds.), *Munchausen syndrome by proxy: Issues in diagnosis and treatment* (pp. 13-38). New York: Lexington Press.

Sanders, M. J. (1996). Narrative family treatment of Munchausen syndrome by proxy: A successful case. *Families, Systems, and Health, 14,* 315-329.

Schreier, H. A. (1996). Repeated false allegations of sexual abuse presenting to sheriffs: When is it Munchausen by proxy? *Child Abuse and Neglect, 20,* 985-991.

Schreier, H.A. (2002). Forensic issues in Munchausen by proxy. In D. H. Schetky and E. P. Benedek (Eds.), *Principles and practice of child and adolescent forensic psychiatry* (pp. 149-160). Washington, DC: American Psychological Association.

Schreier, H. A. and Libow, J. A. (1993). *Hurting for love: Munchausen by proxy syndrome.* New York: Guilford.

Schwartz, S. (2000). *Abnormal psychology: A discovery approach.* Mountain View, CA: Mayfield.

Seidl, T. (1995). Is family preservation, reunification, and successful treatment a possibility? A roundtable. In A. V. Levin and M. S. Sheridan (Eds), *Munchausen syndrome by proxy: Issues in diagnosis and treatment* (pp. 411-422). New York: Lexington Press.

Shabde, N. and Craft, W. A. (1998). Covert video surveillance is acceptable—but only with a rigorous protocol. *British Medical Journal, 316,* 1603-1605.

Sharp, D. (2004). Kathy Bush, FL. Retrieved April 10, 2004 from <AsherMeadow. com>.

Sheridan, M. S. (1989). Social work with Munchausen's by proxy. *Health and Social Work, 14,* 53-58.

Sheridan, M. S. (1992). *Pain in America.* Tuscaloosa: University of Alabama.

Sheridan, M. S. (1995). Munchausen syndrome by proxy in context II: Professional proxy and other analogs. In A. V. Levin and M. S. Sheridan (Eds.), *Munchausen syndrome by proxy: Issues in diagnosis and treatment* (pp. 85-102). New York: Lexington Press.

Sheridan, M. S. (2003). The deceit continues: An updated review of Munchausen syndrome by proxy. *Child Abuse and Neglect, 27,* 431-451.

Shinebourne, E. A. (1996). Covert video surveillance and the principle of double effect: A response to criticism. *Journal of Medical Ethics, 22,* 26-31.

Sidel, R. (1992). *Women and children last: The plight of poor women in affluent America.* New York: Penguin.

Sigal, M. and Altmark, D. (1995). Adult victims. In A. V. Levin and M. S. Sheridan (Eds.), *Munchausen syndrome by proxy: Issues in diagnosis and treatment* (pp. 257-267). New York: Lexington Press.

Sigal, M., Gelkopf, M., and Meadow, R. S. (1989). Munchausen by proxy syndrome: The triad of abuse, self-abuse, and deception. *Comprehensive Psychiatry, 30,* 527-533.

Southall, D. P., Plunkett, M. C. B., Banks, M. W., Falkov, A. F., and Samuels, M. P. (1997). Covert video recordings of life-threatening child abuse: Lessons for child protection. *Pediatrics, 100,* 735-760.

Southall, D. P. and Samuels, M. P. (1996). Guidelines for the multiagency management of patients suspected or at risk of suffering from life-threatening abuse resulting in cyanotic-apnoeic episodes. *Journal of Medical Ethics, 22,* 16-21.

Sperry, L. (1995). *Handbook of diagnosis and treatment of the DSM-IV personality disorders.* New York: Brunner/Mazel.

Stern, P. (1997). *Preparing and presenting expert testimony in child abuse litigation.* Thousand Oaks, CA: Sage.

Surveillance for Lyme disease—United States (2000). *Morbidity and Mortality Weekly Report 49*(SS03), 1-11.

Szajnberg, N. M., Moilanen, I., Kanerva, A., and Tolf, B. (1996). Munchausen-by-proxy syndrome: Countertransference as a diagnostic tool. *Bulletin of the Menninger Clinic, 60,* 229-237.

Thoennes, N. and Tjaden, P. (1990). The extent, nature, and validity of sexual abuse allegations in custody/visitation disputes. *Child Abuse and Neglect, 14,* 151-163.

Thompson, M. K. and Sullivan, M. J. (1995). Community dynamics of working with Munchausen syndrome by proxy in technology-dependent children. *Journal of Home Health Care Practice, 7*(3), 27-35.

Tumlin, K.C. and Geen, R. (2000). The decision to investigate: Understanding state child welfare screening policies and practices. Retrieved May 12, 2000 from <http//newfederalism.urban.org/html/anf_a38.html>.

Warner, J. O. and Hathaway, M. J. (1984). Allergic form of Meadow's syndrome (Munchausen syndrome by proxy). *Archives of Disease in Childhood, 59,* 151-156.

Yorker, B. C. and Kahan, B. B. (1991). The Munchausen syndrome by proxy variant of child abuse in the family courts. *Juvenile and Family Court Journal, 42*(3), 51-58.

Zitelli, B. J., Seltman, M. F., and Shannon, R. M. (1987). Munchausen's syndrome by proxy and its professional participants. *American Journal of Diseases of Children, 141,* 1099-1102.

Index

Page numbers followed by the letter "b" indicate boxed text; those followed by the letter "f" indicate figures.

SCHIZOPHRENIA: INNOVATIONS IN DIAGNOSIS AND TREATMENT by Colin A. Ross. (2004). "Well-documented and clearly explained ... has hugely significant implications for our diagnostic system and for how severely disturbed people are understood and treated." *John Read, PhD, Editor,* Models of Madness: Psychological, Social, and Biological Approaches to Schizophrenia; *Director of Clinical Psychology, The University of Auckland, New Zealand*

EFFECTS OF AND INTERVENTIONS FOR CHILDHOOD TRAUMA FROM INFANCY THROUGH ADOLESCENCE: PAIN UNSPEAKABLE by Sandra B. Hutchison. (2004). "An excellent addition to the healing arts field! The author presents a rich body of research-recent, relevant, and definitive of the many faces of trauma across a wide array of cultures. As enriching and instructional as the research is, the author, as a counselor, does not forget the key focus of addressing the need for healing." *Pat H. NeSmith, PhD, Consultant, Federal Department of Health & Human Services, Head Start Bureau*

REBUILDING ATTACHMENTS WITH TRAUMATIZED CHILDREN: HEALING FROM LOSSES, VIOLENCE, ABUSE, AND NEGLECT by Richard Kagan. (2004). "Dr. Richard Kagan, a recognized expert in working with traumatized children, has written a truly impressive book. Not only does the book contain a wealth of information for understanding the complex issues faced by traumatized youngsters, but it also offers specific interventions that can be used to help these children and their caregivers become more hopeful and resilient. . . . I am certain that this book will be read and reread by professionals engaged in improving the lives of at-risk youth." *Robert Brooks, PhD, Faculty, Harvard Medical School and author of* Raising Resilient Children *and* The Power of Resilience

PSYCHOLOGICAL TRAUMA AND THE DEVELOPING BRAIN: NEUROLOGICALLY BASED INTERVENTIONS FOR TROUBLED CHILDREN by Phyllis T. Stien and Joshua C. Kendall. (2003). "Stien and Kendall provide us with a great service. In this clearly written and important book, they synthesize a wealth of crucial information that links childhood trauma to brain abnormalities and subsequent mental illness. Equally important, they show us how the trauma also affects the child's social and intellectual development. I recommend this book to all clinicians and administrators." *Charles L. Whitfield, MD, Author,* The Truth About Depression *and* The Truth About Mental Illness

CHILD MALTREATMENT RISK ASSESSMENTS: AN EVALUATION GUIDE by Sue Righthand, Bruce Kerr, and Kerry Drach. (2003). "This book is essential reading for clinicians and forensic examiners who see cases involving issues related to child maltreatment. The authors have compiled an impressive critical survey of the relevant research on child maltreatment. Their material is well organized into sections on definitions, impact, risk assessment, and risk management. This book represents a giant step toward promoting evidence-based evaluations, treatment, and testimony." *Diane H. Schetky, MD, Professor of Psychiatry, University of Vermont College of Medicine*

SIMPLE AND COMPLEX POST-TRAUMATIC STRESS DISORDER: STRATEGIES FOR COMPREHENSIVE TREATMENT IN CLINICAL PRACTICE edited by Mary Beth Williams and John F. Sommer Jr. (2002). "A welcome addition to the literature on treating survivors of traumatic events, this volume possesses all the ingredients necessary for even the experienced clinician to master the management of patients with PTSD." *Terence M. Keane, PhD, Chief, Psychology Service, VA Boston Healthcare System; Professor and Vice Chair of Research in Psychiatry, Boston University School of Medicine*

FOR LOVE OF COUNTRY: CONFRONTING RAPE AND SEXUAL HARASSMENT IN THE U.S. MILITARY by T. S. Nelson. (2002). "Nelson brings an important message—that the absence of current media attention doesn't mean the problem has gone away; that only decisive action by military leadership at all levels can break the cycle of repeated traumatization; and that the failure to do so is, as Nelson puts it, a 'power failure'—a refusal to exert positive leadership at all levels to stop violent individuals from using the worst power imaginable." *Chris Lombardi, Correspondent, Women's E-News, New York City*

THE INSIDERS: A MAN'S RECOVERY FROM TRAUMATIC CHILDHOOD ABUSE by Robert Blackburn Knight. (2002). "An important book. . . . Fills a gap in the literature about healing from childhood sexual abuse by allowing us to hear, in undiluted terms, about one man's history and journey of recovery." *Amy Pine, MA, LMFT, psychotherapist and co-founder, Survivors Healing Center, Santa Cruz, California*

WE ARE NOT ALONE: A GUIDEBOOK FOR HELPING PROFESSIONALS AND PARENTS SUPPORTING ADOLESCENT VICTIMS OF SEXUAL ABUSE by Jade Christine Angelica. (2002). "Encourages victims and their families to participate in the system in an effort to heal from their victimization, seek justice, and hold offenders accountable for their crimes. An exceedingly vital training tool." *Janet Fine, MS, Director, Victim Witness Assistance Program and Children's Advocacy Center, Suffolk County District Attorney's Office, Boston*

WE ARE NOT ALONE: A TEENAGE GIRL'S PERSONAL ACCOUNT OF INCEST FROM DISCLOSURE THROUGH PROSECUTION AND TREATMENT by Jade Christine Angelica. (2002). "A valuable resource for teens who have been sexually abused and their parents. With compassion and eloquent prose, Angelica walks people through the criminal justice system—from disclosure to final outcome." *Kathleen Kendall-Tackett, PhD, Research Associate, Family Research Laboratory, University of New Hampshire, Durham*

WE ARE NOT ALONE: A TEENAGE BOY'S PERSONAL ACCOUNT OF CHILD SEXUAL ABUSE FROM DISCLOSURE THROUGH PROSECUTION AND TREATMENT by Jade Christine Angelica. (2002). "Inspires us to work harder to meet kids' needs, answer their questions, calm their fears, and protect them from their abusers and the system, which is often not designed to respond to them in a language they understand." *Kevin L. Ryle, JD, Assistant District Attorney, Middlesex, Massachusetts*

GROWING FREE: A MANUAL FOR SURVIVORS OF DOMESTIC VIOLENCE by Wendy Susan Deaton and Michael Hertica. (2001). "This is a necessary book for anyone who is scared and starting to think about what it would take to 'grow free.' . . . Very helpful for friends and relatives of a person in a domestic violence situation. I recommend it highly." *Colleen Friend, LCSW, Field Work Consultant, UCLA Department of Social Welfare, School of Public Policy & Social Research*

A THERAPIST'S GUIDE TO GROWING FREE: A MANUAL FOR SURVIVORS OF DOMESTIC VIOLENCE by Wendy Susan Deaton and Michael Hertica. (2001). "An excellent synopsis of the theories and research behind the manual." *Beatrice Crofts Yorker, RN, JD, Professor of Nursing, Georgia State University, Decatur*

PATTERNS OF CHILD ABUSE: HOW DYSFUNCTIONAL TRANSACTIONS ARE REPLICATED IN INDIVIDUALS, FAMILIES, AND THE CHILD WELFARE SYSTEM by Michael Karson. (2001). "No one interested in what may well be the major public health epidemic of our time in terms of its long-term consequences for our society can afford to pass up the opportunity to read this enlightening work." *Howard Wolowitz, PhD, Professor Emeritus, Psychology Department, University of Michigan, Ann Arbor*

IDENTIFYING CHILD MOLESTERS: PREVENTING CHILD SEXUAL ABUSE BY RECOGNIZING THE PATTERNS OF THE OFFENDERS by Carla van Dam. (2000). "The definitive work on the subject. . . . Provides parents and others with the tools to recognize when and how to intervene." *Roger W. Wolfe, MA, Co-Director, N. W. Treatment Associates, Seattle, Washington*

POLITICAL VIOLENCE AND THE PALESTINIAN FAMILY: IMPLICATIONS FOR MENTAL HEALTH AND WELL-BEING by Vivian Khamis. (2000). "A valuable book . . . a pioneering work that fills a glaring gap in the study of Palestinian society." *Elia Zureik, Professor of Sociology, Queens University, Kingston, Ontario, Canada*

STOPPING THE VIOLENCE: A GROUP MODEL TO CHANGE MEN'S ABUSIVE ATTITUDES AND BEHAVIORS by David J. Decker. (1999). "A concise and thorough manual to assist clinicians in learning the causes and dynamics of domestic violence." *Joanne Kittel, MSW, LICSW, Yachats, Oregon*

STOPPING THE VIOLENCE: A GROUP MODEL TO CHANGE MEN'S ABUSIVE ATTITUDES AND BEHAVIORS, THE CLIENT WORKBOOK by David J. Decker. (1999).

BREAKING THE SILENCE: GROUP THERAPY FOR CHILDHOOD SEXUAL ABUSE, A PRACTITIONER'S MANUAL by Judith A. Margolin. (1999). "This book is an extremely valuable and well-written resource for all therapists working with adult survivors of child sexual abuse." *Esther Deblinger, PhD, Associate Professor of Clinical Psychiatry, University of Medicine and Dentistry of New Jersey School of Osteopathic Medicine*

"I NEVER TOLD ANYONE THIS BEFORE": MANAGING THE INITIAL DISCLOSURE OF SEXUAL ABUSE RE-COLLECTIONS by Janice A. Gasker. (1999). "Discusses the elements needed to create a safe, therapeutic environment and offers the practitioner a number of useful strategies for responding appropriately to client disclosure." *Roberta G. Sands, PhD, Associate Professor, University of Pennsylvania School of Social Work*

FROM SURVIVING TO THRIVING: A THERAPIST'S GUIDE TO STAGE II RECOVERY FOR SURVIVORS OF CHILDHOOD ABUSE by Mary Bratton. (1999). "A must read for all, including survivors. Bratton takes a lifelong debilitating disorder and unravels its intricacies in concise, succinct, and understandable language." *Phillip A. Whitner, PhD, Sr. Staff Counselor, University Counseling Center, The University of Toledo, Ohio*

SIBLING ABUSE TRAUMA: ASSESSMENT AND INTERVENTION STRATEGIES FOR CHILDREN, FAMILIES, AND ADULTS by John V. Caffaro and Allison Conn-Caffaro. (1998). "One area that has almost consistently been ignored in the research and writing on child maltreatment is the area of sibling abuse. This book is a welcome and required addition to the developing literature on abuse." *Judith L. Alpert, PhD, Professor of Applied Psychology, New York University*

BEARING WITNESS: VIOLENCE AND COLLECTIVE RESPONSIBILITY by Sandra L. Bloom and Michael Reichert. (1998). "A totally convincing argument. . . . Demands careful study by all elected representatives, the clergy, the mental health and medical professions, representatives of the media, and all those unwittingly involved in this repressive perpetuation and catastrophic global problem." *Harold I. Eist, MD, Past President, American Psychiatric Association*

TREATING CHILDREN WITH SEXUALLY ABUSIVE BEHAVIOR PROBLEMS: GUIDELINES FOR CHILD AND PARENT INTERVENTION by Jan Ellen Burton, Lucinda A. Rasmussen, Julie Bradshaw, Barbara J. Christopherson, and Steven C. Huke. (1998). "An extremely readable book that is well-documented and a mine of valuable 'hands on' information. . . . This is a book that all those who work with sexually abusive children or want to work with them must read." *Sharon K. Araji, PhD, Professor of Sociology, University of Alaska, Anchorage*

THE LEARNING ABOUT MYSELF (LAMS) PROGRAM FOR AT-RISK PARENTS: LEARNING FROM THE PAST—CHANGING THE FUTURE by Verna Rickard. (1998). "This program should be a part of the resource materials of every mental health professional trusted with the responsibility of working with 'at-risk' parents." *Terry King, PhD, Clinical Psychologist, Federal Bureau of Prisons, Catlettsburg, Kentucky*

THE LEARNING ABOUT MYSELF (LAMS) PROGRAM FOR AT-RISK PARENTS: HANDBOOK FOR GROUP PARTICIPANTS by Verna Rickard. (1998). "Not only is the LAMS program designed to be educational and build skills for future use, it is also fun!" *Martha Morrison Dore, PhD, Associate Professor of Social Work, Columbia University, New York*

BRIDGING WORLDS: UNDERSTANDING AND FACILITATING ADOLESCENT RECOVERY FROM THE TRAUMA OF ABUSE by Joycee Kennedy and Carol McCarthy. (1998). "An extraordinary survey of the history of child neglect and abuse in America. . . . A wonderful teaching tool at the university level, but should be required reading in high schools as well." *Florabel Kinsler, PhD, BCD, LCSW, Licensed Clinical Social Worker, Los Angeles, California*

CEDAR HOUSE: A MODEL CHILD ABUSE TREATMENT PROGRAM by Bobbi Kendig with Clara Lowry. (1998). "Kendig and Lowry truly . . . realize the saying that we are our brothers' keepers. Their spirit permeates this volume, and that spirit of caring is what always makes the difference for people in painful situations." *Hershel K. Swinger, PhD, Clinical Director, Children's Institute International, Los Angeles, California*

SEXUAL, PHYSICAL, AND EMOTIONAL ABUSE IN OUT-OF-HOME CARE: PREVENTION SKILLS FOR AT-RISK CHILDREN by Toni Cavanagh Johnson and Associates. (1997). "Professionals who make dispositional decisions or who are related to out-of-home care for children could benefit from reading and following the curriculum of this book with children in placements." *Issues in Child Abuse Accusations*

Order a copy of this book with this form or online at:
http://www.haworthpress.com/store/product.asp?sku=5098

MUNCHAUSEN BY PROXY
Identification, Intervention, and Case Management

_____ in hardbound at $59.95 (ISBN: 0-7890-1217-0)

_____ in softbound at $39.95 (ISBN: 0-7890-1218-9)

Or order online and use special offer code HEC25 in the shopping cart.

COST OF BOOKS_____

POSTAGE & HANDLING_____
(US: $4.00 for first book & $1.50
for each additional book)
(Outside US: $5.00 for first book
& $2.00 for each additional book)

SUBTOTAL_____

IN CANADA: ADD 7% GST_____

STATE TAX_____
(NY, OH, MN, CA, IL, IN, & SD residents,
add appropriate local sales tax)

FINAL TOTAL_____
(If paying in Canadian funds,
convert using the current
exchange rate, UNESCO
coupons welcome)

Prices in US dollars and subject to change without notice.

☐ **BILL ME LATER:** (Bill-me option is good on
US/Canada/Mexico orders only; not good to
jobbers, wholesalers, or subscription agencies.)
☐ Check here if billing address is different from
shipping address and attach purchase order and
billing address information.

Signature_____

☐ **PAYMENT ENCLOSED: $**_____

☐ **PLEASE CHARGE TO MY CREDIT CARD.**

☐ Visa ☐ MasterCard ☐ AmEx ☐ Discover
☐ Diner's Club ☐ Eurocard ☐ JCB

Account # _____

Exp. Date_____

Signature_____

NAME_____

INSTITUTION_____

ADDRESS_____

CITY_____

STATE/ZIP_____

COUNTRY_____ COUNTY (NY residents only)_____

TEL_____ FAX_____

E-MAIL_____

May we use your e-mail address for confirmations and other types of information? ☐ Yes ☐ No
We appreciate receiving your e-mail address and fax number. Haworth would like to e-mail or fax special
discount offers to you, as a preferred customer. **We will never share, rent, or exchange your e-mail address
or fax number.** We regard such actions as an invasion of your privacy.

Order From Your Local Bookstore or Directly From
The Haworth Press, Inc.
10 Alice Street, Binghamton, New York 13904-1580 • USA
TELEPHONE: 1-800-HAWORTH (1-800-429-6784) / Outside US/Canada: (607) 722-5857
FAX: 1-800-895-0582 / Outside US/Canada: (607) 771-0012
E-mailto: orders@haworthpress.com

For orders outside US and Canada, you may wish to order through your local
sales representative, distributor, or bookseller.
For information, see http://haworthpress.com/distributors

(Discounts are available for individual orders in US and Canada only, not booksellers/distributors.)
PLEASE PHOTOCOPY THIS FORM FOR YOUR PERSONAL USE.
http://www.HaworthPress.com

BOF04